Advances in Pathogenesis and Therapeutics of Hepatobiliary Diseases

Advances in Pathogenesis and Therapeutics of Hepatobiliary Diseases

Editor

Jinghua Wang

MDPI • Basel • Beijing • Wuhan • Barcelona • Belgrade • Manchester • Tokyo • Cluj • Tianjin

Editor
Jinghua Wang
Institute of Bioscience &
Integrative Medicine
Daejeon University
Daejeon
Korea, South

Editorial Office
MDPI
St. Alban-Anlage 66
4052 Basel, Switzerland

This is a reprint of articles from the Special Issue published online in the open access journal *Biomedicines* (ISSN 2227-9059) (available at: www.mdpi.com/journal/biomedicines/special_issues/Hepatobiliary_Diseases).

For citation purposes, cite each article independently as indicated on the article page online and as indicated below:

LastName, A.A.; LastName, B.B.; LastName, C.C. Article Title. *Journal Name* **Year**, *Volume Number*, Page Range.

ISBN 978-3-0365-7739-5 (Hbk)
ISBN 978-3-0365-7738-8 (PDF)

Contents

About the Editor . . . . **vii**

Jing-Hua Wang
Advances in Pathogenesis and Therapeutics of Hepatobiliary Diseases
Reprinted from: *Biomedicines* **2023**, *11*, 1140, doi:10.3390/biomedicines11041140 1

Georgiana-Diana Cazac, Cristina-Mihaela Lăcătușu, Cătălina Mihai, Elena-Daniela Grigorescu, Alina Onofriescu and Bogdan-Mircea Mihai
Ultrasound-Based Hepatic Elastography in Non-Alcoholic Fatty Liver Disease: Focus on Patients with Type 2 Diabetes
Reprinted from: *Biomedicines* **2022**, *10*, 2375, doi:10.3390/biomedicines10102375 5

Laia Bertran, Ailende Eigbefoh-Addeh, Marta Portillo-Carrasquer, Andrea Barrientos-Riosalido, Jessica Binetti and Carmen Aguilar et al.
Identification of the Potential Molecular Mechanisms Linking RUNX1 Activity with Nonalcoholic Fatty Liver Disease, by Means of Systems Biology
Reprinted from: *Biomedicines* **2022**, *10*, 1315, doi:10.3390/biomedicines10061315 33

Naim Abu-Freha, Bracha Cohen, Sarah Weissmann, Reut Hizkiya, Reem Abu-Hammad and Gadeer Taha et al.
Comorbidities and Outcomes among Females with Non-Alcoholic Fatty Liver Disease Compared to Males
Reprinted from: *Biomedicines* **2022**, *10*, 2908, doi:10.3390/biomedicines10112908 55

Javier Martínez-García, Angie Molina, Gloria González-Aseguinolaza, Nicholas D. Weber and Cristian Smerdou
Gene Therapy for Acquired and Genetic Cholestasis
Reprinted from: *Biomedicines* **2022**, *10*, 1238, doi:10.3390/biomedicines10061238 65

Annarosa Floreani, Daniela Gabbia and Sara De Martin
Update on the Pharmacological Treatment of Primary Biliary Cholangitis
Reprinted from: *Biomedicines* **2022**, *10*, 2033, doi:10.3390/biomedicines10082033 85

Annarosa Floreani, Daniela Gabbia and Sara De Martin
Obeticholic Acid for Primary Biliary Cholangitis
Reprinted from: *Biomedicines* **2022**, *10*, 2464, doi:10.3390/biomedicines10102464 103

Alicja Bauer, Andrzej Habior and Damian Gawel
Diagnostic and Clinical Value of Specific Autoantibodies against Kelch-like 12 Peptide and Nuclear Envelope Proteins in Patients with Primary Biliary Cholangitis
Reprinted from: *Biomedicines* **2022**, *10*, 801, doi:10.3390/biomedicines10040801 115

Selene García-García, Andrea Caballero-Garralda, David Tabernero, Maria Francesca Cortese, Josep Gregori and Francisco Rodriguez-Algarra et al.
Hepatitis B Virus Variants with Multiple Insertions and/or Deletions in the X Open Reading Frame 3′ End: Common Members of Viral Quasispecies in Chronic Hepatitis B Patients
Reprinted from: *Biomedicines* **2022**, *10*, 1194, doi:10.3390/biomedicines10051194 133

Jyun-Yi Wu, Yi-Shan Tsai, Chia-Chen Li, Ming-Lun Yeh, Ching-I Huang and Chung-Feng Huang et al.
Baseline Circulating miR-125b Levels Predict a High FIB-4 Index Score in Chronic Hepatitis B Patients after Nucleos(t)ide Analog Treatment
Reprinted from: *Biomedicines* **2022**, *10*, 2824, doi:10.3390/biomedicines10112824 151

Mélusine Durand, Nicolas Nagot, Quynh Bach Thi Nhu, Amélie Vizeneux, Linh Le Thi Thuy and Huong Thi Duong et al.
Long-Term Persistence of Mitochondrial DNA Instability among HCV-Cured People Who Inject Drugs
Reprinted from: *Biomedicines* **2022**, *10*, 2541, doi:10.3390/biomedicines10102541 . . . . **163**

Benjamin Wei Rong Tay, Daniel Q. Huang, Muthiah Mark, Neo Wee Thong, Lee Guan Huei and Lim Seng Gee et al.
Comparable Outcomes in Early Hepatocellular Carcinomas Treated with Trans-Arterial Chemoembolization and Radiofrequency Ablation
Reprinted from: *Biomedicines* **2022**, *10*, 2361, doi:10.3390/biomedicines10102361 . . . . **171**

About the Editor

Jinghua Wang

Dr. Jing-Hua Wang is an accomplished researcher and educator, currently serving as an assistant professor and principal investigator at the College of Korean Medicine and the Institute of Bioscience & Integrative Medicine (IBIM) at Daejeon University in South Korea. Dr. Wang earned his bachelor's degree in the College of Clinical Chinese Medicine from Anhui University of Chinese Medicine (AUCM), China, and his master's and Ph.D. in the College of Korean Medicine from Daejeon University (DJU), South Korea. He also served as a visiting professor at the Institute of Korean Medicine at Dongguk University from 2013 to 2018. Dr. Wang has nearly two decades of experience in the fields of hepatology, herbal medicine, and the gut microbiome, with his research primarily focused on exploring natural products to alleviate various hepatobiliary diseases. In recognition of his contributions to the field, Dr. Wang was granted a bursary from the European Association for the Study of the Liver (EASL) in 2011. He has also authored 52 SCI papers, holds two patents, and completed twenty-three research projects funded by the Korean government, such as the National Research Foundation of Korea (NRF). Dr. Wang's expertise and contributions to the field make him a valuable member of the academic community, and his work inspires his colleagues and students alike.

biomedicines

MDPI

Editorial

Advances in Pathogenesis and Therapeutics of Hepatobiliary Diseases

Jing-Hua Wang

Liver and Immunology Research Center, Institute of Bioscience & Integrative Medicine, Daejeon University, 75, Daedeok-daero 176 Beon-Gil, Seo-gu, Dunsan-dong, Daejeon 35235, Republic of Korea; ewccwang@gmail.com; Tel.: +82-42-257-6397; Fax: +82-42-257-6398

The hepatobiliary system, comprising the liver, gallbladder, and bile ducts, performs a diverse array of functions that are essential to maintaining homeostasis [1], including digestion, nutrient metabolism, detoxification, coagulation, and immune modulation [2]. Alterations in the normal function of the hepatobiliary system can have serious implications for human health, resulting in a broad range of pathologies spanning from liver disease to bile system disorders.

The Special Issue of *Biomedicines*, entitled "Advances in Pathogenesis and Therapeutics of Hepatobiliary Diseases", presents cutting-edge research findings, innovations, and insights into a wide range of topics related to the hepatobiliary system, such as the molecular mechanisms underlying disease pathogenesis, diagnostic advancements, novel therapeutic approaches, and prevention strategies. The Special Issue comprises seven original articles and four review articles regarding NAFLD, primary biliary cholangitis (PBC), hepatitis B and C, and hepatocellular carcinoma (HCC).

NAFLD is currently a major global health issue. It affects approximately 25% of the global population [3], with the highest prevalence in Western countries (25–30%) [4]. It affects 80–100 million people in the United States, making it the most common type of chronic liver disease [3]. NAFLD is also prevalent in Asia, particularly in Korea (affecting up to 30.3% of adults; men: 41.1%, women: 20.3%) [5]. As a result, many researchers are working to identify methods to prevent and treat NAFLD [6–9]. However, the lack of FDA-approved therapeutic options for NAFLD remains a significant impediment, emphasizing the critical importance of timely and accurate diagnosis [10]. Herein, Cazac et al. offer a comprehensive review of ultrasound-based hepatic elastography as a non-invasive method for diagnosing NAFLD in patients with type 2 diabetes mellitus (T2DM) [11]. They also highlight the limitations of liver biopsy and the need for non-invasive diagnostic tools to assess NAFLD in high-risk patients [11]. Bertran et al. utilized systems biology tools and public databases to identify the potential molecular mechanisms linking RUNX1 and NAFLD, resulting in a promising therapeutic strategy and a novel approach to treating NAFLD [12]. Furthermore, Abu-Freha et al. shed light on an important and relatively under-researched field of study: sex-based differences in NAFLD [13]. They used clinical big data from Clalit Health Services (CHS) in Israel. This discovery would improve our understanding of sex-based differences in NAFLD by highlighting disparities in comorbidities, outcomes, and mortality rates between females and males [13].

Furthermore, cholestatic diseases are significant because they have the potential to cause severe liver damage and long-term complications, emphasizing the importance of early diagnosis and treatment. One review provided a comprehensive overview of cholestatic diseases, including subtypes and causes, as well as the most up-to-date treatment options for cholestatic diseases, including pharmacotherapeutic agents and gene therapy [14]. It is worth noting that the discussion of gene therapy for inherited and acquired cholestasis is insightful and demonstrates the future promise of using gene therapy to address this medical issue [14]. Another review summarized current knowledge

Citation: Wang, J.-H. Advances in Pathogenesis and Therapeutics of Hepatobiliary Diseases. *Biomedicines* **2023**, *11*, 1140. https://doi.org/10.3390/biomedicines11041140

Received: 6 April 2023
Accepted: 7 April 2023
Published: 10 April 2023

regarding pharmacological interventions for the treatment of primary biliary cholangitis (PBC) [15]. As is known, ursodeoxycholic acid (UDCA) is the first-line therapy for PBC and has been proven to normalize liver markers, delay disease progression, and prolong transplant-free survival. Obeticholic acid (OCA) is the only approved second-line treatment for individuals with PBC who do not respond to UDCA. Floreani et al. provided a comprehensive review of the pharmacological properties of OCA, including its mechanism of action, as well as its tolerability and effectiveness in treating PBC patients [16]. Moreover, one cohort study conducted by Bauer and colleagues, comprising 138 PBC patients and 90 non-PBC patients, revealed that the presence of antibodies against the kelch-like 12 (KLHL12) protein is a highly specific marker for diagnosing PBC [17]. When used in conjunction with other markers, it has the potential to significantly enhance the accuracy of PBC diagnosis.

Furthermore, hepatitis B and C also represent major global health issues. According to the World Health Organization (WHO), an estimated 354 million people worldwide are living with viral hepatitis B and C [18]. Infection with HBV and HCV can increase the risk of developing liver fibrosis, cirrhosis, and even liver cancer [19]. Three reports are presented here that are associated with the diagnosis, treatment, and pathogenesis of hepatitis induced by HBV/HCV. A study conducted in Spain found variants with indels in the 3′ end of HBX in most of their chronic hepatitis B (CHB) patients [20]. These variants encoded alternative versions of HBx that have the potential to play a functional role and/or alter transcriptional regulation [20]. This will provide useful insight into the genetic variability of HBV in CHB patients who do not have HCC. Another study investigated the correlation between serum miR-125b levels and liver fibrosis in CHB patients after 12 months of nucleoside analog treatment [21]. The results indicated that there is an inverse relationship between miR-125b levels and the post-treatment FIB-4 index score, but it is not a significant predictor of a higher score. Age, baseline platelet count, and ALT level were all independent predictors of a FIB-index greater than 2.9 post-treatment [21]. The last study investigated the long-term effects of direct-acting antiviral (DAA) regimens on mitochondrial DNA (mtDNA) instability in people who inject drugs (PWID) with chronic HCV [22]. The mtDNA parameters were measured nine months after treatment, and the percentage of deleted mtDNA genomes increased over time due to their replicative advantage over elimination processes [22].

In terms of clinical therapy for HCC, Tay et al. compared the clinical outcomes of trans-arterial chemoembolization (RFA) and radiofrequency ablation (TACE) as initial monotherapy for patients with early-stage HCC [23]. According to their findings, TACE could be considered a potential treatment option for patients who are unsuitable candidates for other therapies [23].

Overall, I anticipate that the collection of articles in this Special Issue will contribute significantly to ongoing efforts to improve the diagnosis, prevention, and treatment of hepatobiliary diseases, resulting in better patient outcomes and overall public health.

Funding: This research was funded by the National Research Foundation of Korea (NRF), grant number 2020R1F1A1074155.

Acknowledgments: I would like to express my sincere appreciation to all of the authors who contributed to this Special Issue. Furthermore, I extend my gratitude to Chang-gue Son at College of Korean Medicine, Daejeon University, for his support.

Conflicts of Interest: The author declares no conflict of interest.

References

1. Ravenscroft, M.M.; Swan, C.H.J. The Hepatobiliary System. In *Gastrointestinal Endoscopy and Related Procedures: A Handbook for Nurses and Assistants*; Ravenscroft, M.M., Swan, C.H.J., Eds.; Springer: Boston, MA, USA, 1984; pp. 127–167. [CrossRef]
2. Hastings, K.L.; Green, M.D.; Gao, B.; Ganey, P.E.; Roth, R.A.; Burleson, G.R. Beyond Metabolism: Role of the Immune System in Hepatic Toxicity. *Int. J. Toxicol.* **2020**, *39*, 151–164. [CrossRef] [PubMed]

3. Younossi, Z.M.; Koenig, A.B.; Abdelatif, D.; Fazel, Y.; Henry, L.; Wymer, M. Global epidemiology of nonalcoholic fatty liver disease—Meta-analytic assessment of prevalence, incidence, and outcomes. *Hepatology* **2016**, *64*, 73–84. [CrossRef]
4. Pouwels, S.; Sakran, N.; Graham, Y.; Leal, A.; Pintar, T.; Yang, W.; Kassir, R.; Singhal, R.; Mahawar, K.; Ramnarain, D. Non-alcoholic fatty liver disease (NAFLD): A review of pathophysiology, clinical management and effects of weight loss. *BMC Endocr. Disord.* **2022**, *22*, 63. [CrossRef] [PubMed]
5. Im, H.J.; Ahn, Y.C.; Wang, J.-H.; Lee, M.M.; Son, C.G. Systematic review on the prevalence of nonalcoholic fatty liver disease in South Korea. *Clin. Res. Hepatol. Gastroenterol.* **2021**, *45*, 101526. [CrossRef] [PubMed]
6. Kosmalski, M.; Frankowski, R.; Ziółkowska, S.; Różycka-Kosmalska, M.; Pietras, T. What's New in the Treatment of Non-Alcoholic Fatty Liver Disease (NAFLD). *J. Clin. Med.* **2023**, *12*, 1852. [CrossRef] [PubMed]
7. Wang, J.-H.; Hwang, S.-J.; Lim, D.-W.; Son, C.-G. Cynanchum atratum Alleviates Non-Alcoholic Fatty Liver by Balancing Lipogenesis and Fatty Acid Oxidation in a High-Fat, High-Fructose Diet Mice Model. *Cells* **2022**, *11*, 23. [CrossRef]
8. Wang, J.-H.; Bose, S.; Shin, N.R.; Chin, Y.-W.; Choi, Y.H.; Kim, H. Pharmaceutical Impact of Houttuynia Cordata and Metformin Combination on High-Fat-Diet-Induced Metabolic Disorders: Link to Intestinal Microbiota and Metabolic Endotoxemia. *Front. Endocrinol.* **2018**, *9*, 620. [CrossRef]
9. Shin, N.R.; Bose, S.; Wang, J.-H.; Ansari, A.; Lim, S.-K.; Chin, Y.-W.; Choi, H.-S.; Kim, H. Flos Lonicera Combined with Metformin Ameliorates Hepatosteatosis and Glucose Intolerance in Association with Gut Microbiota Modulation. *Front. Microbiol.* **2017**, *8*, 2271. [CrossRef]
10. Friesen, C.S.; Chan, S.S.; Wagner, J.B.; Hosey-Cojocari, C.; Csanaky, I.L.; Shakhnovich, V. Critical need for pharmacologic treatment options in NAFLD: A pediatric perspective. *Clin. Transl. Sci.* **2021**, *14*, 781–783. [CrossRef]
11. Cazac, G.-D.; Lăcătușu, C.-M.; Mihai, C.; Grigorescu, E.-D.; Onofriescu, A.; Mihai, B.-M. Ultrasound-Based Hepatic Elastography in Non-Alcoholic Fatty Liver Disease: Focus on Patients with Type 2 Diabetes. *Biomedicines* **2022**, *10*, 2375. [CrossRef]
12. Bertran, L.; Eigbefoh-Addeh, A.; Portillo-Carrasquer, M.; Barrientos-Riosalido, A.; Binetti, J.; Aguilar, C.; Ugarte Chicote, J.; Bartra, H.; Artigas, L.; Coma, M.; et al. Identification of the Potential Molecular Mechanisms Linking RUNX1 Activity with Nonalcoholic Fatty Liver Disease, by Means of Systems Biology. *Biomedicines* **2022**, *10*, 1315. [CrossRef] [PubMed]
13. Abu-Freha, N.; Cohen, B.; Weissmann, S.; Hizkiya, R.; Abu-Hammad, R.; Taha, G.; Gordon, M. Comorbidities and Outcomes among Females with Non-Alcoholic Fatty Liver Disease Compared to Males. *Biomedicines* **2022**, *10*, 2908. [CrossRef] [PubMed]
14. Martínez-García, J.; Molina, A.; González-Aseguinolaza, G.; Weber, N.D.; Smerdou, C. Gene Therapy for Acquired and Genetic Cholestasis. *Biomedicines* **2022**, *10*, 1238. [CrossRef] [PubMed]
15. Floreani, A.; Gabbia, D.; De Martin, S. Update on the Pharmacological Treatment of Primary Biliary Cholangitis. *Biomedicines* **2022**, *10*, 2033. [CrossRef]
16. Floreani, A.; Gabbia, D.; De Martin, S. Obeticholic Acid for Primary Biliary Cholangitis. *Biomedicines* **2022**, *10*, 2464. [CrossRef] [PubMed]
17. Bauer, A.; Habior, A.; Gawel, D. Diagnostic and Clinical Value of Specific Autoantibodies against Kelch-like 12 Peptide and Nuclear Envelope Proteins in Patients with Primary Biliary Cholangitis. *Biomedicines* **2022**, *10*, 801. [CrossRef] [PubMed]
18. World Health Organization. Global Progress Report on HIV, Viral Hepatitis and Sexually Transmitted Infections. Available online: https://www.who.int/publications/i/item/9789240027077 (accessed on 15 July 2021).
19. Wang, J.-H.; Lee, S.-B.; Lee, D.-S.; Son, C.-G. Total Antioxidant Capacity in HBV Carriers, a Promising Biomarker for Evaluating Hepatic Fibrosis: A Pilot Study. *Antioxidants* **2021**, *10*, 77. [CrossRef]
20. García-García, S.; Caballero-Garralda, A.; Tabernero, D.; Cortese, M.F.; Gregori, J.; Rodriguez-Algarra, F.; Quer, J.; Riveiro-Barciela, M.; Homs, M.; Rando-Segura, A.; et al. Hepatitis B Virus Variants with Multiple Insertions and/or Deletions in the X Open Reading Frame 3′ End: Common Members of Viral Quasispecies in Chronic Hepatitis B Patients. *Biomedicines* **2022**, *10*, 1194.
21. Wu, J.-Y.; Tsai, Y.-S.; Li, C.-C.; Yeh, M.-L.; Huang, C.-I.; Huang, C.-F.; Hsu, J.-N.; Hsieh, M.-H.; Chen, Y.-C.; Liu, T.-W.; et al. Baseline Circulating miR-125b Levels Predict a High FIB-4 Index Score in Chronic Hepatitis B Patients after Nucleos(t)ide Analog Treatment. *Biomedicines* **2022**, *10*, 2824. [CrossRef]
22. Durand, M.; Nagot, N.; Nhu, Q.B.; Vizeneux, A.; Thuy, L.L.; Duong, H.T.; Thanh, B.N.; Rapoud, D.; Vallo, R.; Quillet, C.; et al. Long-Term Persistence of Mitochondrial DNA Instability among HCV-Cured People Who Inject Drugs. *Biomedicines* **2022**, *10*, 2541. [CrossRef]
23. Tay, B.W.; Huang, D.Q.; Mark, M.; Thong, N.W.; Guan Huei, L.; Gee, L.S.; Cheng, L.H.; Mei, L.Y.; Thurairajah, P.; Chen, L.J.; et al. Comparable Outcomes in Early Hepatocellular Carcinomas Treated with Trans-Arterial Chemoembolization and Radiofrequency Ablation. *Biomedicines* **2022**, *10*, 2361. [CrossRef] [PubMed]

biomedicines

MDPI

Review

Ultrasound-Based Hepatic Elastography in Non-Alcoholic Fatty Liver Disease: Focus on Patients with Type 2 Diabetes

Georgiana-Diana Cazac [1,2], Cristina-Mihaela Lăcătușu [1,2,*], Cătălina Mihai [3,4], Elena-Daniela Grigorescu [1,*], Alina Onofriescu [1,2] and Bogdan-Mircea Mihai [1,2]

1 Unit of Diabetes, Nutrition and Metabolic Diseases, Faculty of Medicine, "Grigore T. Popa" University of Medicine and Pharmacy, 700115 Iasi, Romania
2 Clinical Center of Diabetes, Nutrition and Metabolic Diseases, "Sf. Spiridon" County Clinical Emergency Hospital, 700111 Iasi, Romania
3 Unit of Medical Semiology and Gastroenterology, Faculty of Medicine,, "Grigore T. Popa", University of Medicine and Pharmacy, 700115 Iasi, Romania
4 Institute of Gastroenterology and Hepatology, "Sf. Spiridon" Emergency Hospital, 700111 Iași, Romania
* Correspondence: cristina.lacatusu@umfiasi.ro (C.-M.L.); elena-daniela-gh-grigorescu@umfiasi.ro (E.-D.G.); Tel.: +40-72-321-1116 (C.-M.L.); +40-74-209-3749 (E.-D.G.)

Abstract: Non-alcoholic fatty liver disease (NAFLD) is the most prevalent liver disease and is the hepatic expression of metabolic syndrome. The development of non-invasive methods for the diagnosis of hepatic steatosis and advanced fibrosis in high-risk patients, especially those with type 2 diabetes mellitus, is highly needed to replace the invasive method of liver biopsy. Elastographic methods can bring significant added value to screening and diagnostic procedures for NAFLD in patients with diabetes, thus contributing to improved NAFLD management. Pharmacological development and forthcoming therapeutic measures that address NAFLD should also be based on new, non-invasive, and reliable tools that assess NAFLD in at-risk patients and be able to properly guide treatment in individuals with both diabetes and NAFLD. This is the first review aiming to outline and discuss recent studies on ultrasound-based hepatic elastography, focusing on NAFLD assessment in patients with diabetes.

Keywords: type 2 diabetes mellitus; non-alcoholic fatty liver disease; transient hepatic elastography; hepatic steatosis; liver fibrosis

Citation: Cazac, G.-D.; Lăcătușu, C.-M.; Mihai, C.; Grigorescu, E.-D.; Onofriescu, A.; Mihai, B.-M. Ultrasound-Based Hepatic Elastography in Non-Alcoholic Fatty Liver Disease: Focus on Patients with Type 2 Diabetes. *Biomedicines* **2022**, *10*, 2375. https://doi.org/10.3390/biomedicines10102375

Academic Editor: Jinghua Wang

Received: 27 August 2022
Accepted: 19 September 2022
Published: 23 September 2022

1. Introduction

Non-alcoholic fatty liver disease (NAFLD) is a chronic liver disorder that is lately becoming a worldwide major public health problem in both adults and children. The high prevalence of metabolic comorbidities such as obesity, dyslipidemia, and diabetes mellitus (DM) that are frequently associated with NAFLD supports the need for increased attention from healthcare providers who should invest in screening and management [1,2].

According to the latest International Diabetes Federation (IDF) Diabetes Atlas data, an estimated 537 million adults worldwide aged 20–79 years are currently living with diabetes, representing 10.5% of all adults in this age group. In 2021, almost 240 million adults had undiagnosed diabetes [3]. Early identification of people with diabetes is key to avoiding or delaying complications and improving quality of life, thus preventing the significant burden on healthcare systems [3].

The estimative global prevalence of NAFLD is 25% of the adult population. More than 50% of persons with type 2 diabetes (T2DM) and 90% of persons with severe obesity have NAFLD [4–6]. Approximately 10 to 15% of NAFLD patients from the United States and Europe have advanced fibrosis. Patients with NAFLD have an increased risk of liver-related death, primarily those with histologically proven non-alcoholic steatohepatitis (NASH) [7]. T2DM doubles the risk of hepatocellular carcinoma [5]. The high prevalence of metabolic syndrome (MS) is independently associated with all-cause, liver-specific, and cardiovascular mortality. Other risk factors leading to the increased prevalence of NAFLD are represented by older age and male sex [5]. The large number of NAFLD patients that are potential candidates for progressive liver disease creates challenges in screening and management, mirroring the evolution of cardiovascular disease development on the background of T2DM, obesity, and insulin resistance [8].

NAFLD covers a spectrum of histological conditions, ranging from simple steatosis (non-alcoholic fatty liver, NAFL) to NASH, which can later progress to liver fibrosis, cirrhosis, or hepatocellular carcinoma (HCC). MS is a predictor of hepatic steatosis [9]. Fibrosis is an important prognostic factor in NAFLD. The fibrosis stage is independently associated with increased overall and liver-specific mortality and with higher rates of liver-related complications and liver transplantation; early studies suggest a higher prevalence of NASH and advanced fibrosis stages among patients with T2DM [9,10].

Experts in the field have recently suggested the introduction of a new acronym, MAFLD (metabolic dysfunction-associated fatty liver disease), which reflects the relevant risk factors for this disease, underlining the association between insulin resistance and MS [11,12].

NAFLD and T2DM display a bidirectional relationship wherein these two pathologies have intricate effects on disease progression. On one hand, NAFLD co-existence increases the incidence of T2DM and the risk of developing micro- and macrovascular complications of diabetes [13–15]. On the other hand, T2DM is recognized as a risk factor for progressive liver disease, leading to advanced fibrosis, cirrhosis-related complications, and increased liver disease mortality [16]. An extensive meta-analysis of 33 studies carried out between 2000 and 2020, including 501,022 individuals and nearly 28,000 cases of incident diabetes, showed that patients with NAFLD had a higher risk of incident diabetes mellitus than those without NAFLD. This risk increased considerably in individuals with advanced liver fibrosis [17]. The co-existence of NAFLD and T2DM acts synergically to increase the risk for other organ complications, with the highest mortality in NAFLD attributed to a worsened cardiovascular risk profile [18]. It is thus becoming evident that the link between NAFLD and diabetes is more complex than previously believed.

Two steps are needed to diagnose NAFLD. The first step is to assess the existence of hepatic steatosis, either by imaging or biopsy, and then to exclude other causes of liver steatosis such as significant alcohol consumption, long-term use of steatogenic medication, or monogenic hereditary disorders [9]. NAFL's only feature is fatty liver infiltration that involves more than 5% of hepatocytes, whereas NASH also features inflammation and evidence of hepatocellular injury, with or without fibrosis, in the absence of alcohol consumption (daily intake of less than 20 g in women and 30 g in men) [9,14].

The European Association for the Study of the Liver (EASL), the European Association for the Study of Diabetes (EASD), and the European Association for the Study of Obesity (EASO) recommend ultrasonography as a first-line screening test for NAFL, whilst liver biopsy represents the essential tool for the diagnosis of NASH [14]. However, the limits of invasive biopsy procedures are acknowledged, and no distinct screening information in the existing guidelines refers to the identification of this metabolic liver disease amongst patients with diabetes.

Therefore, this is the first review aiming to identify and analyze the current elastography-based imaging strategy for NAFLD screening and diagnosis, focusing on its applicability in patients with T2DM. This category of patients has become more and more clinically significant, as the increased prevalence of diabetes and obesity have become important public health issues in recent decades. Among them, non-invasive diagnostic tests such as ultrasound-based hepatic elastography are highly needed to replace liver biopsy, to develop a new protocol for screening patients at risk for NAFLD or those with a history of steatosis diagnosed by hepatic imaging/biopsy, and to non-invasively monitor patients with NAFLD and diabetes and their response to treatment.

2. Common Approaches in NAFLD Assessment

Measures to limit disease progression must be based on the identification of metabolic risk factors (obesity, dyslipidemia, hypertension, and diabetes), on the assessment of anthropometric indices and laboratory tests (fasting blood glucose, oral glucose tolerance test, HbA1c, complete lipid profile, uric acid, and thyroid markers), on the calculation of related biomarkers (homeostatic model assessment for insulin resistance index, estimated glomerular filtration rate, urinary albumin-creatinine ratio), and on imaging techniques [9,19,20].

Liver-related outcomes are influenced by the advanced stage of fibrosis and not steatosis. Commonly used non-invasive tests (NIT) widely available in clinical practice to estimate fibrosis are represented by the fibrosis-4 (FIB-4) index, NAFLD fibrosis score (NFS), and aspartate aminotransferase (AST) [21,22]. By using such NIT in a large cohort of patients with T2DM, Singh et al. identified a high prevalence of fibrosis [23]. In fact, in line with the European guidelines, these scores should be calculated for every patient with NAFLD [14]. Their use can exclude the presence of advanced fibrosis in 50–67% of patients with diabetes [24]. A new prediction model, diabetes liver fibrosis score (DLFS) was recently developed to help identify patients with diabetes at significant risk for liver-related morbidity: DLFS values over 68.9 maximize specificity (98%) and positive predictive value (86%), while values less than 14.5 maximize sensitivity (95%) and negative predictive value (92%) [25]. Other NIT such as AST to platelet ratio index (APRI) or Hepascore had less accuracy predicting cirrhosis in patients with NAFLD and diabetes [26].

Ultrasonography stands at the forefront as a non-invasive method of screening and diagnosing steatosis in patients with diabetes. The lipid deposits in the liver can be detected by ultrasound when steatosis exceeds 30% of the liver parenchyma, which is visualized as a bright liver echotexture (hyperechoic) blurring the deeper structures [16,27]. An ultrasonography-based study showed that 127 out of 204 patients with T2DM had hepatic steatosis on ultrasound, and 87% of those having consented to a liver biopsy had NAFLD confirmed by histology [28]. The Edinburgh Type 2 Diabetes Study, the first study using ultrasound grading compared with magnetic resonance spectroscopy to determine NAFLD prevalence in a population of patients with T2DM, showed that the disadvantage of ultrasound is its inability to differentiate grade 1 or 2 of steatosis [29]. Therefore, the most accurate method to quantify fat is magnetic resonance imaging (MRI); however, MRI is limited by its high costs and lesser availability and is mainly used in clinical trials [21].

The "gold standard" in diagnosing NAFLD is liver biopsy and histologic examination. However, liver biopsy is limited by its invasive nature, potentially prone to complications such as pain, bleeding, or sampling errors [30]. The difficulties in repeating biopsies to assess changes in hepatic steatosis and fibrosis and in performing them on individuals with high abdominal circumferences require alternative non-invasive assessment tools [9,31].

The main purposes of following-up patients with diabetes are to identify patients with MS and risk of NAFLD, to detect individuals with a worsening prognosis, and to monitor them once the therapeutic strategy is implemented [32,33]. While the evidence for novel and innovative therapy approaches for NAFLD in subjects with T2DM is rising, elastography techniques might have a reliable role in monitoring patients with NAFLD and diabetes and their response to treatment [34]. Liver imaging plays an important role in NAFLD assessment in patients with T2DM because no clinical manifestations exist in the early stages of disease and functional tests may be within normal limits [35].

The recent recommendations by the EASL, EASD, and EASO designate clinical scores, serum biomarkers, and the elastographic evaluation of the liver as NIT accepted for the diagnosis and staging of hepatic fibrosis [21]. The American Diabetes Association (ADA) guidelines also suggest the use of transient elastography (TE) and non-invasive biomarkers for risk stratification [36]. The elastographic method evaluates the presence and severity of liver fibrosis according to the etiology of the liver disease and has already been tested in many liver-related conditions [37,38].

3. Ultrasound-Based Hepatic Shear Wave Elastography

Ultrasound-based elastography has found its place among NIT used to screen and assess the severity of NAFLD and is represented by TE, point shear wave elastography (pSWE), and two-dimensional shear wave elastography (2D-SWE) [16]. Within this category, TE is extensively available and can be used as a point-of-care test to estimate liver fibrosis by measuring liver stiffness and hepatic steatosis using controlled attenuation parameter (CAP) measurement [39,40]. The practice guidelines of the Brazilian Society of Hepatology and Brazilian College of Radiology have recently supported the use of elastography, among others, as a tool to assess fibrosis and steatosis in various chronic liver diseases, including NAFLD; due to its accuracy, elastography seems to be a non-invasive and cost-effective alternative to liver biopsy [41].

The screening for undiagnosed non-alcoholic fatty liver disease and non-alcoholic steatohepatitis (SUNN) study suggests that even asymptomatic high-risk individuals should, nevertheless, be screened for NAFLD. Using TE and CAP, Eskridge et al. found that 57% of the study population had steatosis without fibrosis and 16% of them had both steatosis and fibrosis [42]. However, the results of this study likely overestimate the presence of steatosis by using a cut-off value of $\geq$238 dB/m [43]. Even though specialists have not yet reached a consensus on cut-off values, the EASL guidelines suggest that a CAP value >275 dB/m might be used to diagnose hepatic steatosis [44]. A meta-analysis by Petroff et al. found that the optimal cut-offs when using the XL probe are 297, 317, and 333 dB/m for >S0, >S1, and S2, respectively [43]. Another study showed that the cut-off for S $\geq$ S2 of 331 dB/m is accurate for the identification of moderate steatosis [39]. Obesity, diabetes, and arterial hypertension proved to be statistically significant risk factors for NAFLD and NASH development [42]. In line with the results of this study, applying such efficient screening strategies to high-risk individuals may help to properly implement therapy and, over time, reduce the burden of NAFLD.

3.1. Elastography-Based Imaging Techniques to Assess Hepatic Fibrosis

Ultrasound-based shear wave elastographic methods for the assessment of advanced fibrosis in NAFLD are represented by [37,45]:

- TE or vibration-controlled transient elastography (VCTE)
- acoustic radiation force impulse (ARFI) quantification:
  - pSWE (point shear wave elastography)
  - 2D-SWE (two-dimensional shear wave elastography), or 3D-SWE (three-dimensional shear wave elastography) [46].

3.1.1. Transient Elastography

TE is a non-invasive imagistic technique able to stage liver fibrosis by LSM. The use of TE to estimate liver fibrosis severity was first described by Sandrin et al. in 2003 [47]. Besides being recommended as a clinical diagnostic method in many liver-related conditions such as chronic viral hepatitis, cholestatic diseases, alcoholic liver disease, and autoimmune hepatitis, an accumulating body of evidence supports the use of TE for the diagnosis and staging of liver fibrosis in NAFLD [44,48].

TE is a method non-integrated into standard ultrasound-based systems and performed using the Fibroscan® device (Echosens, Paris, France) that is well correlated with histologically diagnosed liver fibrosis in NAFLD. LSM quantification of liver fibrosis is expressed in kilopascals (kPa) [33,49]. TE can use an M probe for normal-weight patients and an XL probe for patients with obesity [50]. The feasibility of TE using both M and XL probes is 93.5% [51].

According to the Baveno VI consensus, TE has enabled the identification of asymptomatic patients with advanced fibrosis (stage F3–F4) at risk for clinical complications. This consensus has proposed the term "compensated advanced chronic liver disease" (cACLD) as an alternative to chronic liver disease in asymptomatic F3–F4 patients, who are at risk of developing severe portal hypertension. Values between 10 and 15 kPa need confirmation of cACLD, and a value >15 kPa is suggestive of cACLD in the absence of clinical signs [52].

The TE technique has acquired widespread use in clinical studies and daily medical activities, ranging from the screening and diagnosis of hepatic steatosis and fibrosis in patients with suspected NAFLD to the assessment of T2DM prevalence among patients with NAFLD and the follow-up protocols searching for improvements after the initiation of pharmacologic and non-pharmacologic treatment [53].

The Rotterdam Study found the highest probabilities of fibrosis among participants with diabetes and steatosis [54]. It is noteworthy that most studies having investigated the prevalence of NAFLD and its risk factors by the TE tool resorted to non-diabetic cohorts for validating their results, so further studies are needed to stratify the diabetes-associated risk, as optimal cut-offs may be influenced by diabetes mellitus or body mass index (BMI) [55]. On the other hand, the risk of developing diabetes may be influenced by a NAFLD-associated status that evolves over time [56]. A cross-sectional study using TE to evaluate fibrosis among various chronic liver disease populations in a tertiary center in Lebanon appreciated that more than 58% of subjects had NAFLD; also, almost 50% of patients had at least one metabolic risk factor and 20% had T2DM [57].

The performance of NAFLD diagnostic tools among patients with T2DM varies according to the assessment methods. In healthy people, TE measurements of Young's modulus range from 4.4 to 5.5 kPa [37]. Ahn et al. found a significantly higher LSM in the diabetes group (11.22 $\pm$ 10.51 kPa) than in the non-diabetes group (8.07 $\pm$ 7.29 kPa), and a higher prevalence of diabetes in patients with NAFLD than in those with chronic viral hepatitis [58]. A cohort study on 283 patients performed by Patel and colleagues revealed 82.5% of them were diagnosed with T2DM and one-fifth with severe obesity; the cut-off values applied for LSM were 8.2 kPa for significant fibrosis, $\geq$9.5 kPa for advanced fibrosis, and >13 kPa for cirrhosis. In this study, 76.5% of patients with BMI values greater than 40 kg/m^2 required the use of the XL probe [59]. XL probes are designed for obese patients to improve the measurability of liver stiffness [60]. According to Garg et al., TE using the XL probe has a lower rate of failure than the M probe in patients with obesity, being able to evaluate hepatic steatosis and fibrosis in almost 60% of the obese persons with a BMI $\leq$ 45 kg/m^2 [30].

In a cross-sectional trial conducted in Vietnam, assessing diabetic patients by TE, a 73.3% prevalence of NAFLD was found among patients with T2DM. The LSM values in patients with F2 (significant fibrosis), F3 (advanced fibrosis), and F4 (cirrhosis) were $\geq$7 kPa, $\geq$8.7 kPa, and 11.5 kPa, respectively. After applying multivariable logistic regression, the investigators found AST and platelets as predictors of advanced fibrosis in patients with T2DM [61]. Therefore, patients with diabetes and increased AST values may be predisposed to increased liver stiffness [62].

The heterogeneity of study results may be influenced by specific BMI and waist circumference cut-off values depending on the country and ethnic origin of patients. The rising rates of obesity, dyslipidemia, hypertension, and MS in people with NAFLD support the need for evaluating MS components in patients with fatty liver, but also for NAFLD screening among patients with metabolic risk factors [63].

Several studies compared the use of TE alone with combined NIT for the detection of fibrosis. The STELLAR study demonstrated that the combined use of two NIT among patients with enhanced liver fibrosis (ELF), NFS, FIB-4, and liver stiffness by TE improved the diagnostic performance by reducing the proportion of patients with advanced fibrosis due to NASH and indeterminate results [64].

Combining clinical scores and serum markers with LSM by TE may facilitate and improve the diagnosis of advanced fibrosis and steatosis [65–67]. The Fibroscan-AST (FAST) score combines LSM and CAP measured by TE with aspartate aminotransferase, having already been validated in large global cohorts [68]. Comparison of NIT to accurately identify advanced fibrosis due to NASH subsequently reduces the need for liver biopsy to assess the fibrosis stage [64]. The implementation of such a strategy may be particularly beneficial in high-risk patients such as those with T2DM.

The development of novel therapeutic strategies to improve NAFLD-related outcomes also requires high-value evaluation methods such as LSM. Unlike liver biopsy, this tool is widely available and reproducible, avoids patient reluctance, and can be repeated to monitor the results of pharmacological treatment [69].

As LSM by TE has become the most investigated and embraced method for evaluating NAFLD, forthcoming years will show whether it may be designated as a future "gold standard" among non-invasive assessment tools. Studies focusing on the estimation of liver stiffness with TE in patients with diabetes and NAFLD are described in Table 1.

Table 1. Diagnostic performance and comparison of results for different fibrosis stages using LSM by transient elastography in patients with NAFLD and T2DM.

Author, Ref.	Year	Country	No. of Patients	No. of NAFLD Patients	No. of Diabetic Patients	Diabetes Duration (Years)	Mean Age (Years)	Mean BMI (kg/m²)	Fibrosis Stage	Cut-Off Level (kPa)
Dai et al. [70]	2022	Taiwan	226	50	226	10 ± 7.8	62.1 ± 10.7	27.3 ± 4.1	F3–4: 50	>7
Trifan et al. [71]	2022	Romania	424	349	424		53.67 ± 11.37	28.07 ± 3.22	F2: 57.14% F3: 11.7% F4: 13.6%	≥8.2 ≥9.7 ≥13.6
Alexopoulos et al. [72]	2021	USA	228 DM	15 5 (TE) unknown NAFLD	228	12.5	58.1	35	F0–1: 40% F2: 20% F3: 40% F4: 0	Unavailable
				Known NAFLD 4 (TE)		15.1	57.9	37.8	F0–1: 25% F2: 25% F3: 50% F4: 0	Unavailable
Cardoso et al. [41]	2021	Brasil	400	173	400	8 (3–15)	64.4	30.4	≥F3: 15%	>9.6
Chhabra et al. [73]	2021	India	200	200	100	–	50.3 ± 11.13	–	F1 F2: 30% F3–F4: 70%	<7 ≥7–8.6 ≥8.7–11.4 ≥11.5
Ciardullo et al. [74]	2021	USA	825	557 steatosis 179 fibrosis	825	9.9 ± 0.75 9.2 ± 2.09 12.9 ± 4.08 10.4 ± 9.23	60.6	31.9 ± 0.47 36.3 ± 1,11 37.5 ± 1.42 38.9 ± 1.45	F0–F1: 76.2% F2: 8.4% F3: 7.7% F4: 7.7%	<8.2 8.2–9.6 9.7–13.5 ≥13.6
Grgurevic et al. [75]	2021	Croatia	454	164	454	–	62.5	30.09	86 45 33	>7.9 ≥9.6 ≥11.5
Gupta et al. [76]	2021	India	250 DM	246 steatosis 205 fibrosis	250	9.6 ± 6.4	51 ± 9	31.4 ± 8	F0: 28.8% F1: 14.8% F2: 18.4% F3: 19.6%	<7 7.1–10 10.1–13 ≥13
Lomonaco et al. [77]	2021	USA	561	70% steatosis 21% fibrosis	561	–	60 ± 11	33.4 ± 6.2	F1: 6.5% F2: 5.6% F3: 6.2% F4: 3%	≥7–8.1 8.2–9.6 9.7–13.5 ≥13.6

Table 1. *Cont.*

Author, Ref.	Year	Country	No. of Patients	No. of NAFLD Patients	No. of Diabetic Patients	Diabetes Duration (Years)	Mean Age (Years)	Mean BMI (kg/m^2)	Fibrosis Stage	Cut-Off Level (kPa)
Makker et al. [78]	2021	USA	85	-	59	15 ± 9	62 ± 11.7	33.1 ± 8.4	F0–1: 76% F2: 12% F3: 5% F4: 7%	≤7 ≥7.5 ≥10 ≥14
Mansour et al. [79]	2021	United Kingdom	466	58 underwent TE, according to FIB-4	466	-	65.22	33.36	43.1% 20.7% 22.4%	>8 8–15 >15
Sagara et al. [80]	2021	Japan	115	67	115	-	59 ± 13.8	26.6 ± 4.7	F2: 25% F3: 20.5% F4: 13.3%	8–9.6 9.7–12.9 ≥13
Trivedi et al. [81]	2021	USA	437	385	124	-	58.4	33.5	52 100 24	≥7 <10 ≥10
Blank et al. [82]	2020	Germany	204	184	203	13 ± 10.3	64.2 ± 10.7	32.6 ± 7.6	Low 125 Intermediate 10 High 46	<7.9/7.2 M/XL probe 7.9–9.6/7.2–9.3 M/XL probe >9.6/9.3 M/XL probe
Lee CH et al. [83]	2020	China	711	711	711	16.6 ± 9.2	59.4 ± 10.3	28.6 ± 4.5	F0/F1: 40.2% F2: 40.3 % ≥F3: 19.5 %	- - ≥9.6
Lee HW et al. [84]	2020	China	611	Baseline 611	611	-	57.7 ± 10.9	-	63.5% 20%	<10 ≥10
				After 3 years 611					56.5% 4.3%	<10 ≥10
Mantovani et al. [85]	2020	Italy	137	37	137	11	69.9 ± 7	28.5 ± 4.7	F2: 17.5% F3: 10.2%	≥7 ≥8.7
Mikolasevic et al. [86]	2020	Croatia	679	M probe 366 XL probe 313	679	-	65.2 ± 11.6	30.75 ± 5.15	F1: 27.6% F2: 29.5% F3: 29.5% F4: 6.7%	- ≥7 ≥9.6/9.3 M/XL probe ≥11.5/11 M/XL probe

Table 1. *Cont.*

Author, Ref.	Year	Country	No. of Patients	No. of NAFLD Patients	No. of Diabetic Patients	Diabetes Duration (Years)	Mean Age (Years)	Mean BMI (kg/m^2)	Fibrosis Stage	Cut-Off Level (kPa)
Sawaf et al. [57]	2020	Lebanon	620	362	128	–	47.8 ± 13.4	26.21 ± 4.3	F0–1: 56.6% F2: 9.3% F3: 6.1% F4: 27.9%	Unavailable
Sporea et al. [87]	2020	Romania	776	534	534	10 ± 2	60.8 ± 8.7	32 ± 6	≤F1: 72.6% ≥F2: 7.8% ≥F3: 11.4% F4: 8.2%	- 8.2 9.7 13.6
Tuong et al. [61]	2020	Vietnam	307	18	307	6.5 (3–10)	58.7 ± 11.3	26.3 ± 3.1	F2: 13% F3: 5.9% F4: 3.6%	≥7 ≥8.7 ≥11.5
Arya et al. [88]	2019	India	19,550	6749	13,498	7.52 ± 4.46	50	40% obese 22% overweight 30% normal 8% underweight	F0: 32% F1: 18% F2: 10% F3: 10% F4: 30%	<5.9 6–6.9 7–8.6 8.7–10.2 >10.3
Demir et al. [89]	2019	Turkey	124	31	124	–	53 ± 7	33.2 ± 6.6	≥F3: 16.9% F4: 8%	9.6–11.49.5/9.3–10.9 M/XL probe F4 ≥ 11.5/≥11 M/XL probe
Fernando et al. [90]	2019	Philippines	704	164	285	4.05 ± 3.63	57.27 ± 13.06	27.58 ± 4.25	F0–1: 44.51% F2: 37.8% F3: 5.49% F4: 12.2%	≥5.8 5.9–9.5 9.6–11.5 >11.5
Jaafar et al. [91]	2019	Lebanon	248	248	73	–	53.7 ± 14.6	29.43 ± 7.59	≤F1: 24.66% F2: 17.81% F3: 7% F4: 47.94%	Unavailable
Kumar NA et al. [92]	2019	India	50	47	50	Newly diagnosed	45 ± 4	40% obese	F1: 34% F2: 10% F3: 22% F4: 22% 12%	<5.8 5.8–6.8 6.8–7.8 7.8–11.8 >11.8

Table 1. *Cont.*

Author, Ref.	Year	Country	No. of Patients	No. of NAFLD Patients	No. of Diabetic Patients	Diabetes Duration (Years)	Mean Age (Years)	Mean BMI (kg/m²)	Fibrosis Stage	Cut-Off Level (kPa)
Lai et al. [93]	2019	Malaysia	557	403	557	15.8 ± 11.7	60.4 ± 11	29.2 ± 5.2	171 57 37	≥8 M/XL probe ≥9.6/9.3 M/XL probe ≥11.5/11 M/XL probe
Lombardi et al. [94]	2019	Italy	394	350	394	12.3 ± 7.5	65 ± 10	31.4 ± 4.7	83	≥7/6.2 M/XL probe
Wong VW-S et al. [95]	2019	France Hong Kong	496	496	300	–	54 ± 12	30.4 ± 5.4	F1: 112/124 F2: 83/96 F3: 84/91 F4: 59/70	6.8/6.1 M/XL probe 8.8/6.9 M/XL probe 11.8/8.8 M/XL probe 16.3/14.8 M/XL probe
Zhao et al. [96]	2018	China	629 DM	–	629	–	47.07 ± 12.2	26.58 ±4.17	–	F1 > 7.4 F2 > 10.6
Kartikayan et al. [97]	2017	India	60	60	60	7.38 ± 4.2	54.12 ± 11.3	26.6 ± 2.42	F1:16.7% F2:20% F3-F4: 34%	Mean: 7.95
Prasetya et al. [98]	2017	Indonesia	186	84 64 TE	186	<5 y: 38 ≥5 y: 46	<40: 4 ≥40: 80	<25: 25 ≥25: 59	F0-F2: 51 F3-F4: 17	<9.6 ≥9.6
Kwok R et al. [99]	2016	China	1918	334	2119	11.6	61.2	29.3	F3: 17.1%/27.2% F4:11.2%/25	≥9.6–11.4/9.3–10.9 M/XL probe ≥11.5/11 M/XL probe
Sobhonslidsuk et al. [62]	2015	Thailand	197	82	137	–	63.8	27.6	22% 5.93%	≥7 ≥8.7
Ahn et al. [58]	2014	South Korea	979	13	165	–	51.9	25.12 ± 3.11	F0–1: 14% F2/3: 18% F4: 31%	<8 8–19 >19
Casey et al. [69]	2012	Australia	74	26	74	12.2 ± 7.2	61.5 ± 8.6	36.1 ± 5.6	≥F2: 35%	≥7.65
de Lédinghen et al. [100]	2012	France	277	20	277 (132 T2DM)	13	63.2 ± 12.1	27.2 ± 4.3	17	>8.7

Abbreviations: NAFLD, non-alcoholic fatty liver disease; BMI, body mass index; kPa, kilopascals; F, fibrosis; S, steatosis; M, medium; L, large; TE, transient elastography; DM, diabetes mellitus; T2DM, type 2 diabetes mellitus; FIB-4, Fibrosis-4 score.

3.1.2. Point Shear Wave Elastography (pSWE)

This technique, based on ARFI, is integrated into conventional ultrasound systems [101,102]. A significant advantage of pSWE is that it can assess liver fibrosis and evaluate the liver parenchyma on the same examination [102].

Shear wave elastography was also used in measuring liver stiffness in a case series of ten patients with diabetes and dyslipidemia in which the safety and effectiveness of saroglitazar in improving NAFLD, a dual PPAR α/γ agonist approved for diabetes in India, were assessed [103].

When the accuracies of LSM by TE, ARFI, and supersonic shears wave (SSI) for the staging of fibrosis were compared on a cohort of patients with NAFLD using liver biopsy as a reference, ARFI performance was found to be better for severe fibrosis and cirrhosis than for mild to moderate fibrosis. As more than half of the selected population had T2DM, variables such as BMI $\geq$30 kg/m^2, waist circumference $\geq$102 cm, or increased intercostal wall thickness may have interfered with and provided unreliable results when ARFI was used, compared with other imaging techniques [104].

However, mixed results are reported in this area. A meta-analysis assessing the diagnostic performance of pSWE vs. TE for staging liver fibrosis found a higher rate of failure in TE measurements using the M probe, more than in pSWE estimations, and obesity appeared to have a lesser influence on the results (11.3% vs. 0.8%) [105]. Giuffrè et al. screened several subjects with obesity having undergone bariatric surgery and reported that LSM is machine-dependent when taking into consideration the skin-to-liver distance (SLD) effect and not just the BMI [106].

While the Ultrasound Liver Elastography Consensus Statement, of the Society of Radiologists, recommends the "rule of four" (5, 9, 13, and 17 kPa) for liver stiffness cut-off values obtained using pSWE or 2D-SWE in NAFLD, no cut-off values specific to the T2DM population exist [107].

There are limited studies on the diagnostic ability of pSWE in patients with NAFLD and diabetes, and some of them included a limited number of patients with diabetes in the selected population. However, intriguing results reported by Meyer et al. using pSWE revealed a relatively high prevalence of liver fibrosis associated with NAFLD, even in patients with type 1 diabetes mellitus (T1DM), with a rate of 16% vs. 31% in T2DM subjects [108].

Existing studies have predominantly involved populations with obesity (adults and children), of which some underwent bariatric surgery [109–111]. Studies focusing on the estimation of liver fibrosis with pSWE in patients with T2DM and NAFLD are described in Table 2.

Table 2. Diagnostic performance and comparison of results for different fibrosis stages using pSWE in patients with NAFLD and T2DM.

Author, Ref.	Year	Country	No. of Patients	No. of NAFLD Patients	No. of Diabetic Patients	Diabetes Duration (Years)	Mean Age (Years)	Mean BMI (kg/m^2)	Fibrosis Stage	Optimal Cut-Off
Shaji et al. [112]	2022	India	140	30	140	1–5	54.53 ± 12.42	27.37 ± 2.73	21.43%	Unavailable
Meyer et al. [108]	2021	Germany	310	49	T1DM: 93	29	53	25.3	- F2–F4: 8% F3–F4: 5%	1.34 m/s 1.55 m/s 1.8
				88	T2DM: 161	14	65	29.6	- F2–F4: 27% F3–F4: 19%	1.34 m/s 1.55 m/s 1.8 m/s
Demirtas et al. [113]	2020	Turkey	108	54	34	–	54.9 ± 7.7	28 ± 2.2	F1 F2 F3	6.19 ± 1.89 kPa 7.6 ± 1.39 kPa 10.03 ± 4.71 kPa
Roy et al. [103]	2020	India	10	10	10 (T2DM)	7–11	59.3	25.21 ± 3.07	N Mild Moderate Severe Unavailable	1–1.5 m/s 1.5–1.75 m/s 1.75–2.1 m/s >2.1 m/s
Roy et al. [114]	2019	India	36	32	36 (T2DM)	6	52	27.75	N: 11.1% Mild: 27.7% Moderate: 52.7% Severe: 8.3%	1–1.5 m/s 1.5–1.75 m/s 1.75–2.1 m/s >2.1 m/s

Abbreviations: NAFLD, non-alcoholic fatty liver disease; T1DM, type 1 diabetes mellitus; T2DM, type 2 diabetes mellitus; BMI, body mass index; F, fibrosis; N, normal.

3.1.3. Two-dimensional Shear Wave Elastography (2D-SWE)

Two-dimensional shear wave elastography, or SSI, is also an ARFI-based technique that seems to be a rapid and reproducible technique that adapts ultrasound imaging to measure liver stiffness [102]. In healthy populations, liver stiffness values found by 2D-SWE range between 4.4 and 4.9 kPa [46].

In the two-center study by Cassinotto et al., the relevant covariates influencing the results of the 2D-SWE method were increased waist circumference, higher BMI values, thicker intercostal wall, and, in some cases, diabetes [104].

MS is associated with high liver stiffness [115]. Moreover, a cross-sectional, one-center Japanese study in people with abdominal obesity (Japanese diagnostic criteria for MS include waist circumference values of ≥85 cm for men and ≥90 cm for women) showed that waist circumference was significantly and independently correlated with liver stiffness measured by 2D-SWE [116]. The advantages of 2D-SWE have become evident in individuals with NAFLD and severe obesity, where its findings showed a higher success rate in comparison with TE, one of the most validated tools available [117]. In patients with clinically severe obesity that were evaluated before and after metabolic surgery by 2D-SWE-based LSM, improved characteristics were seen [118].

A comparison of TE, 2D-SWE, and magnetic resonance elastography (MRE) methods found them to be viable alternatives to liver biopsy for examining hepatic stiffness in 231 NAFLD patients. No differences were found between these techniques in the ability to diagnose the F1–3 stages, but MRE was superior to TE and 2D-SWE in detecting the F4 stage. Patients in this study included more than 60% subjects with diabetes, but no other information about this category was available [119].

In another study, obesity, T2DM, and arterial hypertension were independent predictors of a 2D-SWE value ≥ 8 kPa; patients with T2DM and hypertension exhibited a double risk for a hepatologist referral, while patients with obesity had a threefold risk. Therefore, focusing on patients with these medical conditions may improve NAFLD-related risk stratification [120].

Even though pSWE and 2D-SWE are less available in tertiary hepatology clinics and current evidence in patients with T2DM is limited, they may become a forthcoming routine tool for the screening, diagnostic, and therapeutic follow-up of patients with both NAFLD and diabetes [121].

Studies using the 2D-SWE method to assess liver fibrosis in patients with T2DM and NAFLD are described in Table 3.

Table 3. Diagnostic performance and comparison of results for different fibrosis stages using 2D-SWE in patients with NAFLD and T2DM.

Author, Ref	Year	Country	No. of Patients	No. of NAFLD Patients	No. of Diabetic Patients	Diabetes Duration (Years)	Mean Age (Years)	Mean BMI (kg/m^2)	Fibrosis Stage	Optimal Cut-Off (kPa)
Miyoshi et al. [116]	2021	Japan	318	-	41	–	63.4	22.7	Unavailable	5.79 ± 1.11
Shaheen et al. [120]	2020	United Kingdom	1958	67 (SWE ≥ 8 kPa)	38	–	61	37.2	91.5% 3.4% 5.1%	<8 ≥8 inconclusive

Abbreviations: NAFLD, non-alcoholic fatty liver disease; BMI, body mass index; kPa, kilopascals; SWE, shear wave elastography.

3.2. *Additional Results Obtained by Imaging Methods Complemented with Elastography*

CAP uses ultrasound waves to detect and quantify liver fat by measuring the degree of ultrasound attenuation by hepatic steatosis after the initial attenuation in the adipose tissue within the abdominal wall [87,122]. It is an affordable method that can identify and monitor persons at risk for NAFLD. Fibroscan® software added CAP in 2010, so it can assess both fibrosis by LSM and steatosis by CAP at the same time [123]. CAP is derived from the attenuation of the same ultrasound data used to track the shear wave speed [124]. Several measurement algorithms based on the same principle as CAP are available on other ultrasound systems [124] but are less used in studies on patients with NAFLD.

CAP qualifies today as a standardized non-invasive measure of liver steatosis. The clinical use of CAP is limited due to difficulties in establishing optimal cut-offs for every steatosis grade and to the influence of other conditions such as diabetes. It appears that the steatosis prevalence in a specific population, its etiology, BMI values, and the co-existence of diabetes must be taken into consideration when interpreting CAP [125].

Several studies using LSM and CAP support the use of CAP to screen for NAFLD in patients with T2DM [87,89,99]. However, current guidelines do not yet recommend it as a standard routine method to identify NAFLD among asymptomatic, even though high-risk, populations [9]. It is noteworthy that a large number of studies overestimated the grade of hepatic fat by using lower, inappropriate CAP cut-offs, as described in Table 4 [75,76,83,89,90].

Table 4. Diagnostic performance and comparison of results for different steatosis degrees using CAP in patients with NAFLD and T2DM.

Author, Ref	Year	Country	No. of Patients	No. of NAFLD Patients	No. of Diabetic Patients	Diabetes Duration (Years)	Mean Age (Years)	Mean BMI (kg/m^2)	Steatosis Stage	Optimal Cut-Off (dB/m)
Trifan et al. [71]	2022	Romania	424	424	424	-	55.22 ± 10.88	29.12 ± 5.64	S1: 13.1% S2: 8.4% S3: 78.5%	≥274 ≥290 ≥302
Cardoso et al. [41]	2021	Brasil	400	336	400	8 (3–15)	64.4	30.4	41% 22%	>296 >330
Ciardullo et al. [74]	2021	USA	825	557 steatosis 179 fibrosis	825	10.1 ± 0.67 9.8 ± 1.28 15.8 ± 4.16 9.40 ± 1.14	60.6	29.5 ± 0.4 30.3 ± 0.63 34.1 ± 2.72 35.1 ± 0.66	S0: 26.2% S1: 7.2% S2: 8.3% S3: 58.3%	<274 274–289 290–301 ≥302
Grgurevic et al. [75]	2021	Croatia	454	353	454	-	64	30.09	29 22 302	249–268 269–280 >280
Gupta et al. [76]	2021	India	250 DM	246 steatosis 205 fibrosis	250	9.6 ± 6.4	51 ± 9	31.4 ± 8	S1: - S2: - S3: 85.2%	237–259 260–292 >292
Lee CH et al. [83]	2021	China	766	766	766	16.6 ± 9.2	59.4 ± 10.3	28.6 ± 4.5	Mild: 10.2% Moderate: 27.4% Severe: 62.4%	248–267 268–279 ≥280
Lomonaco el al. [77]	2021	USA	561	70% steatosis 21% fibrosis	561	-	60 ± 11	33.4 ± 6.2	S1: 9% S2: 7% S3: 54%	274–289 290–301 ≥302
Makker et al. [78]	2021	USA	85	81	59	15 ± 9	62 ± 11.7	33.1 ± 8.4	S0: 19% S1: 13% S2: 22% S3: 46%	<238 238 259 290
Trivedi et al. [81]	2021	USA	437	213	124	-	58.4	33.5	113 102	≥248 ≥280
Lee HW et al. [84]	2020	China	611	Baseline 611	611	-	57.7 ± 10.9	-	32% 61%	<248 ≥248
				After 3 years 611					12% 52%	<10 ≥10
Mikolasevic et al. [86]	2020	Croatia	679	568	679	7.15 ± 2.33	65.2 ± 11.6	30.75 ± 5.15	83.6%	≥238

Table 4. *Cont.*

Author, Ref	Year	Country	No. of Patients	No. of NAFLD Patients	No. of Diabetic Patients	Diabetes Duration (Years)	Mean Age (Years)	Mean BMI (kg/m^2)	Steatosis Stage	Optimal Cut-Off (dB/m)
Sawaf et al. [57]	2020	Lebanon	620	131	128	–	47.8 ± 13.4	26.21 ± 4.3	S1: 5.2% S2: 7% S3: 45.5%	Unavailable
Sporea et al. [87]	2020	Romania	776	534	534	10 ± 2	60.8 ± 8.7	32 ± 6	S0: 23.9% S1: 8.9% S2: 6.9% S3: 60.3%	- 274 290 302
Tuong et al. [61]	2020	Vietnam	307	225	307	3	56.5 ± 10.5	25.4 ± 2.8	S0: 26.7% S1: 20.5% S2: 21.8% S3: 31%	- 234–269 270–300 ≥301
Demir et al. [89]	2019	Turkey	124	117	124	–	53 ± 7	33.2 ± 6.6	Mild: 0 Moderate: 29 Severe: 88	222–232 233–289 ≥290
Fernando et al. [90]	2019	Philippines	704	164	285	4.05 ± 3.63	57.27 ± 13.06	27.58 ± 4.25	S0: 3.66% S1: 12.8% S2: 39.02% S3: 44.51%	<221 222–232 233–289 ≥290
Jaafar et al. [91]	2019	Lebanon	248	248	73	–	53.7 ± 14.6	29.43 ± 7.59	≤S1 32.3% S2 18.46% S3 27.7% S4 21.54%	Unavailable
Lombardi et al. [94]	2019	Italy	394	238	394	14 ± 8	67 ± 10	29.6 ± 4.2	171 128	≥248 ≥280
Kwok et al. [99]	2016	China	1918	1309	2119	10.7	60.6	26.2	S1: 5.1% S2: 29.6% S3: 38%	222–232 233–289 ≥290
Ahn et al. [58]	2014	South Korea	979	13	165	-	51.9	25.12 ± 3.11	S1: 15% S2: 17% S3: 26%	239–258 259–292 >292

Abbreviations: NAFLD, non-alcoholic fatty liver disease; BMI, body mass index; kPa, kilopascals; F, fibrosis; S, steatosis.

In the Vietnamese study previously mentioned in the TE section of this paper, steatosis severity was graded using the following CAP cut-off values: S0 (26.7% steatosis) for CAP ≤ 233 dB/m, S1 (20.5% steatosis) for CAP 234–269 dB/m, S2 (21.8% steatosis) for CAP 270–300 dB/m, and S3 (31% steatosis) for CAP > 301 dB/m [61]. This is another example of a study that used an inappropriate CAP cut-off and overestimated the results.

The simultaneous use of LSM and CAP to assess liver fibrosis and steatosis was brought into the spotlight by their implementation in patients with severe obesity that were candidates for bariatric surgery [126]. Only 60% of subjects were eligible for the use of the XL Fibroscan® probe. The results suggested that TE could estimate significant fibrosis (an LSM cut-off value ≥ 9 kPa) and significant hepatic steatosis (CAP ≥ 305 dB/m). The histological findings of patients who underwent liver biopsies appeared to correlate with LSM and CAP results [127].

As previously mentioned, higher estimates of hepatic tissue stiffness are associated with elevated BMI and waist circumference values. Moreover, Sporea et al. found supplementary associations between waist circumference, BMI, elevated AST, HbA1c, severe steatosis, higher CAP values, and advanced fibrosis [87].

The usefulness of CAP in monitoring therapeutic effects is the objective of several studies [34]. Liraglutide was able to reduce CAP-measured hepatic steatosis in addition to its well-known effects on body weight and plasma glucose control [128]. A study investigating, by TE, the effects of the GLP-1 receptor agonist dulaglutide in patients with T2DM was not able to show a reduction of intrahepatic fat, probably due to the short 12-week period of treatment [129]. Another study with a novel thiazolidinedione (lobeglitazone), using CAP by TE and having a primary endpoint of hepatic fat reduction, found improvements in NAFLD in patients with T2DM [130]: a 65% improvement in steatosis, comparable to the PIVENS trial where 69% of NAFLD patients responded to pioglitazone treatment [130,131]. Shimizu et al. assessed the impact of dapagliflozin, an SGLT-2 inhibitor, on liver steatosis and fibrosis: after 24 weeks of therapy, LSM decreased from 9.49 ± 6.05 kPa to 8.01 ± 5.78 kPa and CAP reduced from 314 ± 61 to 290 ± 73 dB/m in the dapagliflozin group [132].

As most studies did not have CAP available when evaluating liver stiffness, and some other studies used only the CAP software to assess NAFLD, we have chosen to address LSM and CAP separately in this paper. Studies using the CAP method to assess liver steatosis in patients with T2DM and NAFLD are described in Table 4.

4. The Place of Elastography-Based Techniques in the Screening Algorithm for NAFLD

As previously mentioned, an accumulating body of evidence supports the systematic use of ultrasound-based elastography for assessing hepatic steatosis and advanced fibrosis in high-risk patients. The appropriate management of patients with NAFLD must rely on accurate identification of fibrosis and steatosis severity [133].

Whether a screening strategy using NIT such as TE for the diagnosis of liver fibrosis is cost-effective is still a matter of debate [134]. Future results of the LiverScreen project, which aims to screen for liver fibrosis in the general population in European countries, will probably answer this question after 2025. If the results of this study help identify groups at high risk for chronic liver disease in the general or high-risk population, particularly in patients with obesity and diabetes, improved prevention of liver complications will perhaps become possible, thus ameliorating the burden on healthcare systems [135].

Until then, alternative non-invasive scores such as NFS or FIB-4 are recommended to rule out advanced fibrosis when TE is unavailable, thus minimizing the costs [136]. Other methods, such as MRE, have better sensitivity and specificity but are limited by cost and availability [44,137]. The selection of NIT for the diagnostic algorithm in low-prevalence populations must be performed by consulting a liver specialist [44].

Preliminary results of an ongoing cross-sectional trial reported that less than 2% of patients with diabetes are screened for liver fibrosis in primary and secondary care. A high proportion of cases in which liver fibrosis was confirmed (80.6%) were identified using serum fibrosis markers associated with TE or liver biopsy [138]. On the other hand, in the cross-sectional study by Park et al., the patients with diabetes benefited from fibrosis screening procedures in primary care, even in the absence of steatosis [139].

Unfortunately, the screening rate is low in this high-risk population, despite the high prevalence of significant liver fibrosis and steatosis among patients with diabetes [138]. Therefore, the systematic implementation of a routine screening algorithm is needed to improve the clinical care of patients with NAFLD and diabetes.

Current practices and guidelines have not yet adopted widespread screening because of the lack of evidence supporting the long-term benefits of screening and a favorable cost-effectiveness ratio [9,139]. This might hinder the identification of population groups at risk for NAFLD. Lomonaco et al. argue that NAFLD represents a public health problem for patients with T2DM by emphasizing the burden of the disease in a population with T2DM unaware of NAFLD that was screened with TE [77]. In line with this, Mansour et al., after demonstrating better identification of NAFLD in this category of patients, advised incorporating FIB-4 and TE as a two-tier assessment approach into the routine annual evaluation of patients with T2DM [79]. However, given the large number of people with diabetes, it is unlikely that clinicians will be able to apply TE to all T2DM patients. Therefore, it is important to identify patients at risk for fatty liver disease progression [99].

Currently, most screening suggestions for people with T2DM include non-invasive scores such as FIB-4 or NFS in association with TE [21,140]; this combination can be used to distinguish between populations at low or high risk for advanced fibrosis (Figure 1).

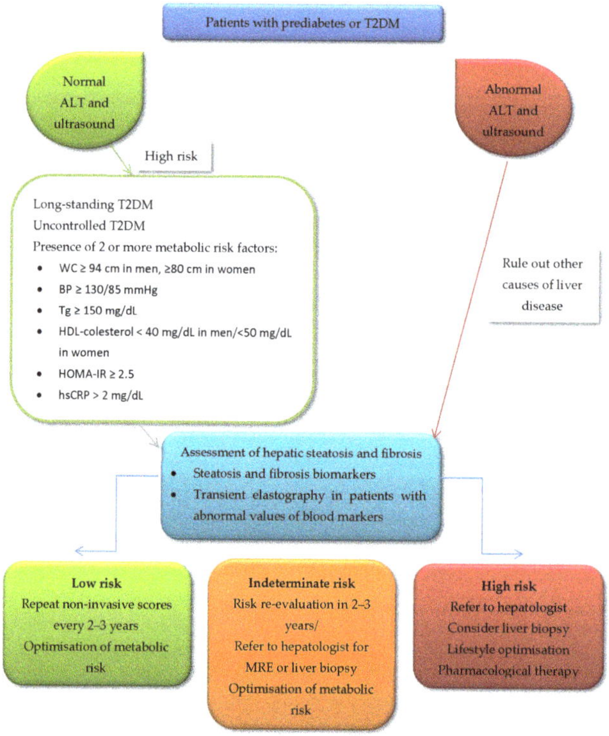

Figure 1. A suggested algorithm to screen patients with T2DM for NAFLD and advanced fibrosis [2,33,63,141]. *Abbreviations:* ALT, alanine aminotransferase; WC, waist circumference; BP, blood pressure; Tg, triglycerides; HOMA-IR, homeostatic model assessment for insulin resistance; hsCRP, high-sensitive C-reactive protein.

5. Gaps in Knowledge

Different researchers have used various cut-offs to study where elastography is positioned in the NAFLD assessment tree. As specific LSM cut-off values to predict fibrosis stages are not yet acknowledged, the method's reliability could be impaired. The spotlight falls on the optimal LSM cut-off values used to define severe fibrosis (F3 or F4 stages). $F \geq 3$ represents advanced fibrosis, while the F4 fibrosis stage usually suggests cirrhosis [142]. Supplementary difficulties arise from some studies not reporting LSM cut-offs that define different fibrosis stages [57,72,91], while others use different stage appellations that are difficult to correlate with the current standard definitions [81,83,89,116]. The age-adapted cut-offs should also be taken into account to improve the method's performance. Finally, some studies suggest that the use of lower cut-off values would optimize their negative predictive value.

As yet, patients with diabetes have not been compared directly with non-diabetic control groups in elastography-based investigation protocols. Hence, the same cut-off points were applied to stratify fibrosis and steatosis as in any other NAFLD patient. However, the diagnostic and prognostic accuracy for NAFLD of non-invasive imaging tools is significantly influenced by the presence of diabetes [143]. This category of methods needs, therefore, further investigation and validation in populations with T2DM, among which advanced fibrosis has a significantly rising prevalence.

When focusing on T2DM patients and trying to gather specific information on this NAFLD at-risk group population, researchers need to find the best methods to fill in these substantial knowledge gaps. There are only a few studies that directly targeted the diabetic population, while most research involved a larger population, among which only a subgroup of subjects had T2DM [71,96]. Because patients at risk for NAFLD may frequently have significant fibrosis, which can be overlooked on common ultrasound, especially when normal liver enzymes are associated, supplementary screening approaches should be considered, either in the general population or only in at-risk individuals represented by patients with obesity, T2DM, and MS [143]. It is, therefore, logical to presume that the utility of novel non-invasive assessment tools for NAFLD is of utmost importance, but we must acknowledge for now that their predictive ability is insufficiently demonstrated in diabetes populations [144]. At present, ADA recommends that all patients with prediabetes/T2DM and increased liver enzymes or steatosis on ultrasound should be evaluated for the presence of NAFLD, while the other guidelines have discordant approaches [36]. No guideline clearly states who should be selected for screening, who should do the screening, and which method is best to use.

Among elastography-based methods, most available evidence supports the use of TE, while pSWE and 2D-SWE, which are less available in liver clinics, feature limited data on patients with diabetes. Several studies are currently using the SWE techniques, but the available proof is not yet sufficient to generate recommendations, and the need to continue dedicated research in this at-risk population is still high.

The lack of technical information also narrows the reproducibility of data using LSM and CAP assessment. Many publications do not specify whether one or more operators were involved, if they were trained certified examiners, or if patients respected the examination protocol requiring, at least, a three-hour fast before undergoing elastography. [37,107]. The success rate depends on the operator's experience, but also other various factors such as age, BMI, visceral fat, or the presence of ascites; the probability of elastography-based methods failing increases in patients who are old, obese, or have ascites [14,37]. The number of exploratory measurements may also differ from one study to the other [37,145].

The method's applicability to NAFLD can be challenging in patients with obesity because of the high rate of failure in measurement and performance without the use of an XL probe. Some of the existing studies had limitations due to not using the XL probe to perform TE examinations on patients with obesity.

As mentioned before, liver biopsy is unsuited for large-scale applications in the diagnosis of NAFLD [143]. Moreover, the applicability of liver biopsies is limited in patients with T2DM and associated cardiovascular disease that need antiplatelet or anticoagulant therapy. However, this method is still required to confirm the results of non-invasive tools in clinical trials. Beyond designing an optimal, cost-effective algorithm for systematic risk stratification, the management of NAFLD in primary care should, therefore, include procedures to accurately estimate and minimize the need for biopsy.

At present, ultrasound-based elastography devices are not accessible in diabetes care clinics, thus requiring a strong collaboration with hepatologists to implement these new, simpler, non-invasive tools and to limit the use of invasive methods in the future. Among steps already taken in this direction, NIMBLE (non-invasive biomarkers of metabolic liver disease) [146] in the USA and LITMUS (liver investigation: testing marker utility in steatohepatitis) [147] in Europe are two projects looking to integrate non-invasive tools into clinical practice and to offer the scientific community data required to receive uniform acceptance.

6. Conclusions

To sum up, the results of recent studies show a high prevalence of NAFLD identified by TE among patients with T2DM. These findings support the need for systematic screening for NAFLD to assess the severity of hepatic steatosis and fibrosis in T2DM patients. Within the group of shear wave elastography-based methods, TE has already acquired a well-deserved place, while ARFI-based techniques have begun to collect scientific evidence supporting their value in NAFLD screening, diagnosis, and monitoring among patients with T2DM.

Priorities of this research field should include the setting of cut-off points adapted to specific situations such as the co-existence of diabetes, assessment of the cost-effectiveness and validation of quality criteria for these imaging methods, the risk stratification based on the fibrosis stage, and evaluation of elastography value in the assessment of therapeutic success. Producing a strategic algorithm to check each of these purposes could help diabetes care specialists and primary care providers. An early diagnosis in high-risk patients and the subsequent implementation of adapted interventions such as lifestyle optimization, lipid-lowering therapy, and antihyperglycemic drugs may have the chance to limit NAFLD and its extrahepatic complications, at least until further effective therapies are developed. Beyond this, supplementary research is needed to completely define all long-term benefits of these ultrasound-based elastography techniques.

Author Contributions: Conceptualization, G.-D.C., C.-M.L. and B.-M.M.; methodology, G.-D.C., C.M. and E.-D.G.; validation, G.-D.C., C.M. and B.-M.M.; formal analysis, C.M., E.-D.G. and A.O.; investigation, C.M., E.-D.G. and A.O.; resources, G.-D.C., C.-M.L., E.-D.G. and A.O.; writing—original draft preparation, G.-D.C., E.-D.G. and A.O.; writing—review and editing, C.-M.L., C.M. and B.-M.M.; visualization, G.-D.C. and C.-M.L.; supervision, B.-M.M.; project administration, C.-M.L. and E.-D.G. All authors have read and agreed to the published version of the manuscript.

Funding: This research received no external funding.

Institutional Review Board Statement: Not applicable.

Informed Consent Statement: Not applicable.

Data Availability Statement: Not applicable.

Conflicts of Interest: The authors declare no conflict of interest.

References

1. Younossi, Z.; Anstee, Q.M.; Marietti, M.; Hardy, T.; Henry, L.; Eslam, M.; George, J.; Bugianesi, E. Global Burden of NAFLD and NASH: Trends, Predictions, Risk Factors and Prevention. *Nat. Rev. Gastroenterol. Hepatol.* **2018**, *15*, 11–20. [CrossRef]
2. Kanwal, F.; Shubrook, J.H.; Adams, L.A.; Pfotenhauer, K.; Wai-Sun Wong, V.; Wright, E.; Abdelmalek, M.F.; Harrison, S.A.; Loomba, R.; Mantzoros, C.S.; et al. Clinical Care Pathway for the Risk Stratification and Management of Patients With Nonalcoholic Fatty Liver Disease. *Gastroenterology* **2021**, *161*, 1657–1669. [CrossRef] [PubMed]

3. IDF Diabetes Atlas. Available online: https://idf.org/e-library/epidemiology-research/diabetes-atlas.html?id=171 (accessed on 26 August 2022).
4. Younossi, Z.M.; Koenig, A.B.; Abdelatif, D.; Fazel, Y.; Henry, L.; Wymer, M. Global Epidemiology of Nonalcoholic Fatty Liver Disease-Meta-Analytic Assessment of Prevalence, Incidence, and Outcomes. *Hepatology* **2016**, *64*, 73–84. [CrossRef] [PubMed]
5. Younossi, Z.M.; Henry, L. Epidemiology of Non-Alcoholic Fatty Liver Disease and Hepatocellular Carcinoma. *JHEP Rep. Innov. Hepatol.* **2021**, *3*, 100305. [CrossRef] [PubMed]
6. Younossi, Z.M.; Golabi, P.; de Avila, L.; Paik, J.M.; Srishord, M.; Fukui, N.; Qiu, Y.; Burns, L.; Afendy, A.; Nader, F. The Global Epidemiology of NAFLD and NASH in Patients with Type 2 Diabetes: A Systematic Review and Meta-Analysis. *J. Hepatol.* **2019**, *71*, 793–801. [CrossRef]
7. Younossi, Z.; Tacke, F.; Arrese, M.; Chander Sharma, B.; Mostafa, I.; Bugianesi, E.; Wai-Sun Wong, V.; Yilmaz, Y.; George, J.; Fan, J. Global Perspectives on Nonalcoholic Fatty Liver Disease and Nonalcoholic Steatohepatitis. *Hepatology* **2019**, *69*, 2672–2682. [CrossRef]
8. Duell, P.B.; Welty, F.K.; Miller, M.; Chait, A.; Hammond, G.; Ahmad, Z.; Cohen, D.E.; Horton, J.D.; Pressman, G.S.; Toth, P.P. Nonalcoholic Fatty Liver Disease and Cardiovascular Risk: A Scientific Statement from the American Heart Association. *Arterioscler. Thromb. Vasc. Biol.* **2022**, *42*, e168–e185. [CrossRef]
9. Chalasani, N.; Younossi, Z.; Lavine, J.E.; Charlton, M.; Cusi, K.; Rinella, M.; Harrison, S.A.; Brunt, E.M.; Sanyal, A.J. The Diagnosis and Management of Nonalcoholic Fatty Liver Disease: Practice Guidance from the American Association for the Study of Liver Diseases. *Hepatology* **2018**, *67*, 328–357. [CrossRef]
10. Ekstedt, M.; Hagström, H.; Nasr, P.; Fredrikson, M.; Stål, P.; Kechagias, S.; Hultcrantz, R. Fibrosis Stage Is the Strongest Predictor for Disease-Specific Mortality in NAFLD after up to 33 Years of Follow-Up. *Hepatology* **2015**, *61*, 1547–1554. [CrossRef]
11. Eslam, M.; Sanyal, A.J.; George, J. International Consensus Panel MAFLD: A Consensus-Driven Proposed Nomenclature for Metabolic Associated Fatty Liver Disease. *Gastroenterology* **2020**, *158*, 1999–2014.e1. [CrossRef]
12. Kang, S.H.; Cho, Y.; Jeong, S.W.; Kim, S.U.; Lee, J.-W. From Nonalcoholic Fatty Liver Disease to Metabolic-Associated Fatty Liver Disease: Big Wave or Ripple? *Clin. Mol. Hepatol.* **2021**, *27*, 257–269. [CrossRef] [PubMed]
13. Hazlehurst, J.M.; Woods, C.; Marjot, T.; Cobbold, J.F.; Tomlinson, J.W. Non-Alcoholic Fatty Liver Disease and Diabetes. *Metabolism* **2016**, *65*, 1096–1108. [CrossRef] [PubMed]
14. European Association for the Study of the Liver (EASL); European Association for the Study of Diabetes (EASD); European Association for the Study of Obesity (EASO). EASL-EASD-EASO Clinical Practice Guidelines for the Management of Non-Alcoholic Fatty Liver Disease. *J. Hepatol.* **2016**, *64*, 1388–1402. [CrossRef]
15. Kitagawa, N.; Hashimoto, Y.; Hamaguchi, M.; Osaka, T.; Fukuda, T.; Yamazaki, M.; Fukui, M. Liver Stiffness Is Associated With Progression of Albuminuria in Adults With Type 2 Diabetes: Nonalcoholic Fatty Disease Cohort Study. *Can. J. Diabetes* **2020**, *44*, 428–433. [CrossRef] [PubMed]
16. Powell, E.E.; Wong, V.W.-S.; Rinella, M. Non-Alcoholic Fatty Liver Disease. *Lancet Lond. Engl.* **2021**, *397*, 2212–2224. [CrossRef]
17. Mantovani, A.; Petracca, G.; Beatrice, G.; Tilg, H.; Byrne, C.D.; Targher, G. Non-Alcoholic Fatty Liver Disease and Risk of Incident Diabetes Mellitus: An Updated Meta-Analysis of 501 022 Adult Individuals. *Gut* **2021**, *70*, 962–969. [CrossRef]
18. Luo, J.; Xu, L.; Li, J.; Zhao, S. Nonalcoholic Fatty Liver Disease as a Potential Risk Factor of Cardiovascular Disease. *Eur. J. Gastroenterol. Hepatol.* **2015**, *27*, 193–199. [CrossRef]
19. Wijarnpreecha, K.; Aby, E.S.; Ahmed, A.; Kim, D. Evaluation and Management of Extrahepatic Manifestations of Nonalcoholic Fatty Liver Disease. *Clin. Mol. Hepatol.* **2021**, *27*, 221–235. [CrossRef]
20. Poustchi, H.; Alaei-Shahmiri, F.; Aghili, R.; Nobarani, S.; Malek, M.; Khamseh, M.E. Hepatic Steatosis and Fibrosis in Type 2 Diabetes: A Risk-Based Approach to Targeted Screening. *Arch. Iran. Med.* **2021**, *24*, 177–186. [CrossRef]
21. Cotter, T.G.; Rinella, M. Nonalcoholic Fatty Liver Disease 2020: The State of the Disease. *Gastroenterology* **2020**, *158*, 1851–1864. [CrossRef]
22. Guan, C.; Fu, S.; Zhen, D.; Yang, K.; An, J.; Wang, Y.; Ma, C.; Jiang, N.; Zhao, N.; Liu, J.; et al. Metabolic (Dysfunction)-Associated Fatty Liver Disease in Chinese Patients with Type 2 Diabetes from a Subcenter of the National Metabolic Management Center. *J. Diabetes Res.* **2022**, *2022*, e8429847. [CrossRef] [PubMed]
23. Singh, A.; Le, P.; Peerzada, M.M.; Lopez, R.; Alkhouri, N. The Utility of Noninvasive Scores in Assessing the Prevalence of Nonalcoholic Fatty Liver Disease and Advanced Fibrosis in Type 2 Diabetic Patients. *J. Clin. Gastroenterol.* **2018**, *52*, 268–272. [CrossRef] [PubMed]
24. Ciardullo, S.; Sala, I.; Perseghin, G. Screening Strategies for Nonalcoholic Fatty Liver Disease in Type 2 Diabetes: Insights from NHANES 2005-2016. *Diabetes Res. Clin. Pract.* **2020**, *167*, 108358. [CrossRef]
25. Singh, A.; Garg, R.; Lopez, R.; Alkhouri, N. Diabetes Liver Fibrosis Score to Detect Advanced Fibrosis in Diabetics with Nonalcoholic Fatty Liver Disease. *Clin. Gastroenterol. Hepatol.* **2022**, *20*, e624–e626. [CrossRef] [PubMed]
26. Bertot, L.C.; Jeffrey, G.P.; de Boer, B.; MacQuillan, G.; Garas, G.; Chin, J.; Huang, Y.; Adams, L.A. Diabetes Impacts Prediction of Cirrhosis and Prognosis by Non-Invasive Fibrosis Models in Non-Alcoholic Fatty Liver Disease. *Liver Int. Off. J. Int. Assoc. Study Liver* **2018**, *38*, 1793–1802. [CrossRef] [PubMed]
27. Lee, Y.; Cho, Y.; Lee, B.-W.; Park, C.-Y.; Lee, D.H.; Cha, B.-S.; Rhee, E.-J. Nonalcoholic Fatty Liver Disease in Diabetes. Part I: Epidemiology and Diagnosis. *Diabetes Metab. J.* **2019**, *43*, 31–45. [CrossRef]

28. Prashanth, M.; Ganesh, H.K.; Vima, M.V.; John, M.; Bandgar, T.; Joshi, S.R.; Shah, S.R.; Rathi, P.M.; Joshi, A.S.; Thakkar, H.; et al. Prevalence of Nonalcoholic Fatty Liver Disease in Patients with Type 2 Diabetes Mellitus. *J. Assoc. Physicians India* **2009**, *57*, 205–210.
29. Williamson, R.M.; Price, J.F.; Glancy, S.; Perry, E.; Nee, L.D.; Hayes, P.C.; Frier, B.M.; Van Look, L.A.F.; Johnston, G.I.; Reynolds, R.M.; et al. Prevalence of and Risk Factors for Hepatic Steatosis and Nonalcoholic Fatty Liver Disease in People with Type 2 Diabetes: The Edinburgh Type 2 Diabetes Study. *Diabetes Care* **2011**, *34*, 1139–1144. [CrossRef]
30. Garg, H.; Aggarwal, S.; Shalimar; Yadav, R.; Datta Gupta, S.; Agarwal, L.; Agarwal, S. Utility of Transient Elastography (Fibroscan) and Impact of Bariatric Surgery on Nonalcoholic Fatty Liver Disease (NAFLD) in Morbidly Obese Patients. *Surg. Obes. Relat. Dis. Off. J. Am. Soc. Bariatr. Surg.* **2018**, *14*, 81–91. [CrossRef]
31. Troelstra, M.A.; Witjes, J.J.; van Dijk, A.-M.; Mak, A.L.; Gurney-Champion, O.; Runge, J.H.; Zwirs, D.; Stols-Gonçalves, D.; Zwinderman, A.H.; Ten Wolde, M.; et al. Assessment of Imaging Modalities Against Liver Biopsy in Nonalcoholic Fatty Liver Disease: The Amsterdam NAFLD-NASH Cohort. *J. Magn. Reson. Imaging JMRI* **2021**, *54*, 1937–1949. [CrossRef]
32. Francque, S.M.; Marchesini, G.; Kautz, A.; Walmsley, M.; Dorner, R.; Lazarus, J.V.; Zelber-Sagi, S.; Hallsworth, K.; Busetto, L.; Frühbeck, G.; et al. Non-Alcoholic Fatty Liver Disease: A Patient Guideline. *JHEP Rep. Innov. Hepatol.* **2021**, *3*, 100322. [CrossRef]
33. Tomah, S.; Alkhouri, N.; Hamdy, O. Nonalcoholic Fatty Liver Disease and Type 2 Diabetes: Where Do Diabetologists Stand? *Clin. Diabetes Endocrinol.* **2020**, *6*, 9. [CrossRef] [PubMed]
34. Negi, C.K.; Babica, P.; Bajard, L.; Bienertova-Vasku, J.; Tarantino, G. Insights into the Molecular Targets and Emerging Pharmacotherapeutic Interventions for Nonalcoholic Fatty Liver Disease. *Metabolism* **2022**, *126*, 154925. [CrossRef]
35. Arab, J.P.; Barrera, F.; Gallego, C.; Valderas, J.P.; Uribe, S.; Tejos, C.; Serrano, C.; Serrano, C.; Huete, Á.; Liberona, J.; et al. High Prevalence of Undiagnosed Liver Cirrhosis and Advanced Fibrosis in Type 2 Diabetic Patients. *Ann. Hepatol.* **2016**, *15*, 721–728. [CrossRef] [PubMed]
36. American Diabetes Association Standards of Medical Care in Diabetes—2022 Abridged for Primary Care Providers. *Clin. Diabetes* **2022**, *40*, 10–38. [CrossRef]
37. Dietrich, C.F.; Bamber, J.; Berzigotti, A.; Bota, S.; Cantisani, V.; Castera, L.; Cosgrove, D.; Ferraioli, G.; Friedrich-Rust, M.; Gilja, O.H.; et al. EFSUMB Guidelines and Recommendations on the Clinical Use of Liver Ultrasound Elastography, Update 2017 (Short Version). *Ultraschall Med.* **2017**, *38*, 377–394. [CrossRef] [PubMed]
38. Srinivasa Babu, A.; Wells, M.L.; Teytelboym, O.M.; Mackey, J.E.; Miller, F.H.; Yeh, B.M.; Ehman, R.L.; Venkatesh, S.K. Elastography in Chronic Liver Disease: Modalities, Techniques, Limitations, and Future Directions. *Radiographics* **2016**, *36*, 1987–2006. [CrossRef] [PubMed]
39. Eddowes, P.J.; Sasso, M.; Allison, M.; Tsochatzis, E.; Anstee, Q.M.; Sheridan, D.; Guha, I.N.; Cobbold, J.F.; Deeks, J.J.; Paradis, V.; et al. Accuracy of FibroScan Controlled Attenuation Parameter and Liver Stiffness Measurement in Assessing Steatosis and Fibrosis in Patients With Nonalcoholic Fatty Liver Disease. *Gastroenterology* **2019**, *156*, 1717–1730. [CrossRef] [PubMed]
40. Marie, S.; Tripp, D.K.K.; Cherrington, N.J. Strategies to Diagnose Non-Alcoholic Steatohepatitis: A Novel Approach to Take Advantage of Pharmacokinetic Alterations. *Drug Metab. Dispos.* **2022**, *50*, 492–499. [CrossRef]
41. Cardoso, C.R.L.; Villela-Nogueira, C.A.; Leite, N.C.; Salles, G.F. Prognostic Impact of Liver Fibrosis and Steatosis by Transient Elastography for Cardiovascular and Mortality Outcomes in Individuals with Nonalcoholic Fatty Liver Disease and Type 2 Diabetes: The Rio de Janeiro Cohort Study. *Cardiovasc. Diabetol.* **2021**, *20*, 193. [CrossRef]
42. Eskridge, W.; Vierling, J.M.; Gosbee, W.; Wan, G.A.; Hyunh, M.-L.; Chang, H.E. Screening for Undiagnosed Non-Alcoholic Fatty Liver Disease (NAFLD) and Non-Alcoholic Steatohepatitis (NASH): A Population-Based Risk Factor Assessment Using Vibration Controlled Transient Elastography (VCTE). *PLoS ONE* **2021**, *16*, e0260320. [CrossRef] [PubMed]
43. Petroff, D.; Blank, V.; Newsome, P.N.; Shalimar; Voican, C.S.; Thiele, M.; de Lédinghen, V.; Baumeler, S.; Chan, W.K.; Perlemuter, G.; et al. Assessment of Hepatic Steatosis by Controlled Attenuation Parameter Using the M and XL Probes: An Individual Patient Data Meta-Analysis. *Lancet Gastroenterol. Hepatol.* **2021**, *6*, 185–198. [CrossRef]
44. Berzigotti, A.; Tsochatzis, E.; Boursier, J.; Castera, L.; Cazzagon, N.; Friedrich-Rust, M.; Petta, S.; Thiele, M. EASL Clinical Practice Guidelines on Non-Invasive Tests for Evaluation of Liver Disease Severity and Prognosis–2021 Update. *J. Hepatol.* **2021**, *75*, 659–689. [CrossRef] [PubMed]
45. Ferraioli, G. Ultrasound Techniques for the Assessment of Liver Stiffness: A Correct Terminology. *Hepatology* **2019**, *69*, 461. [CrossRef] [PubMed]
46. Lupsor-Platon, M. *Noninvasive Evaluation of Fibrosis and Steatosis in Nonalcoholic Fatty Liver Disease by Elastographic Methods*; IntechOpen: London, UK, 2017; ISBN 978-953-51-3924-9.
47. Yoneda, M.; Yoneda, M.; Yoneda, M.; Fujita, K.; Fujita, K.; Inamori, M.; Inamori, M.; Tamano, M.; Tamano, M.; Hiriishi, H.; et al. Transient Elastography in Patients with Non-Alcoholic Fatty Liver Disease (NAFLD). *Gut* **2007**, *56*, 1330–1331. [CrossRef] [PubMed]
48. European Association for Study of Liver; Asociacion Latinoamericana para el Estudio del Higado EASL-ALEH Clinical Practice Guidelines: Non-Invasive Tests for Evaluation of Liver Disease Severity and Prognosis. *J. Hepatol.* **2015**, *63*, 237–264. [CrossRef]
49. Lim, J.K.; Flamm, S.L.; Singh, S.; Falck-Ytter, Y.T. Clinical Guidelines Committee of the American Gastroenterological Association American Gastroenterological Association Institute Guideline on the Role of Elastography in the Evaluation of Liver Fibrosis. *Gastroenterology* **2017**, *152*, 1536–1543. [CrossRef]

50. Roulot, D. Screening for Liver Fibrosis in General or At-Risk Populations Using Transient Elastography. In *Liver Elastography: Clinical Use and Interpretation*; Mueller, S., Ed.; Springer International Publishing: Cham, Switzerland, 2020; pp. 545–550, ISBN 978-3-030-40542-7.
51. Sporea, I.; Şirli, R.; Mare, R.; Popescu, A.; Ivaşcu, S.C. Feasibility of Transient Elastography with M and XL Probes in Real Life. *Med. Ultrason.* **2016**, *18*, 7–10. [CrossRef]
52. De Franchis, R. Baveno VI Faculty Expanding Consensus in Portal Hypertension: Report of the Baveno VI Consensus Workshop: Stratifying Risk and Individualizing Care for Portal Hypertension. *J. Hepatol.* **2015**, *63*, 743–752. [CrossRef]
53. Mantovani, A.; Byrne, C.D.; Bonora, E.; Targher, G. Nonalcoholic Fatty Liver Disease and Risk of Incident Type 2 Diabetes: A Meta-Analysis. *Diabetes Care* **2018**, *41*, 372–382. [CrossRef]
54. Koehler, E.M.; Plompen, E.P.C.; Schouten, J.N.L.; Hansen, B.E.; Darwish Murad, S.; Taimr, P.; Leebeek, F.W.G.; Hofman, A.; Stricker, B.H.; Castera, L.; et al. Presence of Diabetes Mellitus and Steatosis Is Associated with Liver Stiffness in a General Population: The Rotterdam Study. *Hepatology* **2016**, *63*, 138–147. [CrossRef] [PubMed]
55. Hari, A. Ultrasound Elastography-Cornerstone of Non-Invasive Metabolic Dysfunction-Associated Fatty Liver Disease Assessment. *Med. Kaunas Lith.* **2021**, *57*, 516. [CrossRef] [PubMed]
56. Cho, H.J.; Hwang, S.; Park, J.I.; Yang, M.J.; Hwang, J.C.; Yoo, B.M.; Lee, K.M.; Shin, S.J.; Lee, K.J.; Kim, J.H.; et al. Improvement of Nonalcoholic Fatty Liver Disease Reduces the Risk of Type 2 Diabetes Mellitus. *Gut Liver* **2019**, *13*, 440–449. [CrossRef] [PubMed]
57. Sawaf, B.; Ali, A.H.; Jaafar, R.F.; Kanso, M.; Mukherji, D.; Khalife, M.J.; Faraj, W. Spectrum of Liver Diseases in Patients Referred for Fibroscan: A Single Center Experience in the Middle East. *Ann. Med. Surg.* **2020**, *57*, 166–170. [CrossRef] [PubMed]
58. Ahn, J.M.; Paik, Y.-H.; Kim, S.H.; Lee, J.H.; Cho, J.Y.; Sohn, W.; Gwak, G.-Y.; Choi, M.S.; Lee, J.H.; Koh, K.C.; et al. Relationship of Liver Stiffness and Controlled Attenuation Parameter Measured by Transient Elastography with Diabetes Mellitus in Patients with Chronic Liver Disease. *J. Korean Med. Sci.* **2014**, *29*, 1113–1119. [CrossRef] [PubMed]
59. Patel, P.; Hossain, F.; Horsfall, L.U.; Banh, X.; Hayward, K.L.; Williams, S.; Johnson, T.; Bernard, A.; Brown, N.N.; Lampe, G.; et al. A Pragmatic Approach Identifies a High Rate of Nonalcoholic Fatty Liver Disease With Advanced Fibrosis in Diabetes Clinics and At-Risk Populations in Primary Care. *Hepatol. Commun.* **2018**, *2*, 897–909. [CrossRef] [PubMed]
60. Sandrin, L. Liver Stiffness Measurement Using Vibration-Controlled Transient Elastography. In *Liver Elastography: Clinical Use and Interpretation*; Mueller, S., Ed.; Springer International Publishing: Cham, Switzerland, 2020; pp. 29–39, ISBN 978-3-030-40542-7.
61. Tuong, T.T.K.; Tran, D.K.; Phu, P.Q.T.; Hong, T.N.D.; Chu Dinh, T.; Chu, D.T. Non-Alcoholic Fatty Liver Disease in Patients with Type 2 Diabetes: Evaluation of Hepatic Fibrosis and Steatosis Using Fibroscan. *Diagnostics* **2020**, *10*, 159. [CrossRef]
62. Sobhonslidsuk, A.; Pulsombat, A.; Kaewdoung, P.; Petraksa, S. Non-Alcoholic Fatty Liver Disease (NAFLD) and Significant Hepatic Fibrosis Defined by Non-Invasive Assessment in Patients with Type 2 Diabetes. *Asian Pac. J. Cancer Prev. APJCP* **2015**, *16*, 1789–1794. [CrossRef]
63. Eslam, M.; Newsome, P.N.; Sarin, S.K.; Anstee, Q.M.; Targher, G.; Romero-Gomez, M.; Zelber-Sagi, S.; Wai-Sun Wong, V.; Dufour, J.-F.; Schattenberg, J.M.; et al. A New Definition for Metabolic Dysfunction-Associated Fatty Liver Disease: An International Expert Consensus Statement. *J. Hepatol.* **2020**, *73*, 202–209. [CrossRef]
64. Anstee, Q.M.; Lawitz, E.J.; Alkhouri, N.; Wong, V.W.-S.; Romero-Gomez, M.; Okanoue, T.; Trauner, M.; Kersey, K.; Li, G.; Han, L.; et al. Noninvasive Tests Accurately Identify Advanced Fibrosis Due to NASH: Baseline Data From the STELLAR Trials. *Hepatology* **2019**, *70*, 1521–1530. [CrossRef]
65. Chan, W.-K.; Treeprasertsuk, S.; Goh, G.B.-B.; Fan, J.-G.; Song, M.J.; Charatcharoenwitthaya, P.; Duseja, A.; Dan, Y.-Y.; Imajo, K.; Nakajima, A.; et al. Optimizing Use of Nonalcoholic Fatty Liver Disease Fibrosis Score, Fibrosis-4 Score, and Liver Stiffness Measurement to Identify Patients With Advanced Fibrosis. *Clin. Gastroenterol. Hepatol.* **2019**, *17*, 2570–2580.e37. [CrossRef] [PubMed]
66. Petta, S.; Vanni, E.; Bugianesi, E.; Di Marco, V.; Cammà, C.; Cabibi, D.; Mezzabotta, L.; Craxì, A. The Combination of Liver Stiffness Measurement and NAFLD Fibrosis Score Improves the Noninvasive Diagnostic Accuracy for Severe Liver Fibrosis in Patients with Nonalcoholic Fatty Liver Disease. *Liver Int.* **2015**, *35*, 1566–1573. [CrossRef] [PubMed]
67. Petta, S.; Wong, V.W.-S.; Cammà, C.; Hiriart, J.-B.; Wong, G.L.-H.; Vergniol, J.; Chan, A.W.-H.; Di Marco, V.; Merrouche, W.; Chan, H.L.-Y.; et al. Serial Combination of Non-Invasive Tools Improves the Diagnostic Accuracy of Severe Liver Fibrosis in Patients with NAFLD. *Aliment. Pharmacol. Ther.* **2017**, *46*, 617–627. [CrossRef] [PubMed]
68. Newsome, P.N.; Sasso, M.; Deeks, J.J.; Paredes, A.; Boursier, J.; Chan, W.-K.; Yilmaz, Y.; Czernichow, S.; Zheng, M.-H.; Wong, V.W.-S.; et al. FibroScan-AST (FAST) Score for the Non-Invasive Identification of Patients with Non-Alcoholic Steatohepatitis with Significant Activity and Fibrosis: A Prospective Derivation and Global Validation Study. *Lancet Gastroenterol. Hepatol.* **2020**, *5*, 362–373. [CrossRef]
69. Casey, S.P.; Kemp, W.W.; McLean, C.A.; Topliss, D.J.; Adams, L.A.; Roberts, S.K. A Prospective Evaluation of the Role of Transient Elastography for the Detection of Hepatic Fibrosis in Type 2 Diabetes without Overt Liver Disease. *Scand. J. Gastroenterol.* **2012**, *47*, 836–841. [CrossRef]
70. Dai, C.-Y.; Fang, T.-J.; Hung, W.-W.; Tsai, H.-J.; Tsai, Y.-C. The Determinants of Liver Fibrosis in Patients with Nonalcoholic Fatty Liver Disease and Type 2 Diabetes Mellitus. *Biomedicines* **2022**, *10*, 1487. [CrossRef]
71. Trifan, A.; Stratina, E.; Nastasa, R.; Rotaru, A.; Stafie, R.; Zenovia, S.; Huiban, L.; Sfarti, C.; Cojocariu, C.; Cuciureanu, T.; et al. Simultaneously Screening for Liver Steatosis and Fibrosis in Romanian Type 2 Diabetes Mellitus Patients Using Vibration-Controlled Transient Elastography with Controlled Attenuation Parameter. *Diagnostics* **2022**, *12*, 1753. [CrossRef]

72. Alexopoulos, A.-S.; Duffy, R.; Kobe, E.A.; German, J.; Moylan, C.A.; Soliman, D.; Jeffreys, A.S.; Coffman, C.J.; Crowley, M.J. Underrecognition of Nonalcoholic Fatty Liver Disease in Poorly Controlled Diabetes: A Call to Action in Diabetes Care. *J. Endocr. Soc.* **2021**, *5*, bvab155. [CrossRef]
73. Chhabra, S.; Singh, S.P.; Singh, A.; Mehta, V.; Kaur, A.; Bansal, N.; Sood, A. Diabetes Mellitus Increases the Risk of Significant Hepatic Fibrosis in Patients With Non-Alcoholic Fatty Liver Disease. *J. Clin. Exp. Hepatol.* **2022**, *12*, 409–416. [CrossRef]
74. Ciardullo, S.; Monti, T.; Perseghin, G. High Prevalence of Advanced Liver Fibrosis Assessed by Transient Elastography Among U.S. Adults With Type 2 Diabetes. *Diabetes Care* **2021**, *44*, 519–525. [CrossRef]
75. Grgurevic, I.; Salkic, N.; Mustapic, S.; Bokun, T.; Podrug, K.; Marusic, S.; Rahelic, D.; Matic, T.; Skurla, V.; Mikolasevic, I. Liver and Nonliver-Related Outcomes at 2 Years Are Not Influenced by the Results of the FIB-4 Test and Liver Elastography in a Real-Life Cohort of Patients with Type 2 Diabetes. *Can. J. Gastroenterol. Hepatol.* **2021**, *2021*, 5582813. [CrossRef] [PubMed]
76. Gupta, A.; Anoop, S.; Ansari, I.A.; Prakash, S.; Misra, A. High Prevalence of Hepatic Steatosis and Hepatic Fibrosis in Patients with Type 2 Diabetes Mellitus. *Clin. Nutr. ESPEN* **2021**, *46*, 519–526. [CrossRef] [PubMed]
77. Lomonaco, R.; Godinez Leiva, E.; Bril, F.; Shrestha, S.; Mansour, L.; Budd, J.; Portillo Romero, J.; Schmidt, S.; Chang, K.-L.; Samraj, G.; et al. Advanced Liver Fibrosis Is Common in Patients With Type 2 Diabetes Followed in the Outpatient Setting: The Need for Systematic Screening. *Diabetes Care* **2021**, *44*, 399–406. [CrossRef] [PubMed]
78. Makker, J.; Tariq, H.; Kumar, K.; Ravi, M.; Shaikh, D.H.; Leung, V.; Hayat, U.; Hassan, M.T.; Patel, H.; Nayudu, S.; et al. Prevalence of Advanced Liver Fibrosis and Steatosis in Type-2 Diabetics with Normal Transaminases: A Prospective Cohort Study. *World J. Gastroenterol.* **2021**, *27*, 523–533. [CrossRef] [PubMed]
79. Mansour, D.; Grapes, A.; Herscovitz, M.; Cassidy, P.; Vernazza, J.; Broad, A.; Anstee, Q.M.; McPherson, S. Embedding Assessment of Liver Fibrosis into Routine Diabetic Review in Primary Care. *JHEP Rep. Innov. Hepatol.* **2021**, *3*, 100293. [CrossRef]
80. Sagara, M.; Iijima, T.; Kase, M.; Kato, K.; Sakurai, S.; Tomaru, T.; Jojima, T.; Usui, I.; Aso, Y. Serum Levels of Soluble Dipeptidyl Peptidase-4 in Type 2 Diabetes Are Associated with Severity of Liver Fibrosis Evaluated by Transient Elastography (FibroScan) and the FAST (FibroScan-AST) Score, a Novel Index of Non-Alcoholic Steatohepatitis with Significant Fibrosis. *J. Diabetes Complicat.* **2021**, *35*, 107885. [CrossRef]
81. Trivedi, H.D.; Suri, J.; Oh, D.; Schwartz, J.; Goyes, D.; Idriss, R.; Curry, M.P.; Lai, M. The Presence of Diabetes Impacts Liver Fibrosis and Steatosis by Transient Elastography in a Primary Care Population. *Ann. Hepatol.* **2021**, *24*, 100336. [CrossRef]
82. Blank, V.; Petroff, D.; Beer, S.; Böhlig, A.; Heni, M.; Berg, T.; Bausback, Y.; Dietrich, A.; Tönjes, A.; Hollenbach, M.; et al. Current NAFLD Guidelines for Risk Stratification in Diabetic Patients Have Poor Diagnostic Discrimination. *Sci. Rep.* **2020**, *10*, 18345. [CrossRef]
83. Lee, C.-H.; Seto, W.-K.; Ieong, K.; Lui, D.T.W.; Fong, C.H.Y.; Wan, H.Y.; Chow, W.-S.; Woo, Y.-C.; Yuen, M.-F.; Lam, K.S.L. Development of a Non-Invasive Liver Fibrosis Score Based on Transient Elastography for Risk Stratification in Patients with Type 2 Diabetes. *Endocrinol. Metab.* **2021**, *36*, 134–145. [CrossRef]
84. Lee, H.W.; Wong, G.L.-H.; Kwok, R.; Choi, K.C.; Chan, C.K.-M.; Shu, S.S.-T.; Leung, J.K.-Y.; Chim, A.M.-L.; Luk, A.O.-Y.; Ma, R.C.-W.; et al. Serial Transient Elastography Examinations to Monitor Patients With Type 2 Diabetes: A Prospective Cohort Study. *Hepatology* **2020**, *72*, 1230–1241. [CrossRef]
85. Mantovani, A.; Turino, T.; Lando, M.G.; Gjini, K.; Byrne, C.D.; Zusi, C.; Ravaioli, F.; Colecchia, A.; Maffeis, C.; Salvagno, G.; et al. Screening for Non-Alcoholic Fatty Liver Disease Using Liver Stiffness Measurement and Its Association with Chronic Kidney Disease and Cardiovascular Complications in Patients with Type 2 Diabetes. *Diabetes Metab.* **2020**, *46*, 296–303. [CrossRef] [PubMed]
86. Mikolasevic, I.; Domislovic, V.; Turk Wensveen, T.; Delija, B.; Klapan, M.; Juric, T.; Lukic, A.; Mijic, A.; Skenderevic, N.; Puz, P.; et al. Screening for Nonalcoholic Fatty Liver Disease in Patients with Type 2 Diabetes Mellitus Using Transient Elastography-a Prospective, Cross Sectional Study. *Eur. J. Intern. Med.* **2020**, *82*, 68–75. [CrossRef] [PubMed]
87. Sporea, I.; Mare, R.; Popescu, A.; Nistorescu, S.; Baldea, V.; Sirli, R.; Braha, A.; Sima, A.; Timar, R.; Lupusoru, R. Screening for Liver Fibrosis and Steatosis in a Large Cohort of Patients with Type 2 Diabetes Using Vibration Controlled Transient Elastography and Controlled Attenuation Parameter in a Single-Center Real-Life Experience. *J. Clin. Med.* **2020**, *9*, E1032. [CrossRef]
88. Arya, S.; Haria, J.M.; Mishra, A. To Study the Occurrence of Non-Alcoholic Fatty Liver Disease (NAFLD) in Type -II Diabetes Mellitus. *J. Assoc. Physicians India* **2020**, *68*, 51. [PubMed]
89. Demir, M.; Deyneli, O.; Yılmaz, Y. Screening for Hepatic Fibrosis and Steatosis in Turkish Patients with Type 2 Diabetes Mellitus: A Transient Elastography Study. *Turk. J. Gastroenterol.* **2019**, *30*, 266–270. [CrossRef] [PubMed]
90. Fernando, J.N.; Alba, R.L.; Alba, W. Factors Associated with the Severity of Findings on Hepatic Transient Elastography among Persons with Type 2 Diabetes and Fatty Liver. *J. ASEAN Fed. Endocr. Soc.* **2019**, *34*, 134–143. [CrossRef]
91. Jaafar, R.F.; Hajj Ali, A.M.; Zaghal, A.M.; Kanso, M.; Habib, S.G.; Halaoui, A.F.; Daniel, F.; Mokaddem, F.; Khalife, M.J.; Mukherji, D.M.; et al. Fibroscan and Low-Density Lipoprotein as Determinants of Severe Liver Fibrosis in Diabetic Patients with Nonalcoholic Fatty Liver Disease. *Eur. J. Gastroenterol. Hepatol.* **2019**, *31*, 1540–1544. [CrossRef]
92. Kumar, N.A.; Das, S. Fibroscan of Liver in Type 2 Diabetes Mellitus and Its Correlation with Risk Factors. *J. Diabetes Mellit.* **2019**, *9*, 62–68. [CrossRef]
93. Lai, L.-L.; Wan Yusoff, W.N.I.; Vethakkan, S.R.; Nik Mustapha, N.R.; Mahadeva, S.; Chan, W.-K. Screening for Non-Alcoholic Fatty Liver Disease in Patients with Type 2 Diabetes Mellitus Using Transient Elastography. *J. Gastroenterol. Hepatol.* **2019**, *34*, 1396–1403. [CrossRef]

94. Lombardi, R.; Airaghi, L.; Targher, G.; Serviddio, G.; Maffi, G.; Mantovani, A.; Maffeis, C.; Colecchia, A.; Villani, R.; Rinaldi, L.; et al. Liver Fibrosis by FibroScan®Independently of Established Cardiovascular Risk Parameters Associates with Macrovascular and Microvascular Complications in Patients with Type 2 Diabetes. *Liver Int.* **2020**, *40*, 347–354. [CrossRef]
95. Wong, V.W.-S.; Irles, M.; Wong, G.L.-H.; Shili, S.; Chan, A.W.-H.; Merrouche, W.; Shu, S.S.-T.; Foucher, J.; Le Bail, B.; Chan, W.K.; et al. Unified Interpretation of Liver Stiffness Measurement by M and XL Probes in Non-Alcoholic Fatty Liver Disease. *Gut* **2019**, *68*, 2057–2064. [CrossRef] [PubMed]
96. Zhao, H.; Song, X.; Li, Z.; Wang, X. Risk Factors Associated with Nonalcohol Fatty Liver Disease and Fibrosis among Patients with Type 2 Diabetes Mellitus. *Medicine* **2018**, *97*, e12356. [CrossRef] [PubMed]
97. Kartikayan, R.; Vaishnavi Priya, C.; Rajkumar Solomon, T.; Aravind, A.; Caroline Selvi, K.; Balamurali, R.; Ramkumar, G.; Muthukumaran, K.; Kavitha, S.; Anand, A.; et al. Assessment of Liver Stiffness by Transient Elastography in Diabetics with Fatty Liver–A Single Center Cross Sectional Observational Study. *IOSR J. Dent. Med. Sci.* **2017**, *16*, 49–53. [CrossRef]
98. Prasetya, I.B.; Hasan, I.; Wisnu, W.; Rumende, C.M. Prevalence and Profile of Fibrosis in Diabetic Patients with Non-Alcoholic Fatty Liver Disease and the Associated Factors. *Acta Medica Indones.* **2017**, *49*, 91–98.
99. Kwok, R.; Choi, K.C.; Wong, G.L.-H.; Zhang, Y.; Chan, H.L.-Y.; Luk, A.O.-Y.; Shu, S.S.-T.; Chan, A.W.-H.; Yeung, M.-W.; Chan, J.C.-N.; et al. Screening Diabetic Patients for Non-Alcoholic Fatty Liver Disease with Controlled Attenuation Parameter and Liver Stiffness Measurements: A Prospective Cohort Study. *Gut* **2016**, *65*, 1359–1368. [CrossRef]
100. De Lédinghen, V.; Vergniol, J.; Gonzalez, C.; Foucher, J.; Maury, E.; Chemineau, L.; Villars, S.; Gin, H.; Rigalleau, V. Screening for Liver Fibrosis by Using FibroScan(®) and FibroTest in Patients with Diabetes. *Dig. Liver Dis.* **2012**, *44*, 413–418. [CrossRef] [PubMed]
101. Selvaraj, E.A.; Mózes, F.E.; Jayaswal, A.N.A.; Zafarmand, M.H.; Vali, Y.; Lee, J.A.; Levick, C.K.; Young, L.A.J.; Palaniyappan, N.; Liu, C.-H.; et al. Diagnostic Accuracy of Elastography and Magnetic Resonance Imaging in Patients with NAFLD: A Systematic Review and Meta-Analysis. *J. Hepatol.* **2021**, *75*, 770–785. [CrossRef]
102. De Ledinghen, V. Fibrosis Assessment in Patients with NAFLD. In *Liver Elastography: Clinical Use and Interpretation*; Mueller, S., Ed.; Springer International Publishing: Cham, Switzerland, 2020; pp. 123–139. ISBN 978-3-030-40542-7.
103. Roy, S. Clinical Case Series of Decrease in Shear Wave Elastography Values in Ten Diabetic Dyslipidemia Patients Having NAFLD with Saroglitazar 4 Mg: An Indian Experience. *Case Rep. Med.* **2020**, *2020*, 4287075. [CrossRef]
104. Cassinotto, C.; Boursier, J.; de Lédinghen, V.; Lebigot, J.; Lapuyade, B.; Cales, P.; Hiriart, J.-B.; Michalak, S.; Bail, B.L.; Cartier, V.; et al. Liver Stiffness in Nonalcoholic Fatty Liver Disease: A Comparison of Supersonic Shear Imaging, FibroScan, and ARFI with Liver Biopsy. *Hepatology* **2016**, *63*, 1817–1827. [CrossRef]
105. Jiang, W.; Huang, S.; Teng, H.; Wang, P.; Wu, M.; Zhou, X.; Ran, H. Diagnostic Accuracy of Point Shear Wave Elastography and Transient Elastography for Staging Hepatic Fibrosis in Patients with Non-Alcoholic Fatty Liver Disease: A Meta-Analysis. *BMJ Open* **2018**, *8*, e021787. [CrossRef]
106. Giuffrè, M.; Giuricin, M.; Bonazza, D.; Rosso, N.; Giraudi, P.J.; Masutti, F.; Palmucci, S.; Basile, A.; Zanconati, F.; de Manzini, N.; et al. Optimization of Point-Shear Wave Elastography by Skin-to-Liver Distance to Assess Liver Fibrosis in Patients Undergoing Bariatric Surgery. *Diagnostics* **2020**, *10*, E795. [CrossRef] [PubMed]
107. Barr, R.G.; Wilson, S.R.; Rubens, D.; Garcia-Tsao, G.; Ferraioli, G. Update to the Society of Radiologists in Ultrasound Liver Elastography Consensus Statement. *Radiology* **2020**, *296*, 263–274. [CrossRef] [PubMed]
108. Meyer, G.; Dauth, N.; Grimm, M.; Herrmann, E.; Bojunga, J.; Friedrich-Rust, M. Shear Wave Elastography Reveals a High Prevalence of NAFLD-Related Fibrosis Even in Type 1 Diabetes. *Exp. Clin. Endocrinol. Diabetes* **2021**. [CrossRef] [PubMed]
109. Guzmán-Aroca, F.; Frutos-Bernal, M.D.; Bas, A.; Luján-Mompeán, J.A.; Reus, M.; de Dios Berná-Serna, J.; Parrilla, P. Detection of Non-Alcoholic Steatohepatitis in Patients with Morbid Obesity before Bariatric Surgery: Preliminary Evaluation with Acoustic Radiation Force Impulse Imaging. *Eur. Radiol.* **2012**, *22*, 2525–2532. [CrossRef]
110. Corica, D.; Bottari, A.; Aversa, T.; Morabito, L.A.; Curatola, S.; Alibrandi, A.; Ascenti, G.; Wasniewska, M. Prospective Assessment of Liver Stiffness by Shear Wave Elastography in Childhood Obesity: A Pilot Study. *Endocrine* **2022**, *75*, 59–69. [CrossRef]
111. Praveenraj, P.; Gomes, R.M.; Basuraju, S.; Kumar, S.; Senthilnathan, P.; Parathasarathi, R.; Rajapandian, S.; Palanivelu, C. Preliminary Evaluation of Acoustic Radiation Force Impulse Shear Wave Imaging to Detect Hepatic Fibrosis in Morbidly Obese Patients Before Bariatric Surgery. *J. Laparoendosc. Adv. Surg. Tech. A* **2016**, *26*, 192–195. [CrossRef]
112. Shaji, N.; Singhai, A.; Sarawagi, R.; Pakhare, A.P.; Mishra, V.N.; Joshi, R. Assessment of Liver Fibrosis Using Non-Invasive Screening Tools in Individuals With Diabetes Mellitus and Metabolic Syndrome. *Cureus* **2022**, *14*, e22682. [CrossRef]
113. Demirtas, D.; Kocaer, A.S.; Sumbul, H.E. The Role of Liver Elastography Point Quantification in the Assessment of Fibrosis in Non-Alcoholic Fatty Liver Disease and Comparison with Other Non-Invasive Methods. *Akdeniz Med. J.* **2020**. [CrossRef]
114. Roy, S.; Majumder, A. A Retrospective Study to Examine the Correlation of Bioelectrical Impedance Analysis with Shear-Wave Elastography in Indian Patients with Non-Alcoholic Fatty Liver Disease and Diabetes on Background Sodium-Glucose Cotransporter-2 Inhibitor Therapy. *Cureus* **2019**, *11*, e4674. [CrossRef]
115. Castera, L. Noninvasive Evaluation of Nonalcoholic Fatty Liver Disease. *Semin. Liver Dis.* **2015**, *35*, 291–303. [CrossRef]
116. Miyoshi, T.; Hamaguchi, M.; Kitagawa, N.; Hashimoto, Y.; Fukui, M. Correlation between Liver Stiffness by Two-Dimensional Shear Wave Elastography and Waist Circumference in Japanese Local Citizens with Abdominal Obesity. *J. Clin. Med.* **2021**, *10*, 1971. [CrossRef] [PubMed]

117. Chimoriya, R.; Piya, M.K.; Simmons, D.; Ahlenstiel, G.; Ho, V. The Use of Two-Dimensional Shear Wave Elastography in People with Obesity for the Assessment of Liver Fibrosis in Non-Alcoholic Fatty Liver Disease. *J. Clin. Med.* **2021**, *10*, 95. [CrossRef]
118. Jamialahmadi, T.; Jangjoo, A.; Rezvani, R.; Goshayeshi, L.; Tasbandi, A.; Nooghabi, M.J.; Rajabzadeh, F.; Ghaffarzadegan, K.; Mishamandani, Z.J.; Nematy, M. Hepatic Function and Fibrosis Assessment Via 2D-Shear Wave Elastography and Related Biochemical Markers Pre- and Post-Gastric Bypass Surgery. *Obes. Surg.* **2020**, *30*, 2251–2258. [CrossRef] [PubMed]
119. Imajo, K.; Honda, Y.; Kobayashi, T.; Nagai, K.; Ozaki, A.; Iwaki, M.; Kessoku, T.; Ogawa, Y.; Takahashi, H.; Saigusa, Y.; et al. Direct Comparison of US and MR Elastography for Staging Liver Fibrosis in Patients with Nonalcoholic Fatty Liver Disease. *Clin. Gastroenterol. Hepatol.* **2022**, *20*, 908–917.e11. [CrossRef] [PubMed]
120. Shaheen, A.A.; Riazi, K.; Medellin, A.; Bhayana, D.; Kaplan, G.G.; Jiang, J.; Park, R.; Schaufert, W.; Burak, K.W.; Sargious, M.; et al. Risk Stratification of Patients with Nonalcoholic Fatty Liver Disease Using a Case Identification Pathway in Primary Care: A Cross-Sectional Study. *CMAJ Open* **2020**, *8*, E370–E376. [CrossRef]
121. Xie, L.-T.; Yan, C.-H.; Zhao, Q.-Y.; He, M.-N.; Jiang, T.-A. Quantitative and Noninvasive Assessment of Chronic Liver Diseases Using Two-Dimensional Shear Wave Elastography. *World J. Gastroenterol.* **2018**, *24*, 957–970. [CrossRef]
122. Wernberg, C.; Thiele, M.; Balle Hugger, M. Steatosis Assessment with Controlled Attenuation Parameter (CAP) in Various Diseases. In *Liver Elastography*; Sebastian, M., Ed.; Springer: Berlin/Heidelberg, Germany, 2020; pp. 441–457. ISBN 978-3-030-40541-0.
123. Sasso, M.; Beaugrand, M.; de Ledinghen, V.; Douvin, C.; Marcellin, P.; Poupon, R.; Sandrin, L.; Miette, V. Controlled Attenuation Parameter (CAP): A Novel VCTE^{TM} Guided Ultrasonic Attenuation Measurement for the Evaluation of Hepatic Steatosis: Preliminary Study and Validation in a Cohort of Patients with Chronic Liver Disease from Various Causes. *Ultrasound Med. Biol.* **2010**, *36*, 1825–1835. [CrossRef] [PubMed]
124. Ferraioli, G.; Kumar, V.; Ozturk, A.; Nam, K.; de Korte, C.L.; Barr, R.G. US Attenuation for Liver Fat Quantification: An AIUM-RSNA QIBA Pulse-Echo Quantitative Ultrasound Initiative. *Radiology* **2022**, *302*, 495–506. [CrossRef]
125. Karlas, T.; Petroff, D.; Sasso, M.; Fan, J.-G.; Mi, Y.-Q.; de Lédinghen, V.; Kumar, M.; Lupsor-Platon, M.; Han, K.-H.; Cardoso, A.C.; et al. Individual Patient Data Meta-Analysis of Controlled Attenuation Parameter (CAP) Technology for Assessing Steatosis. *J. Hepatol.* **2017**, *66*, 1022–1030. [CrossRef]
126. Naveau, S.; Voican, C.S.; Lebrun, A.; Gaillard, M.; Lamouri, K.; Njiké-Nakseu, M.; Courie, R.; Tranchart, H.; Balian, A.; Prévot, S.; et al. Controlled Attenuation Parameter for Diagnosing Steatosis in Bariatric Surgery Candidates with Suspected Nonalcoholic Fatty Liver Disease. *Eur. J. Gastroenterol. Hepatol.* **2017**, *29*, 1022–1030. [CrossRef]
127. Wan, T.; Köhn, N.; Kröll, D.; Berzigotti, A. Applicability and Results of Liver Stiffness Measurement and Controlled Attenuation Parameter Using XL Probe for Metabolic-Associated Fatty Liver Disease in Candidates to Bariatric Surgery. A Single-Center Observational Study. *Obes. Surg.* **2021**, *31*, 702–711. [CrossRef] [PubMed]
128. Vedtofte, L.; Bahne, E.; Foghsgaard, S.; Bagger, J.I.; Andreasen, C.; Strandberg, C.; Gørtz, P.M.; Holst, J.J.; Grønbæk, H.; Svare, J.A.; et al. One Year's Treatment with the Glucagon-Like Peptide 1 Receptor Agonist Liraglutide Decreases Hepatic Fat Content in Women with Nonalcoholic Fatty Liver Disease and Prior Gestational Diabetes Mellitus in a Randomized, Placebo-Controlled Trial. *J. Clin. Med.* **2020**, *9*, 3213. [CrossRef] [PubMed]
129. Seko, Y.; Sumida, Y.; Tanaka, S.; Mori, K.; Taketani, H.; Ishiba, H.; Hara, T.; Okajima, A.; Umemura, A.; Nishikawa, T.; et al. Effect of 12-Week Dulaglutide Therapy in Japanese Patients with Biopsy-Proven Non-Alcoholic Fatty Liver Disease and Type 2 Diabetes Mellitus. *Hepatol. Res.* **2017**, *47*, 1206–1211. [CrossRef] [PubMed]
130. Lee, Y.; Kim, J.H.; Kim, S.R.; Jin, H.Y.; Rhee, E.-J.; Cho, Y.M.; Lee, B.-W. Lobeglitazone, a Novel Thiazolidinedione, Improves Non-Alcoholic Fatty Liver Disease in Type 2 Diabetes: Its Efficacy and Predictive Factors Related to Responsiveness. *J. Korean Med. Sci.* **2017**, *32*, 60–69. [CrossRef] [PubMed]
131. Sanyal, A.J.; Chalasani, N.; Kowdley, K.V.; McCullough, A.; Diehl, A.M.; Bass, N.M.; Neuschwander-Tetri, B.A.; Lavine, J.E.; Tonascia, J.; Unalp, A.; et al. Pioglitazone, Vitamin E, or Placebo for Nonalcoholic Steatohepatitis. *N. Engl. J. Med.* **2010**, *362*, 1675–1685. [CrossRef]
132. Shimizu, M.; Suzuki, K.; Kato, K.; Jojima, T.; Iijima, T.; Murohisa, T.; Iijima, M.; Takekawa, H.; Usui, I.; Hiraishi, H.; et al. Evaluation of the Effects of Dapagliflozin, a Sodium-Glucose Co-Transporter-2 Inhibitor, on Hepatic Steatosis and Fibrosis Using Transient Elastography in Patients with Type 2 Diabetes and Non-Alcoholic Fatty Liver Disease. *Diabetes Obes. Metab.* **2019**, *21*, 285–292. [CrossRef]
133. Rinella, M.E.; Tacke, F.; Sanyal, A.J.; Anstee, Q.M. Participants of the AASLD/EASL Workshop Report on the AASLD/EASL Joint Workshop on Clinical Trial Endpoints in NAFLD. *Hepatology* **2019**, *70*, 1424–1436. [CrossRef]
134. Fujita, N.; Nishie, A.; Asayama, Y.; Ishigami, K.; Ushijima, Y.; Takayama, Y.; Okamoto, D.; Shirabe, K.; Yoshizumi, T.; Kotoh, K.; et al. Fibrosis in Nonalcoholic Fatty Liver Disease: Noninvasive Assessment Using Computed Tomography Volumetry. *World J. Gastroenterol.* **2016**, *22*, 8949–8955. [CrossRef]
135. Graupera, I.; Thiele, M.; Ma, A.T.; Serra-Burriel, M.; Pich, J.; Fabrellas, N.; Caballeria, L.; de Knegt, R.J.; Grgurevic, I.; Reichert, M.; et al. LiverScreen Project: Study Protocol for Screening for Liver Fibrosis in the General Population in European Countries. *BMC Public Health* **2022**, *22*, 1385. [CrossRef]
136. Harrison, S.A.; Oliver, D.; Arnold, H.L.; Gogia, S.; Neuschwander-Tetri, B.A. Development and Validation of a Simple NAFLD Clinical Scoring System for Identifying Patients without Advanced Disease. *Gut* **2008**, *57*, 1441–1447. [CrossRef]
137. Venkatesh, S.K.; Yin, M.; Takahashi, N.; Glockner, J.F.; Talwalkar, J.A.; Ehman, R.L. Non-Invasive Detection of Liver Fibrosis: MR Imaging Features vs. MR Elastography. *Abdom. Imaging* **2015**, *40*, 766–775. [CrossRef]

138. Dobbie, L.J.; Kassab, M.; Davison, A.S.; Grace, P.; Cuthbertson, D.J.; Hydes, T.J. Low Screening Rates Despite a High Prevalence of Significant Liver Fibrosis in People with Diabetes from Primary and Secondary Care. *J. Clin. Med.* **2021**, *10*, 5755. [CrossRef]
139. Park, S.H.; Lee, J.H.; Jun, D.W.; Kang, K.A.; Kim, J.N.; Park, H.J.; Hong, H.P. Determining the Target Population That Would Most Benefit from Screening for Hepatic Fibrosis in a Primary Care Setting. *Diagnostics* **2021**, *11*, 1605. [CrossRef]
140. Pandyarajan, V.; Gish, R.G.; Alkhouri, N.; Noureddin, M. Screening for Nonalcoholic Fatty Liver Disease in the Primary Care Clinic. *Gastroenterol. Hepatol.* **2019**, *15*, 357–365.
141. Bril, F.; Cusi, K. Management of Nonalcoholic Fatty Liver Disease in Patients With Type 2 Diabetes: A Call to Action. *Diabetes Care* **2017**, *40*, 419–430. [CrossRef]
142. Fang, C.; Lim, A.; Sidhu, P.S. Ultrasound-Based Liver Elastography in the Assessment of Fibrosis. *Clin. Radiol.* **2020**, *75*, 822–831. [CrossRef]
143. Cusi, K.; Isaacs, S.; Barb, D.; Basu, R.; Caprio, S.; Garvey, W.T.; Kashyap, S.; Mechanick, J.I.; Mouzaki, M.; Nadolsky, K.; et al. American Association of Clinical Endocrinology Clinical Practice Guideline for the Diagnosis and Management of Nonalcoholic Fatty Liver Disease in Primary Care and Endocrinology Clinical Settings: Co-Sponsored by the American Association for the Study of Liver Diseases (AASLD). *Endocr. Pract.* **2022**, *28*, 528–562. [CrossRef]
144. Dokmak, A.; Lizaola-Mayo, B.; Trivedi, H.D. The Impact of Nonalcoholic Fatty Liver Disease in Primary Care: A Population Health Perspective. *Am. J. Med.* **2021**, *134*, 23–29. [CrossRef]
145. Sporea, I.; Grădinaru-Taşcău, O.; Bota, S.; Popescu, A.; Şirli, R.; Jurchiş, A.; Popescu, M.; Dănilă, M. How Many Measurements Are Needed for Liver Stiffness Assessment by 2D-Shear Wave Elastography (2D-SWE) and Which Value Should Be Used: The Mean or Median? *Med. Ultrason.* **2013**, *15*, 268–272. [CrossRef]
146. Sanyal, A.J.; Shankar, S.S.; Calle, R.A.; Samir, A.E.; Sirlin, C.B.; Sherlock, S.P.; Loomba, R.; Fowler, K.J.; Dehn, C.A.; Heymann, H.; et al. Non-Invasive Biomarkers of Nonalcoholic Steatohepatitis: The FNIH NIMBLE Project. *Nat. Med.* **2022**, *28*, 430–432. [CrossRef]
147. LITMUS-Liver Investigation: Testing Marker Utility in Steatohepatitis Home Page. Available online: https://litmus-project.eu/ (accessed on 20 August 2022).

biomedicines

MDPI

Article

Identification of the Potential Molecular Mechanisms Linking RUNX1 Activity with Nonalcoholic Fatty Liver Disease, by Means of Systems Biology

Laia Bertran [1], Ailende Eigbefoh-Addeh [1], Marta Portillo-Carrasquer [1], Andrea Barrientos-Riosalido [1], Jessica Binetti [1], Carmen Aguilar [1], Javier Ugarte Chicote [1], Helena Bartra [2], Laura Artigas [2], Mireia Coma [2], Cristóbal Richart [1] and Teresa Auguet [1,*]

[1] Grup de Recerca GEMMAIR (AGAUR)—Medicina Aplicada (URV), Departament de Medicina i Cirurgia, Institut d'Investigació Sanitària Pere Virgili (IISPV), Universitat Rovira i Virgili (URV), 43007 Tarragona, Spain; laia.bertran@urv.cat (L.B.); ailende.eigbefoh-addeh@urv.cat (A.E.-A.); marta.portillo.carrasquer@gmail.com (M.P.-C.); andreitabarri18@gmail.com (A.B.-R.); jessica.binetti@gmail.com (J.B.); caguilar.hj23.ics@gencat.cat (C.A.); ugartecj@gmail.com (J.U.C.); cristobalmanuel.richart@urv.cat (C.R.)

[2] Anaxomics Biotech S.L., 08007 Barcelona, Spain; helena.bartra@anaxomics.com (H.B.); laura.artigas@anaxomics.com (L.A.); mcoma@anaxomics.com (M.C.)

* Correspondence: tauguet.hj23.ics@gencat.cat; Tel.: +34-977-295-833

Citation: Bertran, L.; Eigbefoh-Addeh, A.; Portillo-Carrasquer, M.; Barrientos-Riosalido, A.; Binetti, J.; Aguilar, C.; Ugarte Chicote, J.; Bartra, H.; Artigas, L.; Coma, M.; et al. Identification of the Potential Molecular Mechanisms Linking RUNX1 Activity with Nonalcoholic Fatty Liver Disease, by Means of Systems Biology. *Biomedicines* **2022**, *10*, 1315. https://doi.org/10.3390/biomedicines10061315

Academic Editors: Jinghua Wang and Albrecht Piiper

Received: 13 April 2022
Accepted: 1 June 2022
Published: 3 June 2022

Abstract: Nonalcoholic fatty liver disease (NAFLD) is the most prevalent chronic hepatic disease; nevertheless, no definitive diagnostic method exists yet, apart from invasive liver biopsy, and nor is there a specific approved treatment. Runt-related transcription factor 1 (RUNX1) plays a major role in angiogenesis and inflammation; however, its link with NAFLD is unclear as controversial results have been reported. Thus, the objective of this work was to determine the proteins involved in the molecular mechanisms between RUNX1 and NAFLD, by means of systems biology. First, a mathematical model that simulates NAFLD pathophysiology was generated by analyzing Anaxomics databases and reviewing available scientific literature. Artificial neural networks established NAFLD pathophysiological processes functionally related to RUNX1: hepatic insulin resistance, lipotoxicity, and hepatic injury-liver fibrosis. Our study indicated that RUNX1 might have a high relationship with hepatic injury-liver fibrosis, and a medium relationship with lipotoxicity and insulin resistance motives. Additionally, we found five RUNX1-regulated proteins with a direct involvement in NAFLD motives, which were NFκB1, NFκB2, TNF, ADIPOQ, and IL-6. In conclusion, we suggested a relationship between RUNX1 and NAFLD since RUNX1 seems to regulate NAFLD molecular pathways, posing it as a potential therapeutic target of NAFLD, although more studies in this field are needed.

Keywords: RUNX1; NAFLD; NASH; metabolism; systems biology

1. Introduction

Nonalcoholic fatty liver disease (NAFLD) is a condition characterized by excess fat in the liver, without alcohol implication in the onset of the disease. The term NAFLD comprehends a substantial number of liver conditions, ranging from simple steatosis (SS) to the more aggressive form of nonalcoholic steatohepatitis (NASH), which may lead to cirrhosis and hepatocellular carcinoma [1]. SS is defined as the presence of $\geq$5% hepatic steatosis without evidence of hepatocellular injury in the form of hepatocyte ballooning, inflammation [2], and fibrosis, three remarkable events in NASH pathology. The progress of the disease may vary from individuals, depending on the accumulated fat to the immunological and the oxidant stress responses [3,4].

NAFLD is the most prevalent chronic liver disease, with a global prevalence in adults between 23–25% [5,6]. Nevertheless, nowadays there is no definitive diagnostic test apart from invasive liver biopsy, and no specific approved treatment besides exercise and dietary interventions. Pharmacologic-based therapies for NAFLD are limited, but many clinical trials are in process [7]. For this reason, knowledge about NAFLD pathophysiology is continuously growing.

RUNX1 belongs to the runt-related transcription factor (RUNX) family of genes, and is also known as acute myeloid leukemia 1 [8]. RUNX1 regulates the differentiation of hematopoietic stem cells into mature blood cells [9,10]. It also plays a major role in the development of the neurons that transmit pain [11], and in angiogenesis and inflammation [12]. In addition, RUNX1 involvement in apoptotic processes has been reported on one hand to induce apoptosis and inhibit tumor progression in neuroblastoma [13] and leukaemia [14], while it contrarily seems to present an antiapoptotic effect in pancreatic and ovarian cancer [15,16].

Diseases associated with RUNX1 include platelet disorders with associated myeloid malignancy and blood platelet disease [17]. Related pathways include transport of glucose and other sugars, bile salts, organic acids, metal ions, and amine compounds, as well as transforming growth factor-beta (TGF-β) signaling pathways [18,19]. Recently, Kaur et al. reported a relationship between RUNX1 and NAFLD. Authors related its activity with the progression to NASH, since the interaction of RUNX1 and C-C motif chemokine 2 (CCL2), an important adhesion molecule, mediates the infiltration of pro-inflammatory and pro-angiogenic factors in NASH [20]. Thus, we previously wanted to study the role of RUNX1 mRNA and protein expression in NAFLD in a cohort of women with morbid obesity. We hypothesized that RUNX1 may play a protective role in NAFLD since its expression was enhanced in early stages of the disease and decrease along with the progression to NASH [21]. Given these controversies among our previous results and what was already known, the objective of the present work is to determine the proteins and the potential molecular mechanisms that could establish a link between the activity of RUNX1 and NAFLD pathogenesis by means of systems biology.

2. Materials and Methods

2.1. Bibliographic and Metadata Analysis in Databases

First, we built the molecular description of NAFLD pathophysiology through systematic searches and reviewing the most up-to-date scientific knowledge regarding this pathology (Supplementary Table S1). Accordingly, NAFLD was divided in specific pathophysiological processes–called motives–involved in SS, in NASH, or in both forms (Supplementary Table S1), and the corresponding molecular effectors (or key proteins) playing biological roles in these mechanisms were identified (Supplementary Table S2).

The interactome around RUNX1 was manually curated in order to better fit the mathematical models. Protein relationship databases including TRRUST database (Transcriptional Regulatory Relationships Unravelled by Sentence-based Text-mining) [22], BioGRID (The Biological General Repository for Interaction Datasets) [23], HPRD (Human Protein Reference Database) [24,25], INTACT (IntAct Molecular Interaction Database) [26], KEGG (Kyoto Encyclopedia of Genes and Genomes) [27], REACTOME (Reactome Pathway Database) [28], and available scientific literature were the sources used to identify and curate new direct interactors of RUNX1.

2.2. Mechanistic Model Generation

The compiled information was used to generate a mathematical model that simulate NAFLD pathophysiology by applying Therapeutic Performance Mapping System (TPMS) technology [29], which integrates all available biological, pharmacological, and medical knowledge to simulate human physiology in silico (Supplementary Table S3). Then, we used an artificial neural networks (ANNs) strategy [30,31] to analyze these models in order to establish the functional relationships between RUNX1 and NAFLD, considering the motives both together and individually. ANNs evaluate the relationship among protein sets or regions inside the Anaxomics network, providing a predictive score that quantifies the probability of the existence of a functional relationship between the evaluated regions. Each score is associated with a p-value that describes the probability of the result being a true positive. The ranking score has been divided into five categories: very high (ANN score > 92; $p < 0.01$), high (ANN score = 78–92; p = 0.01–0.05), medium-high (ANN score 71–78; p = 0.05–0.1), medium (ANN score 37–71; p = 0.1–0.25), low (ANN score < 37; >0.25).

Sampling methods-based mathematical models were then generated to determine the potential molecular mechanisms that could justify our hypothesis:

1. Activation of RUNX1 promoting insulin resistance (IR).
2. Activation of RUNX1 promoting lipotoxicity and hepatic injury and liver fibrosis.

TPMS sampling-based methods trace the most probable mechanisms of action (MoA) or paths, both in biological and mathematical terms, which lead from a stimulus (e.g., activation of RUNX1) to a response (e.g., activation of IR) through the biological human protein network. In this way, it identifies the set of possible MoA that achieve a response when the system is stimulated with the specific stimulus. A population of possible solutions was obtained, and this variability was exploited and analysed to obtain a representation with the most represented paths among the set of possible solutions. A detailed description of the applied methodology was described elsewhere [29,32] and in Appendix A.

3. Results

3.1. Functional Relationship between RUNX1 and NAFLD: ANNs Analysis

The possible functional relationship between RUNX1 and NAFLD, defined as the set of proteins included in its molecular characterization, has been evaluated by means of ANNs analysis. To deepen our insights, the analysis has also been performed individually for each pathophysiological motive included in NAFLD characterization: (1) increased body fat, (2) hepatic IR, (3) altered fatty acid metabolism, (4) lipotoxicity, and (5) hepatic injury and liver fibrosis. The first three pathophysiological processes occur in both SS and NASH, while the last two only happen in NASH pathophysiology or participate in the progression of NAFLD to NASH.

In this study, the relationship between RUNX1 and NAFLD or individual NAFLD motives has been evaluated, assuming that a possible functional relationship could indicate a participation of RUNX1 in NAFLD pathophysiology, either in promoting or reverting the process, since ANNs only indicate the existence of a possible relationship but not its direction. As shown in Table 1, the results obtained suggest a medium relationship of RUNX1 with the global NAFLD, considering all motives simultaneously.

Table 1. ANNs score of the relationship between RUNX1 and NAFLD, both globally and for each NAFLD motive.

		SS/NASH	SS/NASH	SS/NASH	NASH	NASH
	NAFLD	**Increased Body Fat**	**Hepatic Insulin Resistance**	**Altered Fatty Acid Metabolism**	**Lipotoxicity**	**Hepatic Injury and Liver Fibrosis**
RUNX1	MEDIUM (67%)	LOW (37%)	MEDIUM (67%)	LOW (22%)	MEDIUM (61%)	HIGH (78%)

When considering the motives separately, however, RUNX1 seems to show a high relationship with hepatic injury and liver fibrosis, and a medium relationship with both lipotoxicity and hepatic IR.

The different columns show the ANNs score obtained for NAFLD globally and for each individual pathophysiological motive, some involved in SS and NASH stages, while others are only implicated in NASH. Category splitting was based on p-value breaks. RUNX1, runt-related transcription factor 1; NAFLD, nonalcoholic fatty liver disease; SS, simple steatosis; NASH, nonalcoholic steatohepatitis. A darker color indicates a higher ANN score.

The MoA of RUNX1 has been built specifically with regards to the pathophysiological motives–hepatic IR, lipotoxicity and hepatic injury & liver fibrosis–due to their high probability of relationship with RUNX1 and the previously known molecular information found in available scientific literature. Figure 1 shows the protein network of direct RUNX1 interactions with NAFLD effector proteins (the activity of which play a known role in the condition).

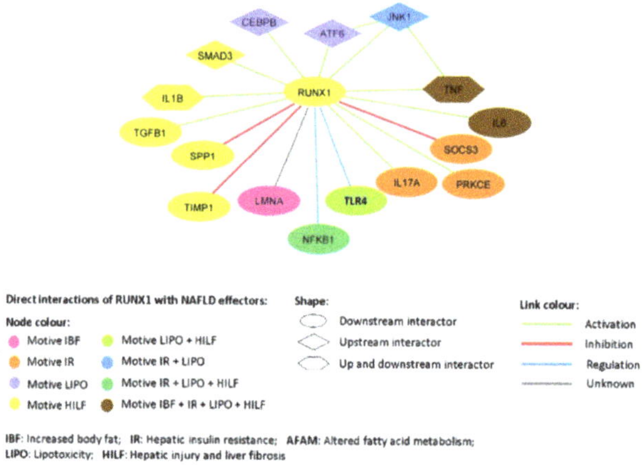

Figure 1. NAFLD effector proteins interacting with RUNX1 at distance 1 (direct link). RUNX1, runt-related protein 1; CEBPB, CCAAT/enhancer-binding protein beta; ATF-6, AMP-dependent transcription factor 6; JNK1, c-Jun N-terminal kinase 1; TNF, tumour necrosis factor; IL6, interleukin 6; SOCS3, suppressor of cytokine signaling 3; PKCE, protein kinase C epsilon type; IL17A, interleukin 17A; TLR4, toll-like receptor 4; NFKB1, nuclear factor kappa B 1; LMNA, lamin-A/C; TIMP1, metalloproteinase inhibitor 1; SPP1, secreted phosphoprotein 1; TFGB1, transforming growth factor beta-1 proprotein; IL1B, interleukin 1 beta; SMAD3, mothers against decapentaplegic homolog 3.

3.2. *Mechanisms of Action of RUNX1*

Then, TPMS sampling methods-based mathematical models were generated simulating NAFLD pathophysiology to identify the key proteins and the most probable paths that link the activation of RUNX1 with the most strongly-related motives according to ANNs analysis (hepatic IR, and lipotoxicity, hepatic injury, and liver fibrosis). To provide new insights on the different disease stages (SS or NASH), we studied two independent MoA, considering whether the motive occurs in early or later stages of the disease: (1) RUNX1 promoting IR and (2) RUNX1 promoting lipotoxicity and hepatic injury and fibrosis, respectively.

3.2.1. Mechanism of Action of RUNX1 Promoting IR

Figure 2 summarizes some of the most interesting pathways that could be regulated by RUNX1 in the context of promotion of IR in NAFLD, including the modulation of genes such as CCAAT/enhancer-binding protein alpha (CEBPA), histone deacetylase 1 (HDAC1), the transcription factor c-JUN, nuclear factor kappa B (NFκB), and some types of protein kinase C (PKCβ and PKCε).

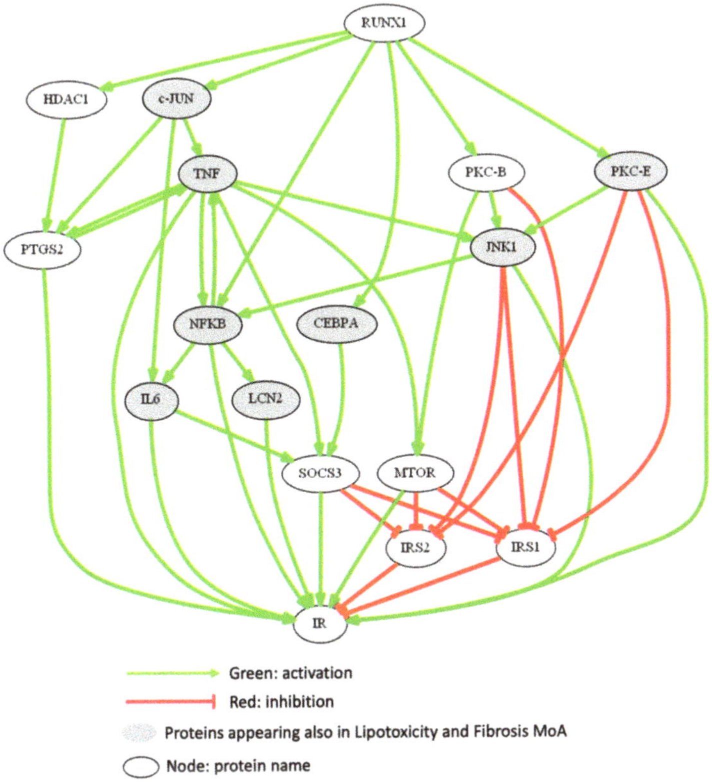

Figure 2. Most represented MoA of RUNX1 promoting IR in NAFLD in the population of TPMS model solutions. Gene names are used in the representations. RUNX1, runt-related protein 1; HDA1C, histone deacetylase 1; PTGS2, prostaglandin G/H synthase 2; c-Jun, protein encoded by JUN gene; TNF, tumour necrosis factor; NFκB, nuclear factor kappa B; IL6, interleukin 6; LCN2, neutrophil gelatinase-associated lipocalin 2; CEBPA, CCAAT/enhancer-binding protein beta; SOCS3, suppressor of cytokine signaling 3; PKC, protein kinase C; JNK1, c-Jun N-terminal kinase 1; MTOR, mammalian target of rapamycin serine/threonine-protein kinase; IRS, insulin receptor substrate. This picture was generated using Graphviz software.

Table 2 shows the IR effector proteins that are regulated by the activation of RUNX1 to promote this motive (considering that the activity values of the proteins in our models range from 1 to -1, only proteins with activation state > 0.1 are shown); the table contains all modulated proteins, not only those highlighted by the most represented paths. RUNX1 could be promoting IR through the regulation of 64.10% of the effector proteins involved in this motive. The IR effector proteins most activated by RUNX1-dependent downstream pathways are, in decreasing order: NFκB, JNK, PKCε, tumour necrosis factor (TNF), inhibitor of nuclear factor kappa B kinase subunit beta (IKBKB), and prostaglandin G/H synthase 2 (PTGS2); while the most inhibited ones are insulin receptor substrate (IRS)-1, phosphatase and tensin homolog (PTEN), IRS2 and sirtuin 1 (SIRT1).

Table 2. IR effector proteins modulated by RUNX1 activation. Causative effect indicates whether the protein is increased/overactivated (1) or reduced/inhibited (–1) in NAFLD.

Gene Name	Protein Name	Causative Effect in NAFLD	MoA Activation by RUNX1
NFKB1	Nuclear factor NF-kappa-B p105 subunit	1	1.000
JNK1	c-Jun N-terminal kinase 1	1	0.992
PKC-E	Protein kinase C epsilon type	1	0.883
TNF	Tumor necrosis factor	1	0.875
IKBKB	Inhibitor of nuclear factor kB kinase subunit beta	1	0.859
PTGS2	Prostaglandin G/H synthase 2	1	0.842
IL17A	Interleukin 17A	1	0.688
MTOR	Serine/threonine-protein kinase mTOR	1	0.684
APOC3	Apolipoprotein C-III	1	0.605
NFKB2	Nuclear factor NF-kappa-B p100 subunit	1	0.543
LCN2	Neutrophil gelatinase-associated lipocalin	1	0.457
SOCS3	Suppressor of cytokine signaling 3	1	0.436
INS	Insulin	1	0.422
NT	Neurotensin	1	0.362
IL6	Interleukin-6	1	0.230
CNR1	Cannabinoid receptor 1	1	0.102
ADIPOQ	Adiponectin	−1	−0.184
NRG4	Pro-neuregulin-4, membrane-bound isoform	−1	−0.305
AKT2	RAC-beta serine/threonine-protein kinase	−1	−0.375
PTPN1	Tyrosine-protein phosphatase non-receptor type 1	−1	−0.436
GSK3	Glycogen synthase kinase-3 alpha	−1	−0.504
SIRT1	Sirtuin 1	−1	−0.868
IRS2	Insulin receptor substrate 2	−1	−0.916
PTEN	Phosphatase and tensin homolog	−1	−0.930
IRS1	Insulin receptor substrate 1	−1	−0.996

NAFLD, nonalcoholic fatty liver disease; NAFLD, nonalcoholic fatty liver disease; RUNX1, runt-related transcription factor 1; MoA, mechanism of action. Green color indicates a positive interaction between the effector protein and RUNX1, while red color indicates a negative one. A more intense color indicates a higher intensity of activation/inhibition.

3.2.2. Mechanism of Action of RUNX1 Promoting Lipotoxicity and Hepatic Injury-Liver Fibrosis

As shown in Figure 3, most of the molecular pathways that may justify the potential role of RUNX1 promoting lipotoxicity and fibrosis-related processes are shared with those involved in the motive IR.

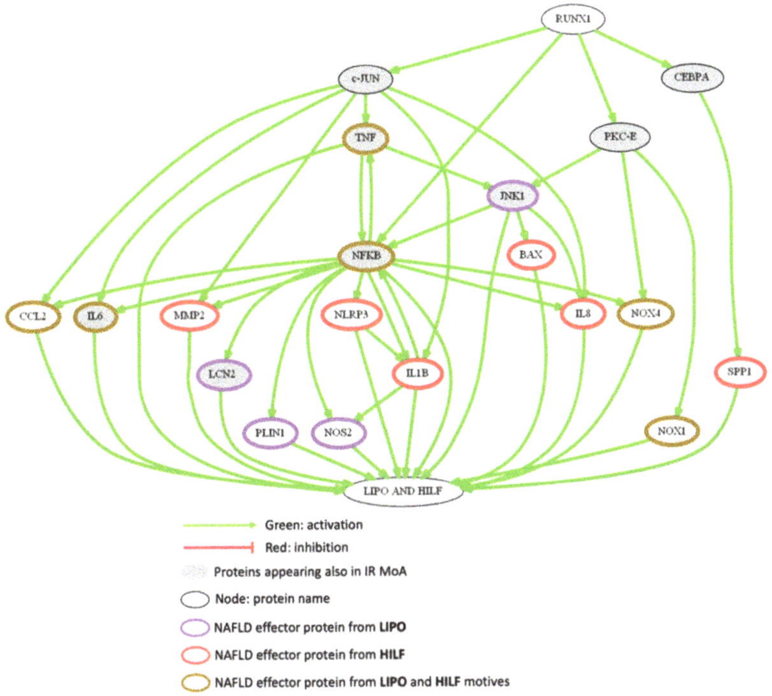

Figure 3. Most represented MoA of RUNX1 promoting lipotoxicity and hepatic injury and fibrosis in NAFLD in the population of TPMS model solutions. Gene names are used in the representations. RUNX1, runt-related protein 1; c-Jun, protein encoded by JUN gene; NFκB, nuclear factor kappa B; PKCε, protein kinase C epsilon; CEBPA, CCAAT/enhancer-binding protein alpha; SPP1, osteopontin; JNK1, c-Jun N-terminal kinase 1; BAX, BCL2 Associated X; CCL2, C-C motif chemokine 2; IL, interleukin; MMP2, matrix metalloproteinase-2; NLRP3, NACHT, LRR and PYD domains-containing protein 3; TLR, toll-like receptor; NOS2, inducible nitric oxide synthase; LCN2, neutrophil gelatinase-associated lipocalin; PLIN1, perlipin; NOX, NADPH oxidase; IR, insulin resistance; LIPO, lipotoxicity; HILF, hepatic injury and liver fibrosis. This picture was generated using Graphviz software.

Table 3 describes the lipotoxicity and fibrosis effector proteins that are regulated by the activation of RUNX1 (considering that the activity values of the proteins in our models range from 1 to −1, only proteins with activation state >0.1 are shown). RUNX1 promotes lipotoxicity and fibrosis by the regulation of 50.88% and 62.07% of the effector proteins involved in these motives, respectively. In total, 17 proteins specific to lipotoxicity, 24 to fibrosis, and 12 involved in both motives are regulated by RUNX1. The proteins most regulated by RUNX1 involved in lipotoxicity-related processes are: JNK1, CEBPB, and IKBKB, and those involved in fibrosis-related processes are mothers against decapentaplegic homolog 3 (SMAD3), angiopoietin-2 (ANGPT2), apoptosis regulator BAX, type-1 angiotensin II receptor (AGTR1), and TGF-β. Effector proteins with a role in both pathophysiological processes most activated by RUNX1 are NFκB, NADPH oxidase (NOX)-1, NOX4, CCL2, and TNF. The proteins most inhibited by RUNX1 are SIRT1 (lipotoxicity) and PTEN (fibrosis). Note that the list of proteins in Table 3 is not limited to those shown in the Figure 3.

Table 3. Lipotoxicity and fibrosis effector proteins modulated when RUNX1 is activated.

Gene Name	Protein Name	Causative Effect in NAFLD	Activation by RUNX1
	LIPOTOXICITY		
JNK1	c-Jun N-terminal kinase 1	1	0.999
CEBPB	CCAAT/enhancer-binding protein beta	1	0.825
IKBKB	Inhibitor of nuclear factor kappa-B kinase subunit beta	1	0.819
MAP3K7	Transforming growth factor beta-activated kinase 1/Mitogen-activated protein kinase 7	1	0.722
NOS2	Nitric oxide synthase, inducible	1	0.667
MTOR	Serine/threonine-protein kinase mTOR	1	0.617
LCN2	Neutrophil gelatinase-associated lipocalin	1	0.609
PLIN1	Perilipin-1	1	0.563
HMOX1	Heme oxygenase 1	1	0.490
MAP3K5	Apoptosis signal-regulating kinase 1/mitogen-activated protein kinase 5	1	0.460
PPARG	Peroxisome proliferator-activated receptor gamma	1	0.402
XBP1	X-box-binding protein 1	1	0.327
UCP2	Mitochondrial uncoupling protein 2	1	0.183
ACC1	Acetyl-CoA carboxylase 1	1	0.113
ADIPOR2	Adiponectin receptor protein 2	−1	−0.600
ADIPOR1	Adiponectin receptor protein 1	−1	−0.633
SIRT1	Sirtuin 1	−1	−0.780
	FIBROSIS		
SMAD3	Mothers against decapentaplegic homolog 3	1	0.859
ANGPT2	Angiopoietin-2	1	0.854
BAX	Apoptosis regulator BAX	1	0.839
AGTR1	Type-1 angiotensin II receptor	1	0.839
TGFB1	Transforming growth factor beta-1	1	0.827
IL1B	Interleukin-1 beta	1	0.693
IL8	Interleukin-8	1	0.683
MMP9	Matrix metalloproteinase-9	1	0.614
FAS	Tumor necrosis factor receptor superfamily member 6	1	0.518
MMP2	72 kDa type IV collagenase	1	0.508
CTGF	Connective tissue growth factor	1	0.497
CASP1	Caspase-1	1	0.472
NLRP3	NACHT, LRR and PYD domains-containing protein 3	1	0.352
AGT	Angiotensinogen	1	0.340
SPP1	Osteopontin	1	0.330
TIMP1	Metalloproteinase inhibitor 1	1	0.282
MYD88	Myeloid differentiation primary response protein MyD88	1	0.277
PDGFA	Platelet-derived growth factor subunit A	1	0.248
LY96	Lymphocyte antigen 96	1	0.224
COL1A1	Collagen alpha-1(I) chain	1	0.209
COL1A2	Collagen alpha-2(I) chain	1	0.124
NR1H4	Bile acid receptor	−1	−0.441
PTEN	Phosphatase and tensin homolog	−1	−0.958

Table 3. *Cont.*

Gene Name	Protein Name	Causative Effect in NAFLD	Activation by RUNX1
	LIPOTOXICITY AND FIBROSIS		
NFKB1	Nuclear factor NF-kappa-B p105 subunit	1	0.999
NOX1	NADPH oxidase 1	1	0.894
NOX4	NADPH oxidase 4	1	0.822
CCL2	C-C motif chemokine 2	1	0.813
TNF	Tumor necrosis factor	1	0.812
CYBB	Cytochrome b-245 heavy chain	1	0.640
NFKB2	Nuclear factor NF-kappa-B p100 subunit	1	0.535
TLR4	Toll-like receptor 4	1	0.501
IL6	Interleukin-6	1	0.342
TLR2	Toll-like receptor 2	1	0.292
TLR9	Toll-like receptor 9	1	0.200
ADIPOQ	Adiponectin	−1	−0.142

NAFLD, nonalcoholic fatty liver disease; RUNX1, runt-related transcription factor 1. Green color indicates a positive interaction between the effector protein and RUNX1, while red color indicates a negative one. A more intense color indicates a higher intensity of activation/inhibition.

3.3. *Overlap between the Mechanistic Pathways Modulated by RUNX1 Activation in IR and Lipotoxicity & Fibrosis Stimulation*

The NAFLD motives that have been studied for the generation of the two MoA in this project seem to be pathophysiologically related to each other since there is an overlap of effector proteins from the three motives, as described in Figure 4.

This high relationship prompted us to explore whether an overlap existed in the pathways regulated by the activation of RUNX1 in promoting these motives, and therefore, to be able to relate them. Thus, we have evaluated the similarities that interrelate the motives at the level of common effector proteins and/or pathways modulated by RUNX1 according to our models.

Common NAFLD effector proteins regulated by RUNX1 downstream mechanisms have been recognized by studying the overlap for the three motives together and studying pairs of motives separately. The proteins that we consider to be RUNX1-regulated with an activation value >0.1 are shown in Table 4. In this sense, cannabinoid receptor 1 (CNR1), which was found to be one of the common effector proteins with the three NAFLD analysed motives, presented an activation value lower than 0.1, and it is for this reason that we stop taking this protein into account from now on.

Values of protein activity in each MoA are displayed. "Causative effect in NAFLD" indicates whether the protein is increased/overactivated (1) or reduced/inhibited (−1) in NAFLD. NAFLD, nonalcoholic fatty liver disease; MoA, mechanism of action; IR, insulin resistance; L&F, lipotoxicity and fibrosis; RUNX1, runt-related transcription factor 1; NFκB, nuclear factor kappa B; TNF, tumour necrosis factor; IL6, interleukin 6; ADIPOQ, adiponectin; NOX, NADPH oxidase; CCL2, C-C motif chemokine 2; CYBB, cytochrome b-245 heavy chain; TLR, toll-like receptor; JNK1, c-Jun N-terminal kinase; IKBKB, inhibitor of nuclear factor kappa B subunit beta; MTOR, mammalian target of rapamycin serine/threonine-protein kinase; LCN2, neutrophil gelatinase-associated lipocalin 2; SIRT1, sirtuin 1; PTEN, phosphatase and tensin homolog. Protein codes were obtained from UniProt database.

As shown in Table 4, overlapping of RUNX1-regulated proteins is observed in all three motives and in each pair. Despite finding six effector proteins that share the three NAFLD motives, only five presented sufficient signal intensity to be considered downstream effector proteins of RUNX1 inducing NAFLD; these are NFκB1, NFκB2, TNF, ADIPOQ, and IL-6.

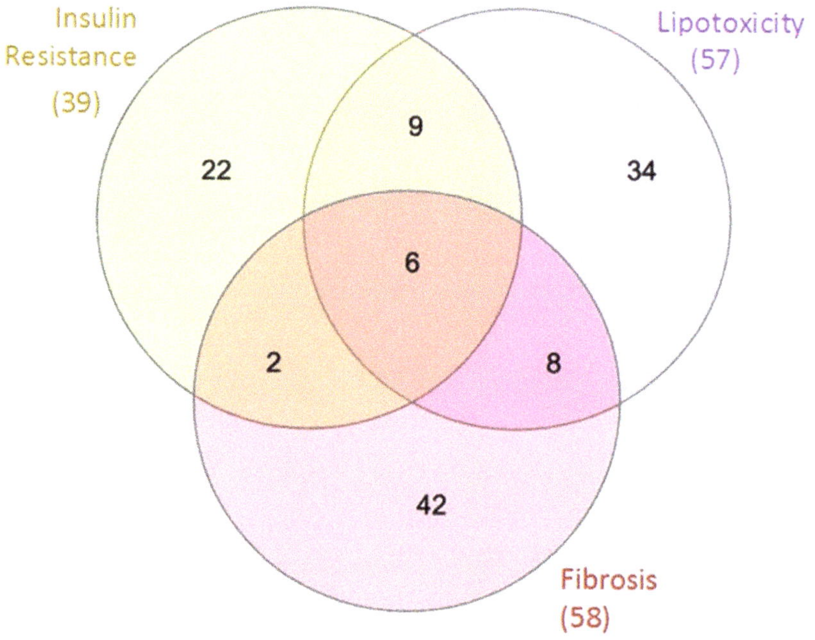

Motives	Overlapping proteins
All	NFKB1, NFKB2, TNF, ADIPOQ, IL6, CNR1
Lipotoxicity and Fibrosis	TLR2, TLR4, TLR9, CYBB, LEP, CCL2, NOX4, NOX1
IR and Fibrosis	PTEN, TGR5
IR and Lipotoxicity	JNK1, SIRT1, IKBKB, MTOR, LCN2, RETN, SFRP5, PPARA, DGAT2

Figure 4. Overlap of effector proteins between the three NAFLD motives evaluated in the project: VENN diagram showing the number of effector proteins overlapping between the three indicated NAFLD motives. There are 39 proteins involved in IR mechanism, 57 in lipotoxicity, and 58 in fibrosis. Concretely, there are 9 proteins involved in IR and lipotoxicity, 6 in lipotoxicity and fibrosis, and only 2 in IR and fibrosis. In this regard, there are six proteins involved in the three motives of NAFLD pathogenesis: NFκB1, NFκB2, TNF, ADIPOQ, IL-6, CNR1. IR, insulin resistance; NFKB, nuclear factor kappa B; TNF, tumour necrosis factor; ADIPOQ, adiponectin; IL6, interleukin 6; CNR1, cannabinoid receptor 1; TLR, toll-like receptor; CYBB, cytochrome b-245 heavy chain; LEP, leptin; CCL2, C-C motif chemokine 2; NOX, NADPH oxidase; PTEN, phosphatase and tensin homolog; TGR5, G protein-coupled bile acid receptor-1; JNK1, c-Jun N-terminal kinase; SIRT1, sirtuin 1; IKBKB, inhibitor of nuclear factor kappa B kinase subunit beta; MTOR, mammalian target of rapamycin serine/threonine-protein kinase; LCN2, neutrophil gelatinase-associated lipocalin 2; RETN, resistin; SFRP5, secreted frizzled-related protein 5; PPARA, peroxisome proliferator-activated receptor alpha; DGAT2, diacylglycerol O-Acyltransferase 2.

Table 4. Effector proteins modulated by RUNX1 activation shared by the three motives: lipotoxicity and fibrosis; IR and lipotoxicity; and IR and fibrosis.

Gene Name	Protein Code	Causative Effect in NAFLD	Activity in IR MoA	Activity in L&F MoA	Present in the Most Represented MoA	
					IR (Figure 2)	L&F (Figure 3)
Common RUNX1-modulated effector proteins in three motives						
NFKB1	P19838	1	1.000	0.999	Yes	Yes
TNF	P01375	1	0.875	0.812	Yes	Yes
NFKB2	Q00653	1	0.543	0.535	-	-
IL6	P05231	1	0.230	0.342	Yes	Yes
ADIPOQ	Q15848	−1	−0.184	−0.142	-	-
Common RUNX1-modulated effector proteins in lipotoxicity and fibrosis						
NOX1	Q9Y5S8	1	-	0.894	-	Yes
NOX4	Q9NPH5	1	-	0.822	-	Yes
CCL2	P13500	1	-	0.813	-	Yes
CYBB	P04839	1	-	0.640	-	-
TLR4	O00206	1	-	0.501	-	-
TLR2	O60603	1	-	0.292	-	-
TLR9	Q9NR96	1	-	0.200	-	-
Common RUNX1-modulated effector proteins in IR and lipotoxicity						
JNK1	P45983	1	0.992	0.999	Yes	Yes
IKBKB	O14920	1	0.859	0.819	-	-
MTOR	P42345	1	0.684	0.617	Yes	-
LCN2	P80188	1	0.457	0.609	Yes	Yes
SIRT1	Q96EB6	−1	−0.868	−0.780	-	-
Common RUNX1-modulated effector proteins in IR and fibrosis						
PTEN	P60484	−1	−0.930	−0.958	-	-

4. Discussion

The novelty of this work lies in the fact that we aimed to perform a high-throughput screening to determine the molecular mechanisms that could establish a link between the activity of RUNX1 and NAFLD pathogenesis.

Until now, the connection between RUNX1 and NAFLD remains uncertain. On one hand, Kaur et al. showed a significant correlation between RUNX1 expression and inflammation, fibrosis, and NASH activity score in patients presenting NASH; they also reported RUNX1 function as a pro-angiogenic factor in SS and NASH [20]. On the other hand, Liu et al. presented low levels of RUNX1 in hepatocellular carcinoma. In this sense, these authors suggested that RUNX1 is a tumour suppressing factor that inhibits angiogenesis [33]. Regarding our previous study, we reported that the mRNA and protein expression of RUNX1 in liver seems to be involved in first steps of NAFLD with a proangiogenic-repairing role; meanwhile, RUNX1 appears to be downregulated in the NASH stage [21]. Since these disagreements, an exhaustive study of the relationship between RUNX1 MoA and NAFLD/NASH pathogenesis need to be performed to clarify this issue. In addition, this study could help to recognize RUNX1 as a potential therapeutic target of NAFLD. Previous reports have suggested that RUNX1 could be a potential therapeutic target of cancers, such as acute myeloid leukaemia, since this protein is an important regulator of haematopoiesis in vertebrates [34,35]. The beneficial effect of the therapeutic amelioration of RUNX1 in patients with nonsmall-cell lung cancer has also been described, since the RUNX1 overexpression is correlated with enhanced metastasis [36]. In addition, RUNX1 have been suggested as a potential therapeutic target to limit the progression of adverse cardiac remodeling and heart failure [37,38]. In this regard, to analyze the potential use of RUNX1 as a therapeutic target of NAFLD should be thoroughly studied. For example, investigating liver targeting through liposomes or bile acids in liver cancer [39] could be possible future strategies to evaluate the role of RUNX1 in the pathogenesis of NAFLD.

In this sense, when we performed an ANN analysis concerning the probability of the relationship between RUNX1 protein and NAFLD motives, our first main finding is that RUNX1 seems to show a medium intensity relationship with both motives–hepatic IR and lipotoxicity–and a high intensity relationship with hepatic injury and liver fibrosis motives, suggesting that this protein probably plays a role in these processes. In this regard, this result matches with Kaur et al., who reported a relevant association between RUNX1 expression and fibrosis and inflammation, two of the main NASH parameters [20]. However, this result contradicts our previous reported hypothesis about the potential protective role of RUNX1 in early stages of NAFLD [21]; in contrast, our current result has shown a low or medium intensity relationship with SS-related parameters. Given that our ANN approach provides the probability of functional relationship–regardless of the activity status (up or downregulation)–and the current conflicting results in the literature, further studies in humans or in vivo are required to clarify these contradictions, although the current available evidence clearly supports an involvement, either by presence or absence, of RUNX1 in NAHLD and NASH.

In the current literature, no direct role of RUNX1 on IR has been described yet. However, as a novelty, we demonstrate in the present study that RUNX1 interacts with proteins involved in this pathophysiological process. IR can be defined as a reduced response of the liver to the effects of insulin, which triggers impaired glucose homeostasis (gluconeogenesis and glucose uptake). IR may exert multiple effects on hepatic metabolism such as increased lipogenesis, increased free fatty acids (FFA) uptake, impaired FFA export, and decreased FFA oxidation. Moreover, outside the liver, IR causes increased serum FFA levels because of failure of insulin to suppress hormone sensitive lipase-mediated lipolysis in adipose tissue [3,40–42]. In this situation, the PKCε, a downstream intermediate of RUNX1 signaling [20], is activated by the accumulation of diacylglycerol and participates in hepatic IR through impairing insulin signaling [43,44]. In addition, it is believed that RUNX1 could also be involved in IR through the transcription of IL-17 [45], a cytokine that leads to neutrophil and monocyte infiltration in the liver, thereby increasing IR [46]. In contrast, RUNX1 has been shown to inhibit the expression of Suppressor of cytokine signaling (SOCS)-3 [47]—an intracellular protein interfering with insulin signaling via ubiquitin-mediated degradation of IRS1 and IRS2 [48]—therefore ameliorating the IR. According to these facts, RUNX1 seems to have a dual role both promoting and/or preventing hepatic IR.

Another crucial event clearly involved in NAFLD progression is the lipotoxicity resulting from an excessive FFA influx to hepatocytes. Hepatic lipotoxicity occurs when the capacity of the hepatocytes to manage and export FFA as triglycerides is overwhelmed [49]. The molecular mechanisms responsible for lipotoxicity in NAFLD include endoplasmic reticulum and oxidative stress and impaired autophagy, processes that in turn activate apoptotic cascades, thus promoting tissue damage and inflammation [49].

Consequently, in conditions of hypoxia induced by steatosis [50] and inflammation, angiogenesis is triggered in chronic liver diseases [51]. It was demonstrated that proangiogenic factors have an early function in NAFLD progression from SS to NASH since proangiogenic treatments reduce not only inflammation but also steatosis [52]. In this regard, RUNX1, a pivotal regulator of hematopoiesis and angiogenesis [12,53], could be activated in order to repair the liver damage in early stages of NAFLD [21,54]. In contrast, RUNX1 activates target genes involved in lipotoxicity [55–58] such as CEBPB [59] and Cyclic AMP-dependent transcription factor (AT6) in a regulatory feed-back loop with the transcription factor AP-1 and JNK [60]. If exposure of hepatocytes to lipotoxicity and liver injury continues, it can induce apoptosis [61] and trigger inflammation by interacting with toll-like receptors (TLRs). Inflammation is a component of the wound healing process that leads to fibrosis, the deposition of extracellular matrix in liver parenchyma [62]. Additionally, RUNX1 may contribute to fibrosis and inflammation by modulation of pro-inflammatory cytokines (IL-1β, IL-6, TNF, etc.) [47,63], tissue inhibitor of metalloproteinase 1 (TIMP-1) [64], osteopontin [65] and TLRs [66], among others. Hence, RUNX1 seems to play a dual role, inducing pro-inflammatory cytokines and triggering liver damage, but at the same time having a protective effect by trying to repair the hepatic damage via angiogenesis-related processes.

The second notable finding of this work was obtained because we performed the TPMS technology to identify the key proteins and the most probable paths that link the activation of RUNX1 with the most strongly related motives according to ANNs analysis. In this regard, we wanted to evaluate IR first, since it is one of the main parameters involved in the first stages of NAFLD [67]. Accordingly, IR effector proteins most activated by RUNX1-dependent downstream pathways are NFκB, JNK, PKCε, TNF, IKBKB, and PTGS2, while the most inhibited ones are IRS1, PTEN, IRS2, and SIRT1.

RUNX1 could activate the PTGS2/cyclooxygenase-2 (COX-2) through its interaction with HDAC1 [68,69]. When PTGS2/COX-2 signaling is activated during inflammation in adipose tissue, it can act as a crucial factor for the promotion of obesity-induced IR and fatty liver [70,71]. According to the inflammatory role of PTGS2/COX-2, this enzyme can be induced by growth factors and different cytokines, such as TNF-α, that play a feed-back regulation role [71]. The cytokine TNF-α, produced by adipocytes and macrophages, is highly activated by the downstream mechanisms of RUNX1, particularly via the interaction with the proto-oncogene c-Jun [60,72] or the activation of NFκB [73]. The IκB kinase (IKBK) complex is the master regulator for activation of the NFκB signaling pathway. The kinase complex comprises the two catalytic subunits, IKK1 (IKBKA) and IKK2 (IKBKB), and the regulatory subunit NEMO (IKBKG), which mediates NFκB activation in response to a number of different stimuli such as RUNX1, by phosphorylating IκB proteins [74]. NFκB plays an important role in the regulation of a wide range of proteins/molecular pathways involved in IR. Its activation can be induced by TNF-α and JNK mechanisms [75,76] and can lead to the up-regulation of TNF-α, IL-6 and neutrophil gelatinase-associated lipocalin (LCN-2), contributing to IR-related processes in NAFLD [48,73,77,78]. In addition, the transcription factor AP-1 aggravates IR by inflammation-related processes, inducing the expression of IL-6 [79,80] and TNF-α [72]. TNF-α could be importantly contributing to the development of IR by inhibition and degradation of the IRS mediated by a serine phosphorylation through different mechanisms: (1) SOCS3 is induced by the NFκB/JNK-mediated activation of TNF-α and IL-6 [81], or via CEBPA activation [82], inducing ubiquitin-mediated degradation of IRS1 and IRS2 [83]; (2) MTOR can be activated by TNF-α or PKCβ pathways [84,85] due to hyperglycemia, leading to phosphorylation of multiple serine residues in IRS1 and IRS2 with their further degradation; (3) JNK1 promotes IRS1 and IRS2 serine phosphorylation [86,87]. The inhibitory effects of JNK1 could be also stimulated by PKCβ and PKCε [88,89]. In this regard, some studies have identified associations of PKC activity with disruption of the insulin-induced signal transduction pathway [90–92].

In contrast, apart from the degradation/silencing of IRS induced by RUNX1, which was explained above, our analysis has also reported the negative effect of RUNX1 in phosphatase and tensin homologue (PTEN) signaling. Decreased PTEN activity would lead to excessive fat deposition in the liver [40]. PTEN physiological functions negatively regulate the activity of phosphatidylinositol 3-kinase (PI3K)/AKT pathway, which in normal conditions induces lipogenesis in hepatocytes, consequently triggering IR [93,94]. PTEN downregulation has been reported to be carried out by mechanisms involving the sequential activation of MTOR and NFκB [95]. On the other hand, we have also reported a strong repression of SIRT1 by RUNX1 action. SIRT1 is an essential negative regulator of pro-inflammatory pathways, mainly through down-modulating NFκB transcriptional activity, decreasing de novo lipogenesis, and increasing fatty acid β-oxidation [96]. Hence, RUNX1-mediated inhibition of SIRT1 interrupts the beneficial effect of this protein, thus promoting IR. In short, the action of all these effector proteins together gives rise to IR mechanisms.

Regarding the second main finding of this work, we wanted to focus the study of the most implicated motives in NASH stage [97]. In this sense, the effector proteins with a role in NASH (lipotoxicity and fibrosis related processes) most activated by RUNX1 are

NFκB, TNF, CCL2, NOX1, and NOX4; the proteins most inhibited by RUNX1 are SIRT1 (lipotoxicity) and PTEN (fibrosis).

NFκB appear to be a relevant regulation core since several RUNX1 interactors regulate its expression [47]. NFκB might be activated by molecular mechanisms such as those explained above (TNF-α/AP-1/JNK pathways). The downstream effects of NFκB activation result in lipotoxicity, hepatocyte injury, inflammation, and fibrosis [40] through upregulated expression of the pro-inflammatory and/or pro-fibrogenic cytokines: CCL2 also called monocyte chemoattractant protein 1 (MCP-1) [98], IL-6 [77] and matrix metalloproteinase-2 (MMP-2) [99]. In particular, higher levels of CCL2 have been identified in NASH subjects in comparison with simple fatty liver [3,100].

Free fatty acids promote hepatic lipotoxicity by stimulating TNF-α expression via a lysosomal pathway, which could be stimulated by the RUNX1/c-Jun link [60,101–104]. JNK-1, also activated by RUNX1 regulated PKCε activation [20,89], leads to the induction of NFκB dependent pathways [105] and the proapoptotic protein BAX [106], resulting in hepatic tissue damage [107].

Additionally, the isoforms NOX1 and NOX4 seem to be upstream regulated by RUNX1. These proteins show a crucial role on both lipotoxicity and fibrosis-related processes, specially by regulating the activation of hepatic stellate cells and apoptosis, which are two important aspects in the fibrogenic process in NASH [108]. Oxidative biomolecular damage and dysregulated redox signaling induce high oxidative stress and thereby liver injury. Moreover, several studies have shown that the inhibition of NOX1 and NOX4 leads to decreased oxidative stress, lipid peroxidation, hepatic injury, inflammation, and fibrosis in NASH [108,109]. RUNX1 could induce NOX4 expression via PKCε [110,111] and NFκB dependent pathways [112], and induce NOX1 only through PKCε activation [111].

Conversely, RUNX1 have shown to inhibit SIRT1 and PTEN. Some studies have reported that liver-specific disruption of SIRT1 not only causes hepatic steatosis but also promotes the progression to an advanced metabolic disorder stage such as lipotoxicity [113]. Additionally, it seems that dysregulations of PTEN expression/activity in hepatocytes represents an important and recurrent molecular mechanism contributing to the development of liver disorders [114], given that further aberrant activation of hepatic stellate and Kupffer cells trigger the development of liver fibrosis and inflammation [95]. In summary, the pathway that constitute these effector proteins gives rise to processes of lipotoxicity and liver damage.

Accordingly, we have reported for the first-time specific MoA that RUNX1 could play a role in NAFLD pathogenesis motives, but this is only an in silico study and needs to be further validated in experimental research.

The last main objective of the present study is to analyze the overlapping proteins between the studied motives involved in NAFLD. In this sense, the shared proteins between IR and lipotoxicity most activated by RUNX1 are JNK1, IKBKB, MTOR, and LCN2, while the most inhibited by RUNX1 is SIRT1. On the other hand, the overlapping proteins observed in lipotoxicity and fibrosis motives that are the most positively modulated by RUNX1 mechanisms are NADPH oxidase NOX1 and NOX4, the chemokine CCL2, the cytochrome CYBB, and the TLRs 2, 4, and 9. The only effector that is shared between IR and fibrosis negatively modulated by RUNX1 is PTEN. Finally, the main contribution of this study is that we found five RUNX1-regulated proteins with a direct involvement in the three main NAFLD motives, which are NFκB 1, NFκB 2, TNF, ADIPOQ, and IL-6. These proteins are indicators of the relevance of their processes in terms of the relationship with RUNX1 mechanisms towards promoting NAFLD. NFκB1 and TNF present a high activation due to RUNX1 activity, as we explained above. In fact, NFκB-dependent pathways seem to definitely be a key element in these MoA due to its high number of up/downstream links, and for its important regulation of a lot of effector proteins of these motives, especially immune response-related proteins that trigger inflammation, fibrosis, or lipotoxicity [96].

On the other hand, in this study, NFκB 2, IL-6, and ADIPOQ present moderated values of activation, which differ from those of NFκB 1 and TNF. NFκB 2 is an important regulator of RUNX1. It was shown that transcription levels of NFκB 2 were increased in RUNX1-deficient cells [115]. Furthermore, IL-6, as we already mentioned, is a pro-inflammatory cytokine that takes part in fibrosis and tissue damage induced by RUNX1 [47]. High TNF-α and IL-6 levels have been found in NAFLD patients, indicating an important role of these cytokines in the disease. In fact, IL-6 reduction was significantly correlated with both weight loss and insulin sensitivity [48]. Conversely, ADIPOQ seems to be downregulated by RUNX1 signaling. It has been shown that significantly up-regulated ADIPOQ expression in white adipose tissue leads to increased serum adiponectin concentrations. Low adiponectin levels are closely related to the severity of liver histology in NAFLD [116].

Our approach, as all modelling approaches, is subjected to limitations. First, it is limited by the current knowledge on the key studied elements, in this case RUNX1 functions and interactors and NAFLD molecular pathophysiology; thus, the models and conclusions are susceptible to being updated over time if prospective data and new information are generated. Nevertheless, TPMS models are built by considering the whole human protein network and a wide range of drug–pathology relationships (Supplementary Table S3); not only limited to the key studied elements, or even to hepatic involvement, they present accuracies against the training set above 80% in the case of ANN models, and above 90% in sampling methods-based models [32]. Thus, systems biology and artificial intelligence approaches allowed us to explore and present mechanistic hypotheses that are in agreement with current knowledge, providing a guide for further pre-clinical investigation in the advancement towards defining treatments for NAFLD. Further studies are needed for confirmation and advancement of these data.

5. Conclusions

NAFLD pathophysiological motives most functionally related to RUNX1, according to an ANNs-based analysis, are hepatic insulin resistance, lipotoxicity, and hepatic injury-liver fibrosis. These three pathophysiological processes are molecularly related, since they share NFκB1, NFκB2, TNF, ADIPOQ, and IL-6 as effector proteins. This connection suggested that RUNX1 could regulate molecular pathways involved in NAFLD pathogenesis, but more studies in this field are needed.

Supplementary Materials: The following supporting information can be downloaded at: https://www.mdpi.com/article/10.3390/biomedicines10061315/s1, Table S1: Condition_MOTIVES; Table S2: Condition_PROTEINS; Table S3: S3 Training set Runx.

Author Contributions: Conceptualization, T.A. and L.B.; methodology, L.A. and M.C.; validation, T.A., L.B. and A.E.-A.; formal analysis, H.B., L.A. and M.C.; investigation, T.A., L.B., A.E.-A., M.P.-C., A.B.-R. and J.U.C.; resources, T.A., L.B., J.B., C.A., J.U.C. and C.R.; data curation, T.A., L.B. and H.B.; writing—original draft preparation, T.A., L.B. and A.E.-A.; writing—review and editing, T.A., L.B., A.E.-A., M.P.-C., A.B.-R., J.B., C.A., J.U.C., H.B., L.A., M.C. and C.R.; visualization, T.A., L.B.; supervision, T.A.; project administration, T.A., C.R.; funding acquisition, T.A. All authors have read and agreed to the published version of the manuscript.

Funding: This research was financed by own funding through the project PV20062N (Teresa Auguet).

Institutional Review Board Statement: Not applicable.

Informed Consent Statement: Not applicable.

Data Availability Statement: Not applicable.

Conflicts of Interest: The authors declare no conflict of interest.

Appendix A

The Sampling Methods

TPMS sampling-based methods [29] generate models like a Multilayer Perceptron of an Artificial Neural Network over the human protein network (where neurons are the proteins, and the edges of the network are used to transfer the information). This methodology can be used for describing with high capability all plausible relationships between an input (or stimulus, in this case RUNX1) and an output (or response, in this case NAFLD motives: IR, lipotoxicity and fibrosis protein effectors).

Although this type of network would generate many possible mechanistic solutions, it can be limited by constraints and restrictions that must be respected: (a) the topology of the protein network, (b) the functional, medical, and biological information stored in Anaxomics' databases, and (c) the available data about the drug (known effects on the target and target biology). Various different approaches and optimization systems can be used for such a purpose, from those based on randomized systems (such as a Montecarlo-based system [30]) to those based on information derived from the topology of the network, in order to solve each parameter of the equation, i.e., the weights associated to the links between the nodes in the human protein network.

The algorithms construct and analyze the regularities of the sampling of different plausible solutions. This information is used to construct feature vectors descriptive of the most probable protein network interaction structure and network activation signal flow derived from the space of plausible protein interaction solutions. The feature vectors are further used as input to supervise machine learning methods as ensembles of classifiers that allow us to infer new clinical and protein level knowledge. K-Fold and leave-one-out cross-validation methods are employed to assess generalization capability.

The mathematical algorithm can be envisioned as an extremely complex multi-parametric function, where each parameter corresponds to the relative weight of a link connecting nodes (genes/proteins) in a graph (protein map). Mathematical models of biological systems have more variables than restrictions (e.g., the number of entries in the training set is always smaller than the number of parameters-link weights-required by the algorithm), so various sets of parameters are equally valid. Therefore, using TPMS sampling-based methods, we could generate populations of solutions that comply with the biological restrictions of the training set.

From this base set of valid mathematical solutions, this approach can be employed to trace back the biological effects on molecules by analyzing the different populations of solutions. This methodology traces the most probable path (in biological and mathematical terms) that leads from the stimulus to the response through the biological network. In other words, it identifies the most probable MoA that achieve a physiological response when the system is stimulated with a specific stimulus. Not all solutions are used for the analysis, as solutions that comply with the general knowledge collated in the training set are preferred. That is, only MoAs that are plausible from the standpoint of currently accepted scientific knowledge are considered. Accuracy is calculated considering the number of restrictions in the training set that the model complies with, and only models with accuracy above 90% are considered.

In this study, the predicted MoAs were aimed at the elucidation of the mechanisms of RUNX1 activity that leads to the promotion of NAFLD motives: (A) IR and (B) lipotoxicity and fibrosis mechanisms. A set of 250 biologically plausible solutions have been calculated, with a mean accuracy of 94%.

References

1. Arciello, M.; Gori, M.; Maggio, R.; Barbaro, B.; Tarocchi, M.; Galli, A.; Balsano, C. Environmental Pollution: A Tangible Risk for NAFLD Pathogenesis. *Int. J. Mol. Sci.* **2013**, *14*, 22052–22066. [CrossRef] [PubMed]
2. Sarwar, R.; Pierce, N.; Koppe, S. Obesity and Nonalcoholic Fatty Liver Disease: Current Perspectives. *DMSO* **2018**, *11*, 533–542. [CrossRef] [PubMed]
3. Larter, C.Z.; Chitturi, S.; Heydet, D.; Farrell, G.C. A Fresh Look at NASH Pathogenesis. Part 1: The Metabolic Movers. *J. Gastroenterol. Hepatol.* **2010**, *25*, 672–690. [CrossRef] [PubMed]
4. Cohen, J.C.; Horton, J.D.; Hobbs, H.H. Human Fatty Liver Disease: Old Questions and New Insights. *Science* **2011**, *332*, 1519–1523. [CrossRef]
5. Cotter, T.G.; Rinella, M. Nonalcoholic Fatty Liver Disease 2020: The State of the Disease. *Gastroenterology* **2020**, *158*, 1851–1864. [CrossRef]

6. Lazarus, J.V.; Mark, H.E.; Anstee, Q.M.; Arab, J.P.; Batterham, R.L.; Castera, L.; Cortez-Pinto, H.; Crespo, J.; Cusi, K.; Dirac, M.A.; et al. Advancing the Global Public Health Agenda for NAFLD: A Consensus Statement. *Nat. Rev. Gastroenterol. Hepatol.* **2022**, *19*, 60–78. [CrossRef]
7. Brunner, K.T.; Henneberg, C.J.; Wilechansky, R.M.; Long, M.T. Nonalcoholic Fatty Liver Disease and Obesity Treatment. *Curr. Obes. Rep.* **2019**, *8*, 220–228. [CrossRef]
8. Okuda, T.; Nishimura, M.; Nakao, M.; Fujitaa, Y. RUNX1/AML1: A Central Player in Hematopoiesis. *Int. J. Hematol.* **2001**, *74*, 252–257. [CrossRef]
9. Ito, Y. Oncogenic Potential of the RUNX Gene Family: 'Overview'. *Oncogene* **2004**, *23*, 4198–4208. [CrossRef]
10. Ichikawa, M.; Yoshimi, A.; Nakagawa, M.; Nishimoto, N.; Watanabe-Okochi, N.; Kurokawa, M. A Role for RUNX1 in Hematopoiesis and Myeloid Leukemia. *Int. J. Hematol.* **2013**, *97*, 726–734. [CrossRef]
11. Chen, C.-L.; Broom, D.C.; Liu, Y.; de Nooij, J.C.; Li, Z.; Cen, C.; Samad, O.A.; Jessell, T.M.; Woolf, C.J.; Ma, Q. Runx1 Determines Nociceptive Sensory Neuron Phenotype and Is Required for Thermal and Neuropathic Pain. *Neuron* **2006**, *49*, 365–377. [CrossRef] [PubMed]
12. Iwatsuki, K.; Tanaka, K.; Kaneko, T.; Kazama, R.; Okamoto, S.; Nakayama, Y.; Ito, Y.; Satake, M.; Takahashi, S.-I.; Miyajima, A.; et al. Runx1 Promotes Angiogenesis by Downregulation of Insulin-like Growth Factor-Binding Protein-3. *Oncogene* **2005**, *24*, 1129–1137. [CrossRef] [PubMed]
13. Hong, M.; He, J.; Li, D.; Chu, Y.; Pu, J.; Tong, Q.; Joshi, H.C.; Tang, S.; Li, S. Runt-Related Transcription Factor 1 Promotes Apoptosis and Inhibits Neuroblastoma Progression in Vitro and in Vivo. *J. Exp. Clin. Cancer Res.* **2020**, *39*, 52. [CrossRef]
14. Liu, S.; Xing, Y.; Lu, W.; Li, S.; Tian, Z.; Xing, H.; Tang, K.; Xu, Y.; Rao, Q.; Wang, M.; et al. RUNX1 Inhibits Proliferation and Induces Apoptosis of t(8;21) Leukemia Cells via KLF4-Mediated Transactivation of P57. *Haematologica* **2019**, *104*, 1597–1607. [CrossRef] [PubMed]
15. Doffo, J.; Bamopoulos, S.A.; Köse, H.; Orben, F.; Zang, C.; Pons, M.; den Dekker, A.T.; Brouwer, R.W.W.; Baluapuri, A.; Habringer, S.; et al. NOXA Expression Drives Synthetic Lethality to RUNX1 Inhibition in Pancreatic Cancer. *Proc. Natl. Acad. Sci. USA* **2022**, *119*, e2105691119. [CrossRef] [PubMed]
16. Xiao, L.; Peng, Z.; Zhu, A.; Xue, R.; Lu, R.; Mi, J.; Xi, S.; Chen, W.; Jiang, S. Inhibition of RUNX1 Promotes Cisplatin-Induced Apoptosis in Ovarian Cancer Cells. *Biochem. Pharmacol.* **2020**, *180*, 114116. [CrossRef]
17. Schlegelberger, B.; Heller, P.G. RUNX1 Deficiency (Familial Platelet Disorder with Predisposition to Myeloid Leukemia, FPDMM). *Semin. Hematol.* **2017**, *54*, 75–80. [CrossRef]
18. Xing, X.; Wang, H.; Niu, T.; Jiang, Y.; Shi, X.; Liu, K. RUNX1 Can Mediate the Glucose and O-GlcNAc-Driven Proliferation and Migration of Human Retinal Microvascular Endothelial Cells. *BMJ Open Diabetes Res. Care* **2021**, *9*, e001898. [CrossRef]
19. RUNX1 Gene-RUNX Family Transcription Factor 1. *GeneCards*. Available online: https://www.genecards.org/cgi-bin/carddisp.pl?gene=RUNX1 (accessed on 2 April 2022).
20. Kaur, S.; Rawal, P.; Siddiqui, H.; Rohilla, S.; Sharma, S.; Tripathi, D.M.; Baweja, S.; Hassan, M.; Vlaic, S.; Guthke, R.; et al. Increased Expression of RUNX1 in Liver Correlates with NASH Activity Score in Patients with Non-Alcoholic Steatohepatitis (NASH). *Cells* **2019**, *8*, 1277. [CrossRef]
21. Bertran, L.; Pastor, A.; Portillo-Carrasquer, M.; Binetti, J.; Aguilar, C.; Martínez, S.; Vives, M.; Sabench, F.; Porras, J.A.; Riesco, D.; et al. The Potential Protective Role of RUNX1 in Nonalcoholic Fatty Liver Disease. *Int. J. Mol. Sci.* **2021**, *22*, 5239. [CrossRef]
22. Han, H.; Cho, J.-W.; Lee, S.; Yun, A.; Kim, H.; Bae, D.; Yang, S.; Kim, C.Y.; Lee, M.; Kim, E.; et al. TRRUST v2: An Expanded Reference Database of Human and Mouse Transcriptional Regulatory Interactions. *Nucleic Acids Res.* **2018**, *46*, D380–D386. [CrossRef]
23. The Biological General Repository for Interaction. *BioGRID*. Available online: https://thebiogrid.org/ (accessed on 23 March 2022).
24. Peri, S.; Navarro, J.D.; Amanchy, R.; Kristiansen, T.Z.; Jonnalagadda, C.K.; Surendranath, V.; Niranjan, V.; Muthusamy, B.; Gandhi, T.K.B.; Gronborg, M.; et al. Development of Human Protein Reference Database as an Initial Platform for Approaching Systems Biology in Humans. *Genome Res.* **2003**, *13*, 2363–2371. [CrossRef]
25. Prasad, T.S.K.; Goel, R.; Kandasamy, K.; Keerthikumar, S.; Kumar, S.; Mathivanan, S.; Telikicherla, D.; Raju, R.; Shafreen, B.; Venugopal, A.; et al. Human Protein Reference Database—2009 Update. *Nucleic Acids Res.* **2009**, *37*, D767–D772. [CrossRef] [PubMed]
26. Orchard, S.; Ammari, M.; Aranda, B.; Breuza, L.; Briganti, L.; Broackes-Carter, F.; Campbell, N.H.; Chavali, G.; Chen, C.; del-Toro, N.; et al. The MIntAct Project—IntAct as a Common Curation Platform for 11 Molecular Interaction Databases. *Nucl. Acids Res.* **2014**, *42*, D358–D363. [CrossRef]
27. Kanehisa, M.; Goto, S. KEGG: Kyoto Encyclopedia of Genes and Genomes. *Nucleic Acids Res.* **2000**, *28*, 27–30. [CrossRef] [PubMed]
28. Griss, J.; Viteri, G.; Sidiropoulos, K.; Nguyen, V.; Fabregat, A.; Hermjakob, H. ReactomeGSA–Efficient Multi-Omics Comparative Pathway Analysis. *Mol. Cell. Proteom.* **2020**, *19*, 2115–2125. [CrossRef] [PubMed]
29. Jorba, G.; Aguirre-Plans, J.; Junet, V.; Segú-Vergés, C.; Ruiz, J.L.; Pujol, A.; Fernández-Fuentes, N.; Mas, J.M.; Oliva, B. In-Silico Simulated Prototype-Patients Using TPMS Technology to Study a Potential Adverse Effect of Sacubitril and Valsartan. *PLoS ONE* **2020**, *15*, e0228926. [CrossRef]
30. Bishop, C.M. *Pattern Recognition and Machine Learning*, 1st ed.; Information Science and Statistics; Springer: New York, NY, USA, 2006; Volume 738.

31. Artigas, L.; Coma, M.; Matos-Filipe, P.; Aguirre-Plans, J.; Farrés, J.; Valls, R.; Fernandez-Fuentes, N.; de la Haba-Rodriguez, J.; Olvera, A.; Barbera, J.; et al. In-Silico Drug Repurposing Study Predicts the Combination of Pirfenidone and Melatonin as a Promising Candidate Therapy to Reduce SARS-CoV-2 Infection Progression and Respiratory Distress Caused by Cytokine Storm. *PLoS ONE* **2020**, *15*, e0240149. [CrossRef] [PubMed]
32. Segú-Vergés, C.; Coma, M.; Kessel, C.; Smeets, S.; Foell, D.; Aldea, A. Application of Systems Biology-Based in Silico Tools to Optimize Treatment Strategy Identification in Still's Disease. *Arthritis Res. Ther.* **2021**, *23*, 126. [CrossRef]
33. Liu, C.; Xu, D.; Xue, B.; Liu, B.; Li, J.; Huang, J. Upregulation of RUNX1 Suppresses Proliferation and Migration through Repressing VEGFA Expression in Hepatocellular Carcinoma. *Pathol. Oncol. Res.* **2020**, *26*, 1301–1311. [CrossRef]
34. Michaud, J.; Simpson, K.M.; Escher, R.; Buchet-Poyau, K.; Beissbarth, T.; Carmichael, C.; Ritchie, M.E.; Schütz, F.; Cannon, P.; Liu, M.; et al. Integrative Analysis of RUNX1 Downstream Pathways and Target Genes. *BMC Genom.* **2008**, *9*, 363. [CrossRef] [PubMed]
35. Thomas, A.L.; Marsman, J.; Antony, J.; Schierding, W.; O'Sullivan, J.M.; Horsfield, J.A. Transcriptional Regulation of RUNX1: An Informatics Analysis. *Genes* **2021**, *12*, 1175. [CrossRef] [PubMed]
36. Chen, Y.; Zhang, L.; Liu, L.; Sun, S.; Zhao, X.; Wang, Y.; Zhang, Y.; Du, J.; Gu, L. Rasip1 Is a RUNX1 Target Gene and Promotes Migration of NSCLC Cells. *CMAR* **2018**, *10*, 4537–4552. [CrossRef] [PubMed]
37. Riddell, A.; McBride, M.; Braun, T.; Nicklin, S.A.; Cameron, E.; Loughrey, C.M.; Martin, T.P. RUNX1: An Emerging Therapeutic Target for Cardiovascular Disease. *Cardiovasc. Res.* **2020**, *116*, 1410–1423. [CrossRef]
38. McCarroll, C.S.; He, W.; Foote, K.; Bradley, A.; Mcglynn, K.; Vidler, F.; Nixon, C.; Nather, K.; Fattah, C.; Riddell, A.; et al. Runx1 Deficiency Protects Against Adverse Cardiac Remodeling After Myocardial Infarction. *Circulation* **2018**, *137*, 57–70. [CrossRef]
39. Shilpi, S.; Shivvedi, R.; Gurnany, E.; Dixit, S.; Khatri, K.; Dwivedi, D.K. Drug Targeting Strategies for Liver Cancer and Other Liver Diseases. *MOJ Drug Des. Dev. Ther.* **2018**, *2*, 171–177. [CrossRef]
40. Byrne, C.D.; Olufadi, R.; Bruce, K.D.; Cagampang, F.R.; Ahmed, M.H. Metabolic Disturbances in Non-Alcoholic Fatty Liver Disease. *Clin. Sci.* **2009**, *116*, 539–564. [CrossRef]
41. Girija, S.M. The Blind Men see the Elephant-the Many Faces of Fatty Liver Disease. *World J. Gastroenterol.* **2008**, *14*, 831–844. [CrossRef]
42. Tacer, K.F.; Rozman, D. Nonalcoholic Fatty Liver Disease: Focus on Lipoprotein and Lipid Deregulation. *J. Lipids* **2011**, *2011*, 783976. [CrossRef]
43. Jornayvaz, F.R.; Shulman, G.I. Diacylglycerol Activation of Protein Kinase Cε and Hepatic Insulin Resistance. *Cell Metab.* **2012**, *15*, 574–584. [CrossRef]
44. Kumashiro, N.; Erion, D.M.; Zhang, D.; Kahn, M.; Beddow, S.A.; Chu, X.; Still, C.D.; Gerhard, G.S.; Han, X.; Dziura, J.; et al. Cellular Mechanism of Insulin Resistance in Nonalcoholic Fatty Liver Disease. *Proc. Natl. Acad. Sci. USA* **2011**, *108*, 16381–16385. [CrossRef] [PubMed]
45. Zhang, F.; Meng, G.; Strober, W. Interactions among the Transcription Factors Runx1, RORγt and Foxp3 Regulate the Differentiation of Interleukin 17–Producing T Cells. *Nat. Immunol.* **2008**, *9*, 1297–1306. [CrossRef] [PubMed]
46. Mukherji, A.; Dachraoui, M.; Baumert, T.F. Perturbation of the Circadian Clock and Pathogenesis of NAFLD. *Metabolism* **2020**, *111*, 154337. [CrossRef] [PubMed]
47. Luo, M.-C.; Zhou, S.-Y.; Feng, D.-Y.; Xiao, J.; Li, W.-Y.; Xu, C.-D.; Wang, H.-Y.; Zhou, T. Runt-Related Transcription Factor 1 (RUNX1) Binds to P50 in Macrophages and Enhances TLR4-Triggered Inflammation and Septic Shock. *J. Biol. Chem.* **2016**, *291*, 22011–22020. [CrossRef]
48. Tilg, H.; Moschen, A.R. Insulin Resistance, Inflammation, and Non-Alcoholic Fatty Liver Disease. *Trends Endocrinol. Metab.* **2008**, *19*, 371–379. [CrossRef]
49. Rada, P.; González-Rodríguez, Á.; García-Monzón, C.; Valverde, Á.M. Understanding Lipotoxicity in NAFLD Pathogenesis: Is CD36 a Key Driver? *Cell Death Dis.* **2020**, *11*, 802. [CrossRef]
50. Farrell, G.C.; Teoh, N.C.; Mccuskey, R.S. Hepatic Microcirculation in Fatty Liver Disease. *Anat. Rec.* **2008**, *291*, 684–692. [CrossRef]
51. Lemoinne, S.; Thabut, D.; Housset, C. Portal Myofibroblasts Connect Angiogenesis and Fibrosis in Liver. *Cell Tissue Res.* **2016**, *365*, 583–589. [CrossRef]
52. Coulon, S.; Legry, V.; Heindryckx, F.; Van Steenkiste, C.; Casteleyn, C.; Olievier, K.; Libbrecht, L.; Carmeliet, P.; Jonckx, B.; Stassen, J.-M.; et al. Role of Vascular Endothelial Growth Factor in the Pathophysiology of Nonalcoholic Steatohepatitis in Two Rodent Models. *Hepatology* **2013**, *57*, 1793–1805. [CrossRef]
53. North, T.E.; de Bruijn, M.F.T.R.; Stacy, T.; Talebian, L.; Lind, E.; Robin, C.; Binder, M.; Dzierzak, E.; Speck, N.A. Runx1 Expression Marks Long-Term Repopulating Hematopoietic Stem Cells in the Midgestation Mouse Embryo. *Immunity* **2002**, *16*, 661–672. [CrossRef]
54. Coulon, S.; Francque, S.; Colle, I.; Verrijken, A.; Blomme, B.; Heindryckx, F.; De Munter, S.; Prawitt, J.; Caron, S.; Staels, B.; et al. Evaluation of Inflammatory and Angiogenic Factors in Patients with Non-Alcoholic Fatty Liver Disease. *Cytokine* **2012**, *59*, 442–449. [CrossRef]
55. Rahman, S.M.; Janssen, R.C.; Choudhury, M.; Baquero, K.C.; Aikens, R.M.; de la Houssaye, B.A.; Friedman, J.E. CCAAT/Enhancer-Binding Protein β (C/EBPβ) Expression Regulates Dietary-Induced Inflammation in Macrophages and Adipose Tissue in Mice. *J. Biol. Chem.* **2012**, *287*, 34349–34360. [CrossRef]

56. Amacher, D.E. The Mechanistic Basis for the Induction of Hepatic Steatosis by Xenobiotics. *Expert Opin. Drug Metab. Toxicol.* **2011**, *7*, 949–965. [CrossRef]
57. Masarone, M.; Rosato, V.; Dallio, M.; Gravina, A.G.; Aglitti, A.; Loguercio, C.; Federico, A.; Persico, M. Role of Oxidative Stress in Pathophysiology of Nonalcoholic Fatty Liver Disease. *Oxidative Med. Cell. Longev.* **2018**, *2018*, 9547613. [CrossRef] [PubMed]
58. Chan, V.; Chan, T.K.; Liu, V.W.S.; Wong, A.C.K. Restriction Fragment Length Polymorphisms Associated with Factor VIII: C Gene in Chinese. *Hum. Genet.* **1988**, *79*, 128–131. [CrossRef] [PubMed]
59. Kantner, H.-P.; Warsch, W.; Delogu, A.; Bauer, E.; Esterbauer, H.; Casanova, E.; Sexl, V.; Stoiber, D. ETV6/RUNX1 Induces Reactive Oxygen Species and Drives the Accumulation of DNA Damage in B Cells. *Neoplasia* **2013**, *15*, 1292–1300. [CrossRef] [PubMed]
60. Whitmore, H.A.B.; Amarnani, D.; O'Hare, M.; Delgado-Tirado, S.; Gonzalez-Buendia, L.; An, M.; Pedron, J.; Bushweller, J.H.; Arboleda-Velasquez, J.F.; Kim, L.A. TNF-α Signaling Regulates RUNX1 Function in Endothelial Cells. *FASEB J.* **2020**, *35*, e21155. [CrossRef] [PubMed]
61. Kanda, T.; Matsuoka, S.; Yamazaki, M.; Shibata, T.; Nirei, K.; Takahashi, H.; Kaneko, T.; Fujisawa, M.; Higuchi, T.; Nakamura, H.; et al. Apoptosis and Non-Alcoholic Fatty Liver Diseases. *World J. Gastroenterol.* **2018**, *24*, 2661–2672. [CrossRef]
62. Petta, S.; Gastaldelli, A.; Rebelos, E.; Bugianesi, E.; Messa, P.; Miele, L.; Svegliati-Baroni, G.; Valenti, L.; Bonino, F. Pathophysiology of Non Alcoholic Fatty Liver Disease. *Int. J. Mol. Sci.* **2016**, *17*, 2082. [CrossRef] [PubMed]
63. O'Hare, M.; Amarnani, D.; Whitmore, H.A.B.; An, M.; Marino, C.; Ramos, L.; Delgado-Tirado, S.; Hu, X.; Chmielewska, N.; Chandrahas, A.; et al. Targeting Runt-Related Transcription Factor 1 Prevents Pulmonary Fibrosis and Reduces Expression of Severe Acute Respiratory Syndrome Coronavirus 2 Host Mediators. *Am. J. Pathol.* **2021**, *191*, 1193–1208. [CrossRef]
64. Bertrand-Philippe, M.; Ruddell, R.G.; Arthur, M.J.P.; Thomas, J.; Mungalsingh, N.; Mann, D.A. Regulation of Tissue Inhibitor of Metalloproteinase 1 Gene Transcription by RUNX1 and RUNX2. *J. Biol. Chem.* **2004**, *279*, 24530–24539. [CrossRef] [PubMed]
65. Liu, K.; Hu, H.; Jiang, H.; Zhang, H.; Gong, S.; Wei, D.; Yu, Z. RUNX1 Promotes MAPK Signaling to Increase Tumor Progression and Metastasis via OPN in Head and Neck Cancer. *Carcinogenesis* **2021**, *42*, 414–422. [CrossRef] [PubMed]
66. Bellissimo, D.C.; Chen, C.; Zhu, Q.; Bagga, S.; Lee, C.-T.; He, B.; Wertheim, G.B.; Jordan, M.; Tan, K.; Worthen, G.S.; et al. Runx1 Negatively Regulates Inflammatory Cytokine Production by Neutrophils in Response to Toll-like Receptor Signaling. *Blood Adv.* **2020**, *4*, 1145–1158. [CrossRef] [PubMed]
67. Manco, M. Insulin Resistance and NAFLD: A Dangerous Liaison beyond the Genetics. *Children* **2017**, *4*, 74. [CrossRef]
68. Guo, H.; Friedman, A.D. Phosphorylation of RUNX1 by Cyclin-Dependent Kinase Reduces Direct Interaction with HDAC1 and HDAC3. *J. Biol. Chem.* **2011**, *286*, 208–215. [CrossRef] [PubMed]
69. Cho, W.; Hong, S.H.; Choe, J. IL-4 and HDAC Inhibitors Suppress Cyclooxygenase-2 Expression in Human Follicular Dendritic Cells. *Immune Netw.* **2013**, *13*, 75. [CrossRef] [PubMed]
70. Hsieh, P.-S.; Jin, J.-S.; Chiang, C.-F.; Chan, P.-C.; Chen, C.-H.; Shih, K.-C. COX-2-Mediated Inflammation in Fat Is Crucial for Obesity-Linked Insulin Resistance and Fatty Liver. *Obesity* **2009**, *17*, 1150–1157. [CrossRef]
71. Chan, P.-C.; Liao, M.-T.; Hsieh, P.-S. The Dualistic Effect of COX-2-Mediated Signaling in Obesity and Insulin Resistance. *Int. J. Mol. Sci.* **2019**, *20*, 3115. [CrossRef]
72. Qiao, Y.; He, H.; Jonsson, P.; Sinha, I.; Zhao, C.; Dahlman-Wright, K. AP-1 Is a Key Regulator of Proinflammatory Cytokine TNFα-Mediated Triple-Negative Breast Cancer Progression. *J. Biol. Chem.* **2016**, *291*, 5068–5079. [CrossRef]
73. Monaco, C.; Andreakos, E.; Kiriakidis, S.; Mauri, C.; Bicknell, C.; Foxwell, B.; Cheshire, N.; Paleolog, E.; Feldmann, M. Canonical Pathway of Nuclear Factor KB Activation Selectively Regulates Proinflammatory and Prothrombotic Responses in Human Atherosclerosis. *Proc. Natl. Acad. Sci. USA* **2004**, *101*, 5634–5639. [CrossRef]
74. Scheidereit, C. IκB Kinase Complexes: Gateways to NF-KB Activation and Transcription. *Oncogene* **2006**, *25*, 6685–6705. [CrossRef] [PubMed]
75. Dhingra, S.; Sharma, A.K.; Arora, R.C.; Slezak, J.; Singal, P.K. IL-10 Attenuates TNF-α-Induced NFκB Pathway Activation and Cardiomyocyte Apoptosis. *Cardiovasc. Res.* **2009**, *82*, 59–66. [CrossRef] [PubMed]
76. Tien, Y.-C.; Lin, J.-Y.; Lai, C.-H.; Kuo, C.-H.; Lin, W.-Y.; Tsai, C.-H.; Tsai, F.-J.; Cheng, Y.-C.; Peng, W.-H.; Huang, C.-Y. *Carthamus Tinctorius* L. Prevents LPS-Induced TNFα Signaling Activation and Cell Apoptosis through JNK1/2–NFκB Pathway Inhibition in H9c2 Cardiomyoblast Cells. *J. Ethnopharmacol.* **2010**, *130*, 505–513. [CrossRef] [PubMed]
77. Cronin, J.G.; Turner, M.L.; Goetze, L.; Bryant, C.E.; Sheldon, I.M. Toll-Like Receptor 4 and MYD88-Dependent Signaling Mechanisms of the Innate Immune System Are Essential for the Response to Lipopolysaccharide by Epithelial and Stromal Cells of the Bovine Endometrium. *Biol. Reprod.* **2012**, *86*, 1–9. [CrossRef] [PubMed]
78. Candido, S.; Maestro, R.; Polesel, J.; Catania, A.; Maira, F.; Signorelli, S.S.; McCubrey, J.A.; Libra, M. Roles of Neutrophil Gelatinase-Associated Lipocalin (NGAL) in Human Cancer. *Oncotarget* **2014**, *5*, 1576–1594. [CrossRef]
79. Schaefer, F.M.; Peng, J.; Hu, W.; Drvarov, O.; Nevzorova, Y.A.; Zhao, G.; Masaoudi, M.A.; Davis, R.J.; Trautwein, C.; Cubero, F.J. Bone Marrow-Derived c-Jun N-Terminal Kinase-1 (JNK1) Mediates Liver Regeneration. *Biochim. Biophys. Acta (BBA)-Mol. Basis Dis.* **2015**, *1852*, 137–145. [CrossRef]
80. Faggioli, L.; Costanzo, C.; Donadelli, M.; Palmieri, M. Activation of the Interleukin-6 Promoter by a Dominant Negative Mutant of c-Jun. *Biochim. Biophys. Acta (BBA)-Mol. Cell Res.* **2004**, *1692*, 17–24. [CrossRef]
81. Torisu, T.; Sato, N.; Yoshiga, D.; Kobayashi, T.; Yoshioka, T.; Mori, H.; Iida, M.; Yoshimura, A. The Dual Function of Hepatic SOCS3 in Insulin Resistance in Vivo. *Genes Cells* **2007**, *12*, 143–154. [CrossRef]

82. Kim, K.; Kim, K.H.; Cheong, J. Hepatitis B Virus X Protein Impairs Hepatic Insulin Signaling Through Degradation of IRS1 and Induction of SOCS3. *PLoS ONE* **2010**, *5*, e8649. [CrossRef]
83. Rui, L.; Yuan, M.; Frantz, D.; Shoelson, S.; White, M.F. SOCS-1 and SOCS-3 Block Insulin Signaling by Ubiquitin-Mediated Degradation of IRS1 and IRS2. *J. Biol. Chem.* **2002**, *277*, 42394–42398. [CrossRef]
84. Laplante, M.; Sabatini, D.M. MTOR Signaling at a Glance. *J. Cell Sci.* **2009**, *122*, 3589–3594. [CrossRef]
85. Tai, H.; Wang, X.; Zhou, J.; Han, X.; Fang, T.; Gong, H.; Huang, N.; Chen, H.; Qin, J.; Yang, M.; et al. Protein Kinase Cβ Activates Fat Mass and Obesity-associated Protein by Influencing Its Ubiquitin/Proteasome Degradation. *FASEB J.* **2017**, *31*, 4396–4406. [CrossRef] [PubMed]
86. Aguirre, V.; Uchida, T.; Yenush, L.; Davis, R.; White, M.F. The C-Jun NH2-Terminal Kinase Promotes Insulin Resistance during Association with Insulin Receptor Substrate-1 and Phosphorylation of Ser307. *J. Biol. Chem.* **2000**, *275*, 9047–9054. [CrossRef] [PubMed]
87. Park, K.; Li, Q.; Rask-Madsen, C.; Mima, A.; Mizutani, K.; Winnay, J.; Maeda, Y.; D'Aquino, K.; White, M.F.; Feener, E.P.; et al. Serine Phosphorylation Sites on IRS2 Activated by Angiotensin II and Protein Kinase C To Induce Selective Insulin Resistance in Endothelial Cells. *Mol. Cell Biol.* **2013**, *33*, 3227–3241. [CrossRef] [PubMed]
88. López-Bergami, P.; Habelhah, H.; Bhoumik, A.; Zhang, W.; Wang, L.-H.; Ronai, Z. Receptor for RACK1 Mediates Activation of JNK by Protein Kinase C. *Mol. Cell* **2005**, *19*, 309–320. [CrossRef] [PubMed]
89. Comalada, M.; Xaus, J.; Valledor, A.F.; López-López, C.; Pennington, D.J.; Celada, A. PKCϵ Is Involved in JNK Activation That Mediates LPS-Induced TNF-α, Which Induces Apoptosis in Macrophages. *Am. J. Physiol.-Cell Physiol.* **2003**, *285*, C1235–C1245. [CrossRef]
90. Kolter, T.; Uphues, I.; Eckel, J. Molecular Analysis of Insulin Resistance in Isolated Ventricular Cardiomyocytes of Obese Zucker Rats. *Am. J. Physiol.-Endocrinol. Metab.* **1997**, *273*, E59–E67. [CrossRef]
91. Naruse, K.; Rask-Madsen, C.; Takahara, N.; Ha, S.; Suzuma, K.; Way, K.J.; Jacobs, J.R.C.; Clermont, A.C.; Ueki, K.; Ohshiro, Y.; et al. Activation of Vascular Protein Kinase C-β Inhibits Akt-Dependent Endothelial Nitric Oxide Synthase Function in Obesity-Associated Insulin Resistance. *Diabetes* **2006**, *55*, 691–698. [CrossRef]
92. Sampson, S.; Cooper, D. Specific Protein Kinase C Isoforms as Transducers and Modulators of Insulin Signaling. *Mol. Genet. Metab.* **2006**, *89*, 32–47. [CrossRef]
93. Matsuda, S.; Kobayashi, M.; Kitagishi, Y. Roles for PI3K/AKT/PTEN Pathway in Cell Signaling of Nonalcoholic Fatty Liver Disease. *Int. Sch. Res. Not.* **2013**, *2013*, 472432. [CrossRef]
94. Huang, X.; Liu, G.; Guo, J.; Su, Z. The PI3K/AKT Pathway in Obesity and Type 2 Diabetes. *Int. J. Biol. Sci.* **2018**, *14*, 1483–1496. [CrossRef] [PubMed]
95. Peyrou, M.; Bourgoin, L.; Foti, M. PTEN in Non-Alcoholic Fatty Liver Disease/Non-Alcoholic Steatohepatitis and Cancer. *Dig. Dis* **2010**, *28*, 236–246. [CrossRef] [PubMed]
96. Ding, R.-B.; Bao, J.; Deng, C.-X. Emerging Roles of SIRT1 in Fatty Liver Diseases. *Int. J. Biol. Sci.* **2017**, *13*, 852–867. [CrossRef] [PubMed]
97. Wasilewska, N.; Lebensztejn, D. Non-Alcoholic Fatty Liver Disease and Lipotoxicity. *Clin. Exp. Hepatol.* **2021**, *7*, 1–6. [CrossRef] [PubMed]
98. Haslinger, B.; Mandl-Weber, S.; Sellmayer, A.; Sitter, T. Hyaluronan Fragments Induce the Synthesis of MCP-1 and IL-8 in Cultured Human Peritoneal Mesothelial Cells. *Cell Tissue Res.* **2001**, *305*, 79–86. [CrossRef]
99. Curran, J.E.; Weinstein, S.R.; Griffiths, L.R. Polymorphic Variants of NFKB1 and Its Inhibitory Protein NFKBIA, and Their Involvement in Sporadic Breast Cancer. *Cancer Lett.* **2002**, *188*, 103–107. [CrossRef]
100. Petta, S.; Muratore, C.; Craxì, A. Non-Alcoholic Fatty Liver Disease Pathogenesis: The Present and the Future. *Dig. Liver Dis.* **2009**, *41*, 615–625. [CrossRef]
101. Feldstein, A.E.; Werneburg, N.W.; Canbay, A.; Guicciardi, M.E.; Bronk, S.F.; Rydzewski, R.; Burgart, L.J.; Gores, G.J. Free Fatty Acids Promote Hepatic Lipotoxicity by Stimulating TNF-α Expression via a Lysosomal Pathway. *Hepatology* **2004**, *40*, 185–194. [CrossRef]
102. Ferraris, S.E.; Isoniemi, K.; Torvaldson, E.; Anckar, J.; Westermarck, J.; Eriksson, J.E. Nucleolar AATF Regulates C-Jun–Mediated Apoptosis. *Mol. Biol. Cell* **2012**, *23*, 4323–4332. [CrossRef]
103. Kagoya, Y.; Yoshimi, A.; Kataoka, K.; Nakagawa, M.; Kumano, K.; Arai, S.; Kobayashi, H.; Saito, T.; Iwakura, Y.; Kurokawa, M. Positive Feedback between NF-KB and TNF-α Promotes Leukemia-Initiating Cell Capacity. *J. Clin. Investig.* **2014**, *124*, 528–542. [CrossRef]
104. Lee, I.-T.; Liu, S.-W.; Chi, P.-L.; Lin, C.-C.; Hsiao, L.-D.; Yang, C.-M. TNF-α Mediates PKCδ/JNK1/2/c-Jun-Dependent Monocyte Adhesion via ICAM-1 Induction in Human Retinal Pigment Epithelial Cells. *PLoS ONE* **2015**, *10*, e0117911. [CrossRef]
105. Liu, C.-J.; Lo, J.-F.; Kuo, C.-H.; Chu, C.-H.; Chen, L.-M.; Tsai, F.-J.; Tsai, C.-H.; Tzang, B.-S.; Kuo, W.-W.; Huang, C.-Y. Akt Mediates 17β-Estradiol and/or Estrogen Receptor-α Inhibition of LPS-Induced Tumor Necresis Factor-α Expression and Myocardial Cell Apoptosis by Suppressing the JNK1/2-NFκB Pathway. *J. Cell. Mol. Med.* **2009**, *13*, 3655–3667. [CrossRef] [PubMed]
106. Tiniakos, D.G.; Vos, M.B.; Brunt, E.M. Nonalcoholic Fatty Liver Disease: Pathology and Pathogenesis. *Annu. Rev. Pathol. Mech. Dis.* **2010**, *5*, 145–171. [CrossRef] [PubMed]
107. Luedde, T.; Schwabe, R.F. NF-KB in the Liver—Linking Injury, Fibrosis and Hepatocellular Carcinoma. *Nat. Rev. Gastroenterol. Hepatol* **2011**, *8*, 108–118. [CrossRef]

108. Ferro, D.; Baratta, F.; Pastori, D.; Cocomello, N.; Colantoni, A.; Angelico, F.; Del Ben, M. New Insights into the Pathogenesis of Non-Alcoholic Fatty Liver Disease: Gut-Derived Lipopolysaccharides and Oxidative Stress. *Nutrients* **2020**, *12*, 2762. [CrossRef] [PubMed]
109. Chen, Z.; Tian, R.; She, Z.; Cai, J.; Li, H. Role of Oxidative Stress in the Pathogenesis of Nonalcoholic Fatty Liver Disease. *Free Radic. Biol. Med.* **2020**, *152*, 116–141. [CrossRef] [PubMed]
110. Xu, H.; Goettsch, C.; Xia, N.; Horke, S.; Morawietz, H.; Förstermann, U.; Li, H. Differential Roles of PKCα and PKCε in Controlling the Gene Expression of Nox4 in Human Endothelial Cells. *Free. Radic. Biol. Med.* **2008**, *44*, 1656–1667. [CrossRef] [PubMed]
111. Sattayakhom, A.; Chunglok, W.; Ittarat, W.; Chamulitrat, W. Study Designs to Investigate Nox1 Acceleration of Neoplastic Progression in Immortalized Human Epithelial Cells by Selection of Differentiation Resistant Cells. *Redox Biol.* **2014**, *2*, 140–147. [CrossRef]
112. Manea, A.; Tanase, L.I.; Raicu, M.; Simionescu, M. Transcriptional Regulation of NADPH Oxidase Isoforms, Nox1 and Nox4, by Nuclear Factor-KB in Human Aortic Smooth Muscle Cells. *Biochem. Biophys. Res. Commun.* **2010**, *396*, 901–907. [CrossRef]
113. Milacic, M.; Haw, R.; Rothfels, K.; Wu, G.; Croft, D.; Hermjakob, H.; D'Eustachio, P.; Stein, L. Annotating Cancer Variants and Anti-Cancer Therapeutics in Reactome. *Cancers* **2012**, *4*, 1180–1211. [CrossRef]
114. Valls, R.; (Anaxomics Biotech, Barcelona, Spain); Pujol, A.; (Anaxomics Biotech; Institute for Research in Biomedicine and Barcelona Supercomputing Center, Barcelona, Spain); Farrés, J.; (Anaxomics Biotech, Barcelona, Spain); Artigas, L.; (Anaxomics Biotech, Barcelona, Spain); Mas, J.M.; (Anaxomics Biotech, Barcelona, Spain). Anaxomics' Methodologies–Understanding the Complexity of Biological Processes. Personal communication (Protocol), 2013.
115. Croft, D.; Mundo, A.F.; Haw, R.; Milacic, M.; Weiser, J.; Wu, G.; Caudy, M.; Garapati, P.; Gillespie, M.; Kamdar, M.R.; et al. The Reactome Pathway Knowledgebase. *Nucl. Acids Res.* **2014**, *42*, D472–D477. [CrossRef] [PubMed]
116. Stark, C.; Breitkreutz, B.-J.; Reguly, T.; Boucher, L.; Breitkreutz, A.; Tyers, M. BioGRID: A General Repository for Interaction Datasets. *Nucleic Acids Res.* **2006**, *34*, D535–D539. [CrossRef] [PubMed]

biomedicines

MDPI

Article

Comorbidities and Outcomes among Females with Non-Alcoholic Fatty Liver Disease Compared to Males

Naim Abu-Freha [1,2,*,†], Bracha Cohen [3,†], Sarah Weissmann [2,3], Reut Hizkiya [2,4], Reem Abu-Hammad [2], Gadeer Taha [5] and Michal Gordon [3]

1 The Institute of Gastroenterology and Hepatology, Soroka University Medical Center, Beer-Sheva 84101, Israel
2 The Faculty of Health Sciences, Ben-Gurion University of the Negev, Beer-Sheva 84101, Israel
3 Soroka Clinical Research Center, Soroka University Medical Center, Beer-Sheva 84101, Israel
4 Internal Medicine Division, Soroka University Medical Center, Beer-Sheva 84101, Israel
5 Department of Gastroenterology, Rambam Health Care Campus, Haifa 31096, Israel
* Correspondence: abufreha@yahoo.de or naimaf@clalit.org.il; Tel.: +972-8-640-2251; Fax: +972-8-623-3083
† These authors contributed equally to this work.

Abstract: Sex-based medicine is an important emerging discipline within medicine. We investigated the clinical characteristics, complications, and outcomes of Nonalcoholic Fatty Liver Disease (NAFLD) in females compared to males. Demographics, comorbidities, malignancy, complications, outcomes, and all-cause mortality of NAFLD patients older than 18 years were analyzed. The data were extracted using the MDClone platform from "Clalit" in Israel. A total of 111,993 (52.8%) of the study subjects were females with an average age of 44.4 ± 14.7 years compared to 39.62 ± 14.9 years in males, $p < 0.001$. Significantly higher rates of hypertension, diabetes mellitus, obesity, dementia, and thyroid cancer and lower rates of ischemic heart disease (22.3% vs. 27.3%, $p < 0.001$) were found among females. Females had a higher rate of cirrhosis, 2.3% vs. 1.9%, $p < 0.001$, and a lower rate of hepatocellular carcinoma, 0.4% vs. 0.5%, $p < 0.001$. In the multivariate analysis, a relationship between age, diabetes mellitus, and cirrhosis development were found among males and females. A lower age-adjusted mortality rate was found among females, 94.5/1000 vs. 116/1000 among males. In conclusion, older age at diagnosis, higher rates of hypertension, diabetes mellitus, obesity, cirrhosis, and a lower age-adjusted all-cause mortality rate were found among females with NAFLD.

Keywords: fatty liver; cirrhosis; females; gender; liver

Citation: Abu-Freha, N.; Cohen, B.; Weissmann, S.; Hizkiya, R.; Abu-Hammad, R.; Taha, G.; Gordon, M. Comorbidities and Outcomes among Females with Non-Alcoholic Fatty Liver Disease Compared to Males. *Biomedicines* **2022**, *10*, 2908. https://doi.org/10.3390/biomedicines10112908

Academic Editor: Jinghua Wang

Received: 7 October 2022
Accepted: 9 November 2022
Published: 12 November 2022

1. Introduction

Non-Alcoholic Fatty Liver Disease (NAFLD) is the most common liver disease, affecting around 25–30% of the population in some countries, with the highest prevalence in the Middle East and South America and the lowest in Africa [1–3]. The prevalence is increased among older people as well as those diagnosed with diabetes or obesity, possibly even reaching 60% of these populations [1]. As a common chronic liver disease, NAFLD frequently causes cirrhosis [4]. Moreover, a large part of chronic liver disease complications such as hepatocellular carcinoma (HCC), liver transplantation, and mortality result from NAFLD [5].

Sex-based medicine is a relatively new and important field of research that has emerged in the last decade. The impact of sex on illnesses can manifest as differences in prevalence, disease course, and outcomes. In the gastroenterology and hepatology field, significant sex-based differences have been found in colorectal cancer development and incidence, anatomical site, survival, indications and upper endoscopy findings [6–8]. Sex-related differences in epidemiology, disease progression, and treatment strategies of liver diseases have also been reported [9]. Drug toxicity and drug-dose gender gaps have been widely reported between males and females. Women have higher rates of autoimmune hepatitis (70–90% of cases are women), primary biliary cholangitis, and hepatocellular carcinoma. Women, however, have lower rates of primary sclerosing cholangitis, with a male:female ratio of 7:3 [9]. Sex differences have also been found regarding alcohol consumption and alcohol-associated liver disease: the prevalence of severe alcohol use disorder was reported in 18.3% of men and 9.7% of women in the USA, with women developing more severe alcohol-associated liver disease at lower levels of exposure compared to their male counterparts [10].

Hepatocellular carcinoma (HCC) is one of the feared complications of chronic liver diseases, and significant sex-related differences have been previously reported. HCC is a liver neoplasm with a multifaceted nature of causes, risk factors and genetic alterations [11,12]. Females present with HCC at an older age and with a higher number of HCC and hypertension cases in their family histories than males [13,14]. In addition, females with HCC were more likely to undergo HCC surveillance, have smaller tumor sizes at diagnosis, and have less vascular involvement [13,14].

Only scant data were published regarding sex-related disparities of NAFLD patients, and it is a relatively under-researched field [15]. On average, females make up a higher percentage of NAFLD cases than males [15]. Sex-related differences have been found in adolescents, with a higher prevalence of NAFLD (16.3% vs. 10.1%) and central obesity (33.2% vs. 9.9%) reported among females [16]. In general, the prevalence of NAFLD is higher among men and postmenopausal women than among women of reproductive age, possibly suggesting a hormonal protective role [17].

This study aimed to investigate and determine the disparities in comorbidities (particularly metabolic syndrome), laboratory data, liver-related outcomes, and mortality of female patients with NAFLD compared to males with NAFLD. Understanding these disparities is crucial for the diagnosis, follow-up, treatment, and surveillance of patients with NAFLD.

2. Materials and Methods

2.1. The Materials Study Design and Patients

This was a retrospective study that included patients aged 18 years or older diagnosed with NAFLD between the years 2000 and 2021. NAFLD patients were identified by having an ICD 10 code of K76.0 at any time in their chronic disease list (according to community data or hospital data). A total of 9353 patients with liver-related comorbidities including alcoholic liver disease, hepatitis B, and hepatitis C were excluded from our population. The sample of NAFLD patients was then subdivided according to sex.

2.2. Data Collection

The data was extracted from Clalit Health Services (CHS) using Clalit's data-sharing platform powered by MDClone (https://www.mdclone.com (accessed on 7 October 2022)). CHS is the largest health maintenance organization in Israel, with about 4.7 million insured residents.

Demographics, laboratory data, complications, outcomes, and mortality data were retrospectively collected from NAFLD patients. Laboratory data included complete blood count, alanine transaminase (ALT), aspartate transaminase (AST), bilirubin, albumin, and international normalized ratio (INR), taken from blood samples at or nearest to the time of diagnosis. In addition, the Fib-4 and APRI scores were calculated at the time of diagnosis. Comorbidities including metabolic syndrome, cancer, and other common diseases were collected from computerized files according to the specific ICD-10 codes. Outcomes including cirrhosis, hepatocellular carcinoma, liver transplantation, and all-cause mortality were collected according to the ICD-10 codes as well. All collected data were compared between males and females.

2.3. Statistical Analysis

Data are presented as mean ± standard deviation (SD) for continuous variables and as a percentage (%) of the total for categorical variables. Univariate analyses were performed using independent T-tests for continuous variables and chi-square tests for categorical variables. We used logistic regression models to examine the multivariate relationships between risk factors and the odds of death. Before introducing the variables into the model, multicollinearity of the variables was examined using the Variance Inflation Factor (VIF) statistic. The variables found to be significant in the univariate analysis were introduced into the multivariate model one after the other, and included age at diagnosis, gender, diabetes mellitus, cirrhosis, hepatocellular carcinoma, and esophageal varices. We calculated the all-cause mortality death rate among the groups, subdivided by age. The all-cause mortality death rate was age-adjusted using a general population control group from Clalit (452,012 people). All statistical analyses were performed using IBM SPSS version 26 (Chicago, IL, USA). *p*-values less than 0.05 were considered statistically significant. The study was carried out in accordance with the principles of the Helsinki Declaration. The study protocol was approved by the Institutional Helsinki Committee, approval number 198-21-SOR.

3. Results

3.1. Patients

The baseline characteristics, comorbidities, and malignancy rates among NAFLD patients are presented in Table 1. A higher percentage of our cohort was female (n = 111,993, 52.8%). Females were diagnosed at an older age, 44.4 ± 14.7 years, compared to males, 39.62 ± 14.9 years, $p < 0.001$. Higher rates of hypertension, diabetes mellitus, obesity, and dementia were observed among female NAFLD patients, 60.7% vs. 53.5%, 24.7% vs. 21.6%, 64.2% vs. 52.7%, 5.2% vs. 2.9%, respectively, $p < 0.001$. However, lower rates of ischemic heart disease and chronic renal failure were found among females, 22.3% vs. 27.3%, 11.2% vs. 14.8%, respectively, $p < 0.001$. A higher rate of thyroid carcinoma and a lower rate of kidney carcinoma were observed among females, 1% vs. 0.4%, $p < 0.001$, and 0.6% vs. 1% $p < 0.001$. No significant difference regarding other malignancies was found between the two populations. We found that NAFLD was diagnosed before most other metabolic syndrome-related diseases. A total of 99.5% of patients were diagnosed with diabetes mellitus after being diagnosed with NAFLD (0.5% of males and 0.5% of females were diagnosed with diabetes before NAFLD ($p = 0.966$). Only 8% of males and 8.5% of females were diagnosed with obesity before NAFLD, compared to 92% of males and 91.5% of females who were diagnosed after being diagnosed with NAFLD, $p = 0.001$. Hypertension, dyslipidemia, CIHD, and CVA were also diagnosed more commonly among males after NAFLD diagnosis compared to females.

Table 1. Baseline characteristics, comorbidities, and malignancy among the study groups.

	Males with NAFLD 99,962 (%)	**Females with NAFLD 111,993 (%)**	
Age at diagnosis, mean, years ± SD	39.62 ± 14.9	44.4 ± 14.7	<0.001
Age	59.5 ± 15.9	64.95 ± 15.3	<0.001
Age group			<0.001
<50 years	74,233 (74.3)	71,167 (63.5)	
≥50 years	25,729 (25.7)	40,826 (34.7)	
Ethnicity, Arabs	15,154 (15.5)	18,936 (17.3)	<0.001
BMI	29 ± 5.2	30.4 ± 6.6	<0.001
CIHD	27,293 (27.3)	25,007 (22.3)	<0.001
COPD	10,181 (10.2)	11,275 (10.1)	0.372
Asthma	11,302 (11.3)	18,919 (16.9)	<0.001
CRF	14,822 (14.8)	12,511 (11.2)	<0.001
Hypertension	53,255 (53.3)	67,947 (60.7)	<0.001
Diabetes Mellitus	21,562 (21.6)	27,701 (24.7)	<0.001

Table 1. *Cont.*

	Males with NAFLD 99,962 (%)	Females with NAFLD 111,993 (%)	
Dyslipidemia	68,309 (68.3)	79,045 (70.6)	<0.001
Obesity	52,704 (52.7)	71,873 (64.2)	<0.001
CVA	3181 (3.2)	3542 (3.2)	0.798
Dementia	2874 (2.9)	5828 (5.2)	<0.001
Vitamin B12 deficiency anemia	1178 (1.2)	1534 (1.4)	<0.001
Folic acid deficiency	24,208 (24.2)	30,760 (27.5)	<0.001
Iron deficiency anemia	18,267 (18.3)	38,916 (34.7)	<0.001
Cancers			
Lung cancer	1047 (1)	954 (0.9)	<0.001
Prostate	3469 (1.6)	—	
CRC	1740 (1.7)	1993 (1.8)	0.497
Stomach	350 (0.4)	313 (0.3)	0.004
Breast	68 (0.1)	5481 (4.9)	<0.001
Pancreas	257 (0.3)	294 (0.3)	0.807
Uterus	—	900 (0.8)	<0.001
Kidney	951 (1)	647 (0.6)	<0.001
Non-Hodgkin lymphoma	736 (0.7)	812 (0.7)	0.762
Hodgkin lymphoma	248 (0.2)	246 (0.2)	0.175
Melanoma	1713 (1.7)	1744 (1.6)	0.005
Basal cell carcinoma	11,546 (11.6)	13,103 (11.7)	0.284
Thyroid carcinoma	368 (0.4)	1175 (1)	<0.001

BMI = Body Mass Index, CIHD = Chronic Ischemic, CVA = Cerebrovascular Accident, COPD = Chronic Obstructive Pulmonary Disease, CRF = Chronic Renal Failure, CRC = Colorectal cancer.

3.2. Laboratory Results among the Study Groups

The laboratory results are summarized in Table 2. Significant differences between females and males were found regarding several lab values: AST (30.7 ± 36 vs. 33.8 ± 39, $p < 0.001$), ALT (34.2 ± 38.6 vs. 47.14 ± 52.9, $p < 0.001$) GGT (51.89 ± 84 vs. 61.45 ± 100, $p < 0.001$) and albumin (4.22 ± 1.4 vs. 4.42 ± 1.76, $p < 0.001$). In addition, lower values of APRI (0.36 ± 0.66 vs. 0.44 ± 0.83, $p < 0.001$) but higher FIB-4 levels were found among females (1 ± 1 vs. 0.96 ± 1.1, $p < 0.001$). All statistical analyses were performed using IBM SPSS version 26 (Chicago, USA). *p*-values less than 0.05 were considered statistically significant.

Table 2. Laboratory values of females and males included in the study.

Variable	Males 99,962 (47.2)	Females 111,993 (52.8)	*p*-Value
Hemoglobin	14.7 ± 1.38	13.0 ± 1.24	<0.001
WBC	7.8 ± 2.9	7.4 ± 3.1	<0.001
PLT	238 ± 66	266 ± 74	<0.001
AST	33.8 ± 39	30.7 ± 36	<0.001
ALT	47.1 ± 52.9	34.2 ± 38.6	<0.001
GGT	61.45 ± 100	51.89 ± 84	<0.001
Bilirubin	0.5 ± 0.56	0.4 ± 0.4	<0.001

Table 2. *Cont.*

Variable	Males 99,962 (47.2)	Females 111,993 (52.8)	*p*-Value
Creatinine	0.95 ± 0.37	0.73 ± 0.29	<0.001
Albumin	4.42 ± 1.76	4.22 ± 1.4	<0.001
Vitamin D	50 ± 23.55	47 ± 25.5	<0.001
Vitamin B12	318 ± 158	352 ± 185	<0.001
Folic Acid	17.6 ± 36.3	19.5 ± 45	<0.001
CRP	3.97 ± 18.6	3.40 ± 16.18	<0.001
Iron	86.6 ± 34	71.5 ± 30	<0.001
Ferritin	177.1 ± 305	89.8 ± 170	<0.001
Calcium	9.47 ± 0.46	9.44 ± 0.48	<0.001
Sodium	140.12 ± 3.2	140.07 ± 3.4	<0.001
INR	1.05 ± 0.34	1.02 ± 0.33	<0.001
APRI	0.44 ± 0.83	0.36 ± 0.66	<0.001
FIB-4	0.96 ± 1.1	1 ± 1.0	<0.001

All values presented as mean ± SD. WBC = White Blood Cells, PLT = Platelets, ALT = Alanine Aminotransferase, AST = Aspartate Aminotransferase, GGT = Gamma-Glutamyl Transferase, INR = International Normalized Ratio, APRI = AST to Platelet Ratio Index.

3.3. Liver-Related Outcomes and All Cause-Mortality

The liver-related outcomes and all-cause mortality rates are summarized in Table 3. More females were diagnosed with cirrhosis (2.3% vs. 1.9%, $p < 0.001$), but at an older age compared to males (65.9 ± 12.3 years vs. 63.4 ± 13.7 years, $p < 0.001$, respectively). Lower rates of HCC and liver transplantation were found among females (0.4% vs. 0.5%, $p < 0.001$, 0.07% vs. 0.11%, $p < 0.003$, respectively). No statistical difference was found regarding esophageal varices, esophageal variceal bleeding, spontaneous bacterial peritonitis, and hepatorenal syndrome between males and females. There was a significantly higher rate of all-cause mortality among females compared to males (11.4% vs. 10.2%, $p < 0.001$). The age-adjusted mortality rate was calculated in our cohort using a reference control group of non-NAFLD patients. The all-cause age-adjusted mortality rate was lower among females compared to males (94.5 patients per 1000 female NAFLD patients compared to 116 patients per 1000 male NAFLD patients). The cirrhosis and all-cause mortality rates according to age group are presented in Tables 4 and 5. A lower rate of liver transplantation was performed in females compared to males (0.07% vs. 0.11%, $p = 0.003$).

Table 3. Liver-related outcomes and all-cause mortality rates among females and males with NAFLD.

	Males with NAFLD 99,962 (%)	Females with NAFLD 111,993 (%)	
Cirrhosis	1901 (1.9)	2528 (2.3)	<0.001
Age at cirrhosis	63.4 ± 13.7	65.9 ± 12.3	<0.001
HCC	492 (0.5)	451 (0.4)	0.002
Age of HCC	68.39 ± 11	69.33 ± 12	0.227
Esophageal varices	603 (0.6)	675 (0.6)	0.988
Esophageal variceal bleeding	326 (0.3)	321 (0.3)	0.1
SBP	146 (0.1)	157 (0.1)	0.721
Hepatorenal syndrome	136 (0.1)	148 (0.1)	0.806
Liver transplantation	112 (0.11)	81 (0.07)	0.003
Age at liver transplantation	54.96 ± 11.6	55.14 ± 12.4	0.920

Table 3. *Cont.*

	Males with NAFLD 99,962 (%)	Females with NAFLD 111,993 (%)	
Death	10,219 (10.2)	12,744 (11.4)	<0.001
Age at death	74.4 ± 12.8	77.5 ± 11.7	<0.001
Number of hospitalizations From diagnosis, mean ± SD	3.99 ± 6.6	4.65 ± 6.5	<0.001
Length of hospitalization mean ± SD	3.67 ± 11	3.6 ± 9.4	0.154

Table 4. Cirrhosis rate according to age group among females and males with NAFLD.

Cirrhosis	Females, n = 111,993			Males, n = 99,962		
Age Group Years	Patient Number (%)	Cirrhosis Number	Cirrhosis Rate per 1000	Patient Number	Cirrhosis Number	Cirrhosis Rate per 1000
18–24	647 (0.6)	1	1.5	716 (0.7)	3	4.2
25–34	4371 (3.9)	13	3	5837 (5.8)	15	2.6
35–44	9271 (8.3)	37	4	15,690 (15.7)	60	3.8
45–54	13,739 (12.3)	112	8.2	18,729 (18.7)	126	6.7
55–64	22,945 (20.5)	336	14.6	18,758 (18.8)	317	16.9
65–74	30,479 (27.2)	755	24.8	21,580 (21.6)	552	25.6
75+	30,541 (27.3)	1274	41.7	18,652 (18.7)	828	44.4
Total	111,993	2528	22.6	99,962	1901	19

Table 5. Age-adjusted mortality rates among females and males with NAFLD.

Mortality	Females, n = 111,993			Males, n = 99,962		
Age Group Years	Patient Number (%)	Death Number	Death Rate per 1000	Patient Number (%)	Death Number	Death Rate per 1000
18–24	647 (0.6)	3	4.6	716 (0.7)	2	2.8
25–34	4371 (3.9)	22	5	5837 (5.8)	23	3.9
35–44	9271 (8.3)	48	5.2	15,690 (15.7)	110	7
45–54	13,739 (12.3)	170	12.4	18,729 (18.7)	255	13.6
55–64	22,945 (20.5)	626	27.3	18,758 (18.8)	830	44.2
65–74	30,479 (27.2)	2037	66.8	21,580 (21.6)	2021	93.7
75+	30,541 (27.3)	9839	332.2	18,652 (18.7)	6978	364.1
Total	111,993	12,744	113.8	99,962	10,219	102.2

3.4. Factors Associated with Cirrhosis and All-Cause Mortality

The multivariate analysis regarding cirrhosis development among males and females is presented in Table 6. A relationship between age, diabetes mellitus, and cirrhosis was found among males and females with NAFLD. A significant relationship between obesity and cirrhosis was found among males but not females.

A multivariate model for the risk of death among NAFLD patients included in our study is shown in Table 7. Age at diagnosis, gender, diabetes mellitus, cirrhosis hepatocellular carcinoma, and esophageal varices were found to be risk factors for death among NAFLD patients in the univariate and multivariate analyses, with odds ratios of 1.125, 1.382, 2.648, 4.016, 9.086 and 2.021, $p < 0.001$, respectively.

Table 6. Univariate and multivariate analyses of risk factors for cirrhosis among NAFLD patients.

	Multivariate Analysis—Males			Multivariate Analysis—Females		
	OR	95% CI	*p*-Value	OR	95% CI	*p*-Value
Age at diagnosis	1.038	1.035–1.042	<0.001	1.032	1.029–1.035	<0.001
Diabetes Mellitus	3.331	3.005–3.692	<0.001	3.403	3.117–3.714	<0.001
Obesity	1.126	1.021–1.241	0.017	0.960	0.880–1.048	0.363
Hypertension	1.032	0.910–1.171	0.620	1.000	0.894–1.120	0.996

Table 7. Univariate and multivariate analyses of risk factors for death among NAFLD patients.

	Univariate Analysis			Multivariate Analysis		
	OR	95% CI	*p*-Value	OR	95% CI	*p*-Value
Age at diagnosis	1.128	1.126–1.130	<0.001	1.125	1.124–1.127	<0.001
Gender (female)	1.128	1.097–1.159	<0.001	1.382	1.336–1.429	<0.001
Diabetes Mellitus	5.069	4.927–5.215	<0.001	2.648	2.562–2.737	<0.001
Cirrhosis	8.271	7.784–8.788	<0.001	4.016	3.690–4.372	<0.001
Hepatocellular Carcinoma	18.761	16.333–21.550	<0.001	9.086	7.646–10.797	<0.001
Esophageal Varices	10.249	9.172–11.453	<0.001	2.021	1.734–2.357	<0.001

4. Discussion

This study included more than 200,000 NAFLD patients (52.8% female). We found (1) females were diagnosed with NAFLD at an older mean age than males, (2) females had higher rates of comorbidities including metabolic syndrome, hypertension, diabetes mellitus, and obesity than their male counterparts, (3) females had a higher rate of thyroid carcinoma but no significant difference in rates of other cancers, (4) female patients had higher rates of cirrhosis than males and had higher all-cause mortality rates than males, (5) age and diabetes were found to be predictors for cirrhosis among males and females, but obesity was found to be a predictor for cirrhosis only among males, not females, and finally, (6) diabetes mellitus, cirrhosis, and HCC were found to be predictors of death among female NAFLD patients.

Sex-related differences in the context of NAFLD could be attributed to several factors: differences in body structure, behavioral risk factors, comorbidities, metabolic factors, genetics, and hormonal effects.

The body structures of females and males are inherently different. Differences in fat storage, fat metabolism, and health risks of obesity among females and males have been noted [18]. All of these differences could influence the prevalence of NAFLD among females and may have an impact on the clinical course and complications of the disease.

Behavioral risk factors such as smoking, alcohol and food consuming habits could also have an impact on the development of NAFLD. These differences in habits could be co-factors for NAFLD development and progression. Smoking, alcohol use, and fast food consumption are more common among males compared to females [19–24]. Despite these differences, the prevalence of NAFLD, cirrhosis development, and all-cause mortality are more common among females, possibly indicating other factors are more dominant influencers of NAFLD among females.

NAFLD is considered as the hepatic manifestation of metabolic syndrome and has a strong relationship with obesity. The chronological relationship between NAFLD and comorbidities is still unclear. In particular, the impact each has on the other, and the causal relationship between the two are still unknown. In our study, the rates of diabetes mellitus, hypertension, and obesity were higher among females than males. Most likely, diabetes mellitus and obesity influence the rate of disease progression of cirrhosis and all-cause mortality rates. In our study, diabetes mellitus was found to be a predictor for cirrhosis among both males and females, while obesity was found to be a predictor for cirrhosis among males only.

Several animal studies have demonstrated sexually dimorphic hepatic genes associated with NAFLD. These genes, related to lipid metabolism, drug metabolism, and glucose homeostasis, impact the severity of cirrhosis and inflammation and are risk factors for the onset, progression, and treatment response of NAFLD [17].

Another critical factor that could contribute to sex differences in NAFLD is the hormonal differences between males and females. Estrogen is a vital sex hormone that not only regulates the female reproductive system but also contributes to several biological functions and protection from different diseases.

In a rodent model, the peak serum tumor necrosis factor-alpha (TNF-a), a proinflammatory cytokine, in the liver was twice as high in rodents who received estrogen compared to controls. This study concluded that estrogen sensitizes Kupffer cells to lipopolysaccharide (LPS), resulting in increased toxic mediator production [25]. This pro-inflammatory and toxic mediator production could also affect the progression of liver diseases such as NAFLD. Hormonal, inflammatory, and oxidative stress factors are part of a complex cascade of NAFLD pathogenesis with sex-related differences [17].

Our results show females are diagnosed with NAFLD about five years later than their male counterparts. This could be explained by the protective estrogen effect from NAFLD, which is lost in postmenopausal women. This is consistent with increasing NAFLD rates with age in women [26,27]. Our findings supported this theory: 34.7% of our female patients were diagnosed with NAFLD at age fifty or older, compared to 25.7% of males.

With regard to comorbidities, we found higher rates of diabetes mellitus, hypertension, and obesity among female NAFLD patients but a lower rate of ischemic heart disease. This finding could be related to the protective effect of estrogen on cardiovascular disease incidence among women [27].

Our study found a higher rate of thyroid malignancy and a lower rate of HCC among females compared to males. Previous studies showed disparities in HCC among females compared to males in terms of undergoing HCC surveillance, tumor size at diagnosis, and vascular involvement [13,14]. Previous studies showed that older age, male sex, the severity of compensated cirrhosis at presentation, and sustained activity of liver disease are important predictors of HCC [28–30].

Our study demonstrated that higher rates of cirrhosis development in females, despite an older age at diagnosis and shorter exposure to the steatosis process in females. Hormonal effects and comorbidities such as diabetes and obesity may influence the progression of fibrosis. Whether or not sex is a risk factor for the progression of fibrosis is a controversial issue with conflicting findings across differently designed studies [27]. However, adjusting the cirrhosis rate according to the different age groups, we found a slightly lower rate of cirrhosis among most of the female age groups.

The all-cause age-adjusted mortality rate was lower among females in our study. In addition, a lower rate of HCC was found among females, though there was no significant difference in other complications such as esophageal varices and hepatorenal syndrome. Lower rates of HCC in females may account for the decreased rate of the all-cause mortality.

One of this study's limitations is the lack of availability of data on liver-specific causes of mortality. This makes it difficult to understand the difference in mortality rate, as it is possibly related to other comorbidities. Nevertheless, in the multivariate analysis, the factors with a significant impact on death were age at diagnosis, gender, diabetes mellitus, cirrhosis, and HCC.

To summarize, significant differences were found between females and males in terms of comorbidities, liver-related outcomes, and all-cause mortality rates. Understanding these differences in depth is crucial for prevention, early diagnosis, interventions, and treatment of NAFLD. Special consideration may be required for females in order to decrease the rate of cirrhosis and all-cause mortality. Additional studies are needed before specific interventions can be carried out; however, the practical implication of the present study lie in increasing awareness about the disparities between NAFLD development and outcomes in males and females.

This study is further strengthened by the use of national-based cohort data with a large number of included patients. However, some limitations should be mentioned. The retrospective design of the study design based on an electronic health file database prevented our ability to differentiate between NAFLD and NASH and there was no data regarding liver biopsy or fibrosis grade available.

5. Conclusions

In conclusion, significant differences were found between males and females with NAFLD regarding the age of diagnosis, comorbidities, liver-related complications and all-cause mortality.

Author Contributions: Conceptualization, N.A.-F., M.G. and G.T.; Methodology, N.A.-F., R.H., R.A.-H. and G.T.; Software, B.C.; S.W. and M.G., Validation, B.C., S.W. and M.G.; Formal Analysis, N.A.-F., B.C. and S.W.; Investigation, S.W., R.H., R.A.-H. and G.T., Resources, B.C., S.W. and M.G.; Data Curation, B.C., S.W., R.H. and R.A.-H.; Writing—Original Draft Preparation, N.A.-F.; Writing—Review and Editing, B.C., S.W., R.H., R.A.-H., G.T. and M.G.; Supervision, N.A.-F.; Project Administration, N.A.-F. All authors have read and agreed to the published version of the manuscript.

Funding: This research received no external funding.

Institutional Review Board Statement: The protocol for this research has been approved by the local Helsinki committee, the Soroka Helsinki committee, and it conforms to the provisions of the Declaration of Helsinki, approval number 198-21-SOR.

Informed Consent Statement: Patient consent was waived due to the retrospective design of the study.

Data Availability Statement: No additional data are available.

Conflicts of Interest: The authors declare no conflict of interest.

References

1. Rinella, M.E. Nonalcoholic fatty liver disease: A systematic review. *JAMA* **2015**, *313*, 2263–2273. [CrossRef] [PubMed]
2. Younossi, Z.M.; Koenig, A.B.; Abdelatif, D.; Fazel, Y.; Henry, L.; Wymer, M. Global epidemiology of nonalcoholic fatty liver disease-Meta-analytic assessment of prevalence, incidence, and outcomes. *Hepatology* **2016**, *64*, 73–84. [CrossRef] [PubMed]
3. Li, J.; Zou, B.; Yeo, Y.H.; Feng, Y.; Xie, X.; Lee, D.H.; Fujii, H.; Wu, Y.; Kam, L.Y.; Ji, F.; et al. Prevalence, incidence, and outcome of non-alcoholic fatty liver disease in Asia, 1999-2019: A systematic review and meta-analysis. *Lancet Gastroenterol. Hepatol.* **2019**, *4*, 389–398. [CrossRef]
4. Tailakh, M.A.; Poupko, L.; Kayyal, N.; Alsana, A.; Estis-Deaton, A.; Etzion, O.; Fich, A.; Yardni, D.; Abu-Freha, N. Liver Cirrhosis, Etiology and Clinical Characteristics Disparities Among Minority Populations. *J. Immigr. Minor. Health* **2021**, *24*, 1122–1128. [CrossRef] [PubMed]
5. Kumar, R.; Priyadarshi, R.N.; Anand, U. Non-alcoholic Fatty Liver Disease: Growing Burden, Adverse Outcomes and Associations. *J. Clin. Transl. Hepatol.* **2020**, *8*, 76–86. [CrossRef] [PubMed]
6. White, A.; Ironmonger, L.; Steele, R.; Ormiston-Smith, N.; Crawford, C.; Seims, A. A review of sex-related differences in colorectal cancer incidence, screening uptake, routes to diagnosis, cancer stage and survival in the UK. *BMC Cancer* **2018**, *18*, 906. [CrossRef]
7. Kim, S.; Paik, H.; Yoon, H.; Lee, J.E.; Kim, N.; Sung, M. Sex- and gender-specific disparities in colorectal cancer risk. *World J. Gastroenterol.* **2015**, *21*, 5167–5175. [CrossRef]
8. Abu-Freha, N.; Gat, R.; Philip, A.; Yousef, B.; Ben Shoshan, L.; Yardeni, D.; Nevo-Shor, A.; Novack, V.; Etzion, O. Indications and Findings of Upper Endoscopies in Males and Females, Are They the Same or Different? *J. Clin. Med.* **2021**, *10*, 1620. [CrossRef]

9. Buzzetti, E.; Parikh, P.M.; Gerussi, A.; Tsochatzis, E. Gender differences in liver disease and the drug-dose gender gap. *Pharmacol. Res.* **2017**, *120*, 97–108. [CrossRef]
10. Kezer, C.A.; Simonetto, D.A.; Shah, V.H. Sex Differences in Alcohol Consumption and Alcohol-Associated Liver Disease. *Mayo Clin. Proc.* **2021**, *96*, 1006–1016. [CrossRef]
11. Villanueva, A. Hepatocellular Carcinoma. *N. Engl. J. Med.* **2019**, *380*, 1450–1462. [CrossRef] [PubMed]
12. El-Serag, H.B.; Rudolph, K.L. Hepatocellular carcinoma: Epidemiology and molecular carcinogenesis. *Gastroenterology* **2007**, *132*, 2557–2576. [CrossRef] [PubMed]
13. Wu, E.M.; Wong, L.L.; Hernandez, B.Y.; Ji, J.F.; Jia, W.; Kwee, S.A.; Kalathil, S. Gender differences in hepatocellular cancer: Disparities in nonalcoholic fatty liver disease/steatohepatitis and liver transplantation. *Hepatoma Res.* **2018**, *4*, 66. [CrossRef] [PubMed]
14. Ladenheim, M.R.; Kim, N.G.; Nguyen, P.; Le, A.; Stefanick, M.L.; Garcia, G.; Nguyen, M.H. Sex differences in disease presentation, treatment and clinical outcomes of patients with hepatocellular carcinoma: A single-centre cohort study. *BMJ Open Gastroenterol.* **2016**, *3*, e000107. [CrossRef]
15. Lonardo, A.; Nascimbeni, F.; Ballestri, S.; Fairweather, D.; Win, S.; Than, T.A.; Abdelmalek, M.F.; Suzuki, A. Sex Differences in Nonalcoholic Fatty Liver Disease: State of the Art and Identification of Research Gaps. *Hepatology* **2019**, *70*, 1457–1469. [CrossRef]
16. Ayonrinde, O.T.; Olynyk, J.K.; Beilin, L.J.; Mori, T.A.; Pennell, C.E.; de Klerk, N.; Oddy, W.H.; Shipman, P.; Adams, L.A. Gender-specific differences in adipose distribution and adipocytokines influence adolescent nonalcoholic fatty liver disease. *Hepatology* **2011**, *53*, 800–809. [CrossRef]
17. Salvoza, N.C.; Giraudi, P.J.; Tiribelli, C.; Rosso, N. Sex differences in non-alcoholic fatty liver disease: Hints for future management of the disease. *Explor. Med.* **2020**, *1*, 51–74. [CrossRef]
18. Power, M.L.; Schulkin, J. Sex differences in fat storage, fat metabolism, and the health risks from obesity: Possible evolutionary origins. *Br. J. Nutr.* **2008**, *99*, 931–940. [CrossRef]
19. Syamlal, G.; Mazurek, J.; Dube, S. Gender differences in smoking among U.S. working adults. *Am. J. Prev. Med.* **2014**, *47*, 467–475. [CrossRef]
20. Lariscy, J.; Hummer, R.; Rath, J.; Villanti, A.; Hayward, M.; Vallone, D. Race/ethnicity, nativity, and tobacco use among U.S. young adults: Results from a nationally representative survey. *Nicotine Tob. Res.* **2013**, *15*, 1417–1426. [CrossRef]
21. Castetbon, K.; Vernay, M.; Malon, A.; Salanave, B.; Deschamps, V.; Roudier, C.; Oleko, A.; Szego, E.; Hercberg, S. Dietary intake, physical activity and nutritional status in adults: The French nutrition and health survey (ENNS, 2006–2007). *Br. J. Nutr.* **2009**, *102*, 733–743. [CrossRef] [PubMed]
22. Wansink, B.; Cheney, M.M.; Chan, N. Exploring comfort food preferences across age and gender. *Physiol. Behav.* **2003**, *79*, 739–747. [CrossRef]
23. Ribas-Barba, L.; Serra-Majem, L.; Salvador, G.; Jover, L.; Raidó, B.; Ngo, J.; Plasencia, A. Trends in dietary habits and food consumption in Catalonia, Spain (1992–2003). *Public Health Nutr.* **2007**, *10*, 1340–1353. [CrossRef] [PubMed]
24. Wilsnack, R.W.; Vogeltanz, N.D.; Wilsnack, S.C.; Harris, T.R.; Ahlström, S.; Bondy, S.; Csémy, L.; Ferrence, R.; Ferris, J.; Fleming, J.; et al. Gender differences in alcohol consumption and adverse drinking consequences: Cross-cultural patterns. *Addiction* **2000**, *95*, 251–265. [CrossRef] [PubMed]
25. Ikejima, K.; Enomoto, N.; Iimuro, Y.; Ikejima, A.; Fang, D.; Xu, J.; Forman, D.T.; Brenner, D.A.; Thurman, R.G. Estrogen increases sensitivity of hepatic Kupffer cells to endotoxin. *Am. J. Physiol.* **1998**, *274*, G669–G676. [CrossRef]
26. Yang, J.D.; Abdelmalek, M.F.; Pang, H.; Guy, C.D.; Smith, A.D.; Diehl, A.M.; Suzuki, A. Gender and menopause impact severity of fibrosis among patients with nonalcoholic steatohepatitis. *Hepatology* **2014**, *59*, 1406–1414. [CrossRef]
27. Ballestri, S.; Nascimbeni, F.; Baldelli, E.; Marrazzo, A.; Romagnoli, D. NAFLD as a sexual dimorphic disease: Role of gender and reproductive status in the development and progression of nonalcoholic fatty liver disease and inherent cardiovascular risk. *Adv. Ther.* **2017**, *34*, 1291–1326. [CrossRef]
28. Fattovich, G.; Stroffolini, T.; Zagni, I.; Donato, F. Hepatocellular carcinoma in cirrhosis: Incidence and risk factors. *Gastroenterology* **2004**, *127* (Suppl. 1), S35–S50. [CrossRef]
29. Yang, J.D.; Hainaut, P.; Gores, G.J.; Amadou, A.; Plymoth, A.; Roberts, L.R. A global view of hepatocellular carcinoma: Trends, risk, prevention and management. *Nat. Rev. Gastroenterol. Hepatol.* **2019**, *16*, 589–604. [CrossRef]
30. Androutsakos, T.; Bakasis, A.D.; Pouliakis, A.; Gazouli, M.; Vallilas, C.; Hatzis, G. Single Nucleotide Polymorphisms of Toll-like Receptor 4 in Hepatocellular Carcinoma-A Single-Center Study. *Int. J. Mol. Sci.* **2022**, *23*, 9430. [CrossRef]

biomedicines

Review

Gene Therapy for Acquired and Genetic Cholestasis

Javier Martínez-García [1], Angie Molina [1], Gloria González-Aseguinolaza [1,2,3], Nicholas D. Weber [3,*] and Cristian Smerdou [1,2,*]

[1] Division of Gene Therapy and Regulation of Gene Expression, Cima Universidad de Navarra, 31008 Pamplona, Spain; jmartinez.71@alumni.unav.es (J.M.-G.); amolinad@unav.es (A.M.); ggonzalez@vivet-therapeutics.com (G.G.-A.)
[2] Instituto de Investigación Sanitaria de Navarra (IdISNA), 31008 Pamplona, Spain
[3] Vivet Therapeutics S.L., 31008 Pamplona, Spain
* Correspondence: nweber@vivet-therapeutics.com (N.D.W.); csmerdou@unav.es (C.S.); Tel.: +34-948194700 (N.D.W. & C.S.)

Abstract: Cholestatic diseases can be caused by the dysfunction of transporters involved in hepatobiliary circulation. Although pharmacological treatments constitute the current standard of care for these diseases, none are curative, with liver transplantation being the only long-term solution for severe cholestasis, albeit with many disadvantages. Liver-directed gene therapy has shown promising results in clinical trials for genetic diseases, and it could constitute a potential new therapeutic approach for cholestatic diseases. Many preclinical gene therapy studies have shown positive results in animal models of both acquired and genetic cholestasis. The delivery of genes that reduce apoptosis or fibrosis or improve bile flow has shown therapeutic effects in rodents in which cholestasis was induced by drugs or bile duct ligation. Most studies targeting inherited cholestasis, such as progressive familial intrahepatic cholestasis (PFIC), have focused on supplementing a correct version of a mutated gene to the liver using viral or non-viral vectors in order to achieve expression of the therapeutic protein. These strategies have generated promising results in treating PFIC3 in mouse models of the disease. However, important challenges remain in translating this therapy to the clinic, as well as in developing gene therapy strategies for other types of acquired and genetic cholestasis.

Keywords: cholestatic diseases; gene therapy; AAV; PFIC

Citation: Martínez-García, J.; Molina, A.; González-Aseguinolaza, G.; Weber, N.D.; Smerdou, C. Gene Therapy for Acquired and Genetic Cholestasis. *Biomedicines* **2022**, *10*, 1238. https://doi.org/10.3390/biomedicines10061238

Academic Editor: Jinghua Wang

Received: 29 April 2022
Accepted: 24 May 2022
Published: 26 May 2022

1. Cholestatic Diseases

Cholestatic diseases are based on bile dysfunction due to defects affecting bile synthesis or secretion. These processes involve a wide range of enzymes and membrane transporters involved in hepatobiliary circulation. According to its origin, cholestasis can be classified into two main groups: acquired cholestasis and genetic cholestasis [1].

1.1. Acquired Cholestasis

Most cholestatic diseases are acquired, presenting a dysregulation of the hepatobiliary transporters as a consequence of an adaptive and protective response to bile acid (BA) accumulation in the liver. This regulation is multifactorial, involving different elements such as hormones, BAs, proinflammatory cytokines, and drugs. These different factors mediate the activation of transcription factors that regulate the expression of export pumps, which promote the reduction of intracellular BAs by their excretion in the urine, resulting in the detoxification of the liver [2]. Acquired cholestatic diseases include primary biliary cholangitis (PBC), primary sclerosing cholangitis (PSC), intrahepatic cholestasis of pregnancy (ICP), biliary atresia, drug-induced cholestasis, and inflammation-mediated cholestasis [1,3].

PBC and PSC are classified as autoimmune diseases of the hepatobiliary system, characterized by the presence of antimitochondrial antibodies, portal inflammation, and an immune-mediated destruction of intra- and extra-hepatic bile ducts [4,5]. Clinical manifestations vary widely, from asymptomatic to end-stage biliary cirrhosis. The pathogenesis of the disease is multifactorial, involving genetic, epigenetic, and environmental factors [4,6].

ICP, which is the most common disorder of the hepatobiliary system, is characterized by high serum BA levels in the third trimester of pregnancy that cause severe pruritus. In the development of this cholestatic disorder, high levels of gestational hormones, such as estrogen and progesterone, play a major causative role, while genetic factors may also be involved. Although symptoms disappear after childbirth, the biliary disorder can often recur during future pregnancies [7].

Biliary atresia is a rare liver disease affecting the bile ducts, resulting in the main cause of neonatal cholestasis. The etiology of this biliary disorder is unknown. In some cases, the origin is thought to be due to an exacerbated autoimmune response in the bile duct epithelium as a consequence of a viral infection or due to toxin-induced injury after birth [8]. In other cases, it is thought to be due to a malformation of the bile ducts during gestation. However, it is known that an early diagnosis allows for better outcomes after surgery [9].

Finally, drug- and inflammation-induced cholestasis are closely related. Both drugs and proinflammatory agents can induce cholestasis following inhibition of hepatobiliary transporters but rarely result in severe liver injury. These types of cholestasis have an immunological origin mediated by proinflammatory cytokines directed against the bile duct epithelium that can alter BA secretion [10].

1.2. Inherited Cholestasis

Genetic cholestasis, which represents a minority of all cholestatic disorders, includes different types of progressive familial intrahepatic cholestasis (PFIC) associated with mutations in relevant channel transporters of the hepatobiliary system. PFIC is a heterogeneous group of autosomal recessively inherited monogenic disorders with a low incidence of 1:50,000–100,000 births worldwide, representing approximately 15% of all cases of neonatal cholestasis [11]. These cholestatic syndromes are characterized by an early onset of the disease, usually in infancy, associated with clinical manifestations such as pruritus, jaundice, malabsorption of fat and fat-soluble vitamins, and hepatomegaly [11]. PFIC is associated with several liver complications, such as portal hypertension and cirrhosis, and can progress to end-stage liver disease and liver failure between childhood and adulthood. Depending on the type of PFIC, extrahepatic clinical manifestations or hepatocellular carcinoma (HCC) may occur [12]. The most common biochemical features of this group of hepatobiliary diseases are increased serum BAs and bilirubin [11]. Depending on their genetic origin, PFICs can be classified into six types. Mutations in *ATP8B1*, *ABCB11*, *ABCB4*, tight junction protein 2 (*TJP2*), *NR1H4*, and Myosin VB (*MYO5B*) genes are known to be the cause of PFIC 1-6 types, respectively (Figure 1). In PFIC1, mutations in the familial intrahepatic cholestasis 1 (*FIC1*) gene cause the loss of the asymmetric distribution of phospholipid content in the canalicular membrane, leading to membrane destabilization and reduced BA transport, resulting in their accumulation in hepatocytes, causing cholestasis. Mutations in the *ABCB11* gene can result in PFIC2 due to the absence of a functional bile salt export pump (BSEP) protein, which also leads to toxic accumulation of BA in hepatocytes. In PFIC3, mutations in *ABCB4* cause multidrug resistance protein 3 (MDR3, ABCB4) deficiency, which results in low levels of phosphatidylcholine (PC) in the bile, which is needed to form micelles and neutralize the toxicity of hydrophobic BAs, resulting in damage to the epithelium of bile canaliculi. Mutations in *TJP2* lead to the misdistribution of claudin tight junction in canaliculi, resulting in bile leakage and subsequently in PFIC4. PFIC5 is due to mutations in the *NR1H4* gene that cause deficiency in farnesoid X receptor (FXR), resulting in a reduction of BSEP and ABCB4 expression and the accumulation of toxic BAs in the hepatocytes. Finally, mutations in *MYO5B* interfere with the processing of normal intracellular trafficking of BSEP, reducing its expression and activity at the canalicular membrane, which results in the accumulation of toxic BAs in hepatocytes, giving rise to PFIC6 [13].

Different disease characteristics such as the age of onset, severity, and the manifestation of specific complications and serum markers vary between PFIC types [12,13].

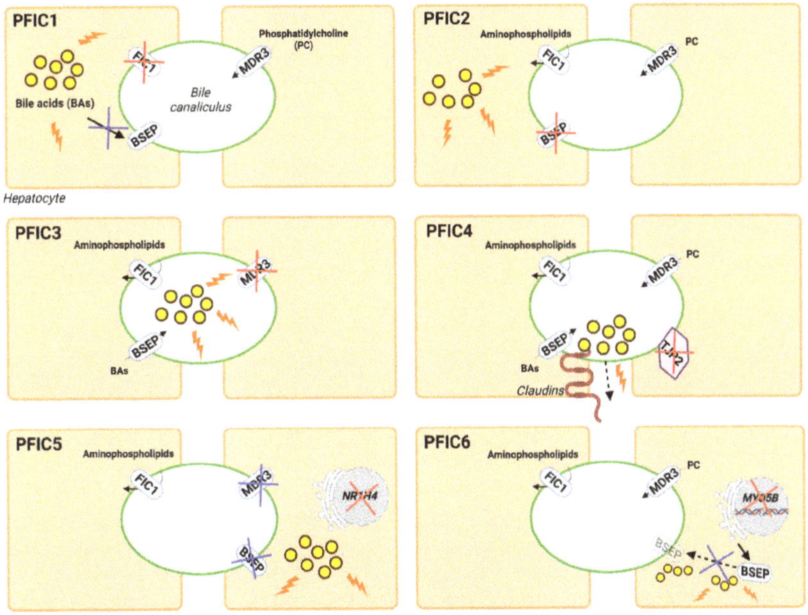

Figure 1. Genetic classification and pathogenesis of PFIC. The diagrams show the genes and functions altered in each type of PFIC. The main deficient proteins for each type of PFIC are indicated by red crosses, while derived alterations in other proteins or pathways are indicated by blue crosses. Damage due to the abnormal accumulation of BAs is shown as yellow circles with orange lightnings.

The role of BSEP in the functioning of the hepatobiliary system is very important, as mutations in different genes involved in BA metabolism and transport, such as *ABCB11*, *NR1H4*, and *MYO5B* causing its deficiency, cause PFIC [14–16]. In addition, depending on the severity of the disease, inherited intrahepatic cholestasis resulting from mutations in *ATP8B1* or *ABCB11* can be classified as either PFIC1 or 2, respectively, or benign recurrent intrahepatic cholestasis (BRIC) 1 or 2, respectively. Sometimes it is clinically difficult to discern between PFIC and BRIC because, in both cases, patients may present mild cholestasis with long-term complications [17]. In addition, some missense mutations in less conserved regions of the *ABCB11* and *ABCB4* genes promote the development of more moderate variants of cholestasis such as BRIC2, ICP, cholesterol cholelithiasis, drug-induced cholestasis, adult biliary cirrhosis, transient neonatal cholestasis, and others [18,19]. In addition, mutations in cholangiocyte transporter genes (e.g., the cystic fibrosis transmembrane conductance regulator (*CFTR*) gene) can cause cholestasis. In fact, a direct association between cystic fibrosis and cholestatic conditions, such as bile duct complications, gallstones, and primary sclerosing cholangitis, has been observed due to mutations in *CFTR* [20]. Other genetic multisystemic diseases associated with cholestatic disorders include Alagille syndrome (ALGS) and cerebrotendinous xanthomatosis (CTX). ALGS arises due to mutations in genes involved in the Notch signaling pathway, such as *JAG1* and *NOTCH2*, and the majority of patients present cholestasis and a deficiency of bile ducts [21]. CTX is caused by mutations in the *CYP27A1* gene, resulting in impaired BA biosynthesis and the accumulation of toxic metabolites. Although liver damage is not common in all CTX patients, some cases of severe infantile cholestasis have been reported [22].

2. Current Treatments

2.1. Surgical Procedures: Hurdles and Limitations

Currently, therapeutic approaches for cholestatic disorders are limited, with liver transplantation being the only curative strategy for the more severe syndromes [23,24]. However, liver transplantation has numerous limitations, such as organ failure, donor shortage, limited organ viability, the requirement of life-long immunosuppression, and immunological rejection [25]. For inherited diseases, such as some types of PFIC, liver transplantation is considered for end-stage patients with severe complications, such as hepatocellular carcinoma (HCC), hepatic steatosis, and liver cirrhosis. Orthotopic transplantation successfully improves cholestasis and related symptoms in 3–5 years [12,26]. However, liver transplant has been shown to be associated with the development of circulating anti-BSEP antibodies in a small fraction of transplanted PFIC2 patients, resulting in the rejection of the transplanted organ [27,28]. Moreover, this approach is only partially effective for cholestatic diseases with extrahepatic manifestations, such as PFIC1.

A therapeutic alternative prior to liver transplantation is surgical treatment aiming to interrupt the enterohepatic circulation, including procedures, such as partial internal biliary diversion (PIBD), ileal exclusion, and partial external biliary diversion (PEBD), that lead to lower BA levels, less pruritus, and even reversal of hepatic fibrosis [29,30]. However, complications such as stoma bag-associated difficulties (e.g., dehydration or leakage) have been reported [30]. For treatment of hereditary cholestatic diseases, biliary diversion has been found to be more effective in PFIC2 patients with residual BSEP activity, while for PFIC3 patients it is usually done late in the disease process, making it hard to prevent disease progression [31,32]. Therefore, there is an urgent need to seek alternative therapeutic approaches to liver transplants and surgical approaches. However, there is room for hope since the increased understanding of the mechanisms leading to genetic and acquired cholestatic diseases has opened the window to develop new drug and gene therapies for the treatment of these disorders.

2.2. Pharmacological Therapies

Drug therapies are considered first-line treatments for cholestatic diseases. The main strategies in the pipeline are based on FXR agonists and inhibitors of BA uptake transporters in the enterohepatic circulation [33,34].

2.2.1. FXR Agonists

In recent years, the use of selective FXR agonists, such as ursodeoxycholic acid (UDCA), has been the first option to treat cholestatic disorders. UDCA, a hydrophilic BA, reduces the hydrophobic pool of toxic BAs in hepatocytes as well as the detergent properties of bile in the bile canaliculi (Figure 2A). Currently, beneficial effects of UDCA have been reported in patients with ICP, PBC, and PFIC3, especially at the early stages of these diseases [35,36], although approximately 50% of the PFIC3 and PBC patients did not respond or had an incomplete response [19,37]. It has also been observed that PFIC3 patients with milder forms of ABCB4 deficiency respond better to UDCA treatment [38]. In contrast, this treatment fails to offer any symptomatic improvement for the majority of patients with PFIC2 or PSC [39,40]. On the other hand, UDCA-derived BAs such as 24-norursodeoxycholic acid (Nor-UDCA) or its taurine conjugate (TUDCA) have also shown potential as therapeutic agents for these liver diseases [35]. Nor-UDCA has shown improvement in serum disease biomarkers such as transaminases and alkaline phosphatase (ALP) levels in patients with PSC [41], although larger studies are needed to establish its real efficacy [42]. Currently, there is one clinical trial evaluating its use in PSC patients (NCT01755507). A recent study has shown that TUDCA was able to normalize serum ALP values in PBC patients [43]. Another FXR agonist with therapeutic potential in the treatment of cholestatic diseases is the semi-synthetic BA, obeticholic acid (OCA). Two phase II studies in PBC and PSC patients demonstrated the safety and beneficial effect of OCA in reducing serum ALP levels [44,45] and, in fact, OCA has been approved as an alternative treatment for patients with PBC who do not respond to UDCA [46]. In addition, a recent study showed that OCA was able to reduce liver damage in a mouse model of PFIC2 [47]. Despite these promising results, its use in cholestatic patients has been associated with severe pruritus, which would make it difficult to be approved as a therapy for PFIC, in which pruritus is one of the main symptoms of concern [48]. Similarly, the non-steroidal FXR agonist cilofexor, which has been reported to lead to significant improvements in cholestasis markers in PSC patients [49], may cause pruritus in a dose-dependent manner as a side effect and is not recommended for certain cholestatic disorders [50].

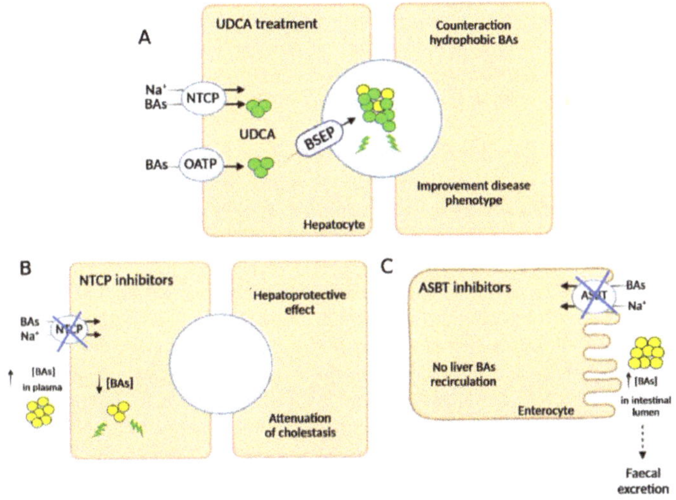

Figure 2. Pharmacological treatments for cholestatic diseases. (**A**) Mechanisms of action of UDCA, which favors the presence of hydrophilic BAs over hydrophobic BAs in bile, decreasing the toxic effect of "detergent bile" in cholestatic patients. (**B**) NTCP transporter inhibitors block the entry of BAs into hepatocytes. (**C**) ASBT inhibitors prevent the reabsorption of BAs in enterocytes, decreasing their entrance into the enterohepatic recirculation. Inhibitions are indicated with blue crosses. BA, bile acid (yellow circles).

Altogether, these data indicate that the identification and development of new and more efficient FXR agonists represents a very interesting area of investigation for the improved clinical management of cholestatic diseases (Table 1) [51,52].

2.2.2. Inhibitors of Bile Acid Uptake Transporters

Recently, there has been great interest in developing drugs that are able to interrupt the enterohepatic circulation in a non-invasive manner for cholestatic disorders. The four transporters that allow circulation of BAs between the liver and intestine are the apical bile salt transporter (ASBT, also known as IBAT for ileal bile acid transporter), BSEP, the sodium-taurocholate cotransporter polypeptide (NTCP) and the basolateral organic solute transporter (OST) [1]. The inhibition of BSEP and OST transporters is not an option as this would result in toxic accumulation of BAs in hepatocytes and enterocytes, respectively [53,54]. In contrast, pharmacological inhibition of the hepatic transporter NTCP results in a well-tolerated increase of BAs in plasma and a subsequent decrease in the liver (Figure 2B) [55]. In fact, recent studies have shown the hepatoprotective effect of NTCP inhibition, resulting in attenuation of cholestasis [56]. ASBT inhibitors prevent the reabsorption of BAs in enterocytes and their recirculation to the liver, favoring their excretion in feces (Figure 2C). ASBT antagonists currently being tested in clinical trials include odevixibat (A4250, Albireo, Boston, MA, USA), maralixibat (LUM001, Mirum Pharmaceuticals, Foster City, CA, USA), elobixibat (A3309, Albireo), linerixibat (GSK2330672, Glaxo

Smith Kline, Brentford, United Kingdom) and volixibat (SHP626, Mirum Pharmaceuticals) (Table 1) [57,58]. Several preclinical studies and clinical trials have shown high safety profiles for all these compounds with limited adverse effects outside the gastrointestinal tract and a high specificity for ASBT when orally administered. The observed therapeutic effects include a decrease of BAs in the liver and serum, reduction in pruritus, liver inflammation, and liver fibrosis [57,58]. In 2021, odevixibat was approved for clinical use in PFIC patients by the US Food and Drug Administration (FDA) and European Medicines Agency (EMA). Moreover, its safety and efficacy for treatment of other cholestatic diseases, such as ALGS, are being evaluated [59]. Maralixibat has also been evaluated in PBC and PSC, but clinical trials were discontinued because this treatment did not improve pruritus compared to placebo [60]. Recently, maralixibat was approved for clinical use for ALGS patients by the FDA [61]. However, its use for other cholestatic diseases, such as PFIC1-4, is currently under evaluation by the EMA [62].

2.2.3. Other Pharmacotherapeutic Agents

Further additional pharmacotherapeutic approaches for the treatment of cholestatic disorders are being explored. Peroxisome proliferator-activated receptor (PPAR) agonists and fibroblast growth factor (FGF) analogues have been shown to be effective for diseases such as PBC and PSC [63]. Activators of FXR transcriptional regulators, such as sirtuin 1, have been shown to alleviate cholestatic liver injury in mice with BA-induced cholestasis by increasing the hydrophilic character of the hepatic BA composition and decreasing plasma BA concentration [64]. The use of antifibrogenic and anti-inflammatory therapeutic agents, such as inhibitors of histone deacetylases and phosphodiesterase 5, led to reduced fibrosis and liver damage in a PFIC3 mouse model [65]. Finally, ABC transporter enhancers, such as ivacaftor, may rescue the functionality of canalicular membrane transporters implicated in cholestatic disorders, including BSEP. Thus, PFIC2 patients may benefit from this type of pharmacological treatment [66]. The use of fibrates, such as the PPAR agonists bezafibrate, fenofibrate, and elafibranor (Table 1), could also be beneficial for the treatment of PBC patients who do not respond to UDCA [67].

Table 1. Drug therapy for cholestatic diseases in clinical trials.

		Drug Name	Indication	Current Status	Clinical Trial	Sponsor [Reference]
FXR agonists	Bile acids	UDCA (Actigall/Ursodiol/Ursofalk)	ICP	Phase III Phase IV	NCT01576458 NCT01510860	Turku University Hospital [68] Pharma GmbH [69]
			PBC	Approved		Sanofi-Synthelabo [70]
			PFIC3			[71]
		Nor-UDCA	PSC	Phase II	NCT01755507	Pharma GmbH [41]
		TUDCA (Taurolite)	PBC	Phase III	NCT01857284	Beijing Friendship Hospital [43]
		OCA (INT-747/Ocaliva)	PBC	Phase II Phase III	NCT00570765 NCT01473524	Intercept Pharmaceuticals [44,45,72,73]
			PSC	Phase II	NCT02177136	
	Non-bile acids	Cilofexor (CILO)	PSC	Phase I/II	NCT02943460	Gilead Sciences [49]
		Tropifexor (LJN452)	PBC	Phase II	NCT02516605	Novartis Pharmaceuticals [74]
		EDP-305	PBC	Phase II	NCT03394924	Enanta Pharmaceuticals

Table 1. *Cont.*

	Drug Name	Indication	Current Status	Clinical Trial	Sponsor [Reference]
ASBT inhibitors	Odevixibat (A4250)	ALGS	Phase III	NCT04674761	Albireo [75,76]
		PFIC	Approved		
	Maralixibat (LUM001)	ALGS	Approved		Mirum Pharmaceuticals, Inc. [61]
		PFIC	Phase III	NCT02057718 NCT03905330	
	Linerixibat (GSK2330672)	PBC	Phase III	NCT02966834 NCT04167358	GlaxoSmithKline [77,78]
	Volixibat (SHP626)	ICP PBC PSC	Phase II	NCT04718961 NCT05050136 NCT04663308	Mirum Pharmaceuticals, Inc.
Other pharmacotherapeutic agents	Aldafermin (NGM282)	PBC	Phase II	NCT02026401	NGM Biopharmaceuticals, Inc. [79]
		PSC		NCT02704364	
	Bezafibrate	PBC	Phase III	NCT01654731	Hôpitaux de Paris [80]
	Elafibranor	PBC	Phase II	NCT03124108	Genfit [81]
	Seladelpar (MBX-8025)	PBC	Phase III	NCT03602560	CymaBay Therapeutics, Inc. [82]

Although the pharmacological strategies mentioned above significantly improved the pathology of cholestatic diseases and the quality of life of the patients [63], they do not represent a definitive cure for hepatobiliary dysfunction. For this reason, the development of new strategies, such as cell and gene therapy, that allow stable, long-term correction of these diseases is highly desired. In the following section, we will focus on gene therapy strategies tested in preclinical models of cholestatic diseases.

3. Gene Therapy

Gene therapy involves the addition, removal, or modification of the genetic material of an individual in order to treat a disease [83]. Its efficacy depends on successful delivery to target cells, for which vectors (viral and non-viral) are utilized. Viral vectors are based on modified viruses, such as adenoviruses (Adv), adeno-associated viruses (AAV), retroviruses, and lentiviruses, among others, which have proven to be very effective for gene delivery, although they present some drawbacks such as immunogenicity and limitations in cargo size. Non-viral vectors, such as polymeric or lipid nanoparticles (LNP), unlike viral vectors, do not achieve delivery to the cell nucleus and induce much more transient transgene expression, but have a better safety profile, are not limited by packaging restrictions, and offer several advantages in manufacturability and shelf-life. Recently, non-viral vectors have shown a high degree of efficacy as demonstrated by the COVID-19 vaccines based on messenger RNA (mRNA)-containing LNPs [84].

Gene therapy has emerged as a promising approach to achieve safe, stable, and efficient long-term correction for a wide range of genetic diseases [85], including monogenic liver disorders, for which liver transplantation remains the only cure [86], as well as acquired liver diseases [87]. Viral and non-viral vectors have shown promising therapeutic results in numerous clinically relevant animal models, as well as in a large number of clinical trials [88,89]. The fact that more than a dozen gene therapy products have been approved by the FDA and EMA, albeit only three for liver gene therapy, is a promising sign for the future application of this technology for liver disorders [90,91].

3.1. *Gene Therapy for Acquired Cholestasis*

Since no definitive treatment has yet been developed for some acquired hepatic cholestasis, such as PBC and PSC, there is a great need to identify novel therapeutic alternatives that can reduce fibrogenesis and potentially prevent the development of chronic liver injury, making genetic-based treatments an attractive strategy to achieve sustained long-term therapeutic effects.

To generate animal models of acquired cholestatic disorders, interventions including bile duct ligation (BDL) and the induction of cholestasis by drugs, such as estrogens and carbon tetrachloride (CCL_4), have been utilized [92]. The development of cholestasis involves several processes including: cellular apoptosis, production of proinflammatory cytokines, and fibrogenesis that ultimately leads to biliary impairment [93].

Gene therapy approaches for acquired cholestasis have been addressed to mitigate liver damage by reducing apoptosis and fibrosis and improving bile formation (Figure 3). Next, we will describe the most relevant gene therapy strategies described so far.

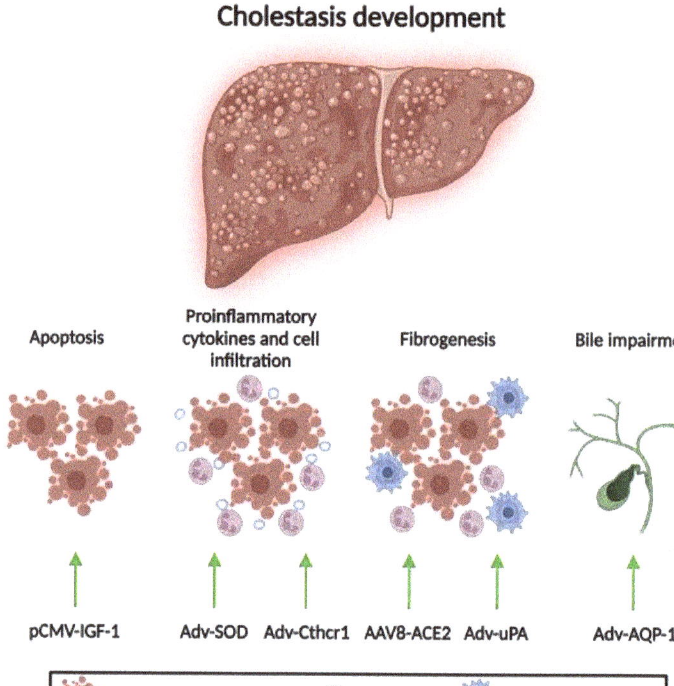

Figure 3. Gene therapy approaches for acquired cholestatic diseases. Different gene therapy strategies have resulted in an alleviation of liver disorders according to their anti-apoptotic, anti-inflammatory, and anti-fibrotic properties, respectively. Adv, adenoviral vector; AAV8, adeno-associated vector with serotype 8; ACE2, angiotensin-converting enzyme; AQP-1, aquaporin; Cthrc-1, collagen triple helix repeat containing-1; HNF4a, hepatocyte nuclear factor 4 alpha; IGF, insulin-like growth factor; SOD, superoxide dismutase; uPA, urokinase-plasminogen activator. This figure was created using BioRender.com.

3.1.1. Apoptosis Attenuation

One of the main targets for gene therapy of acquired liver disorders is the reduction of hepatocyte apoptosis. Hydrodynamic-based gene delivery to the liver of an insulin-like growth factor 1 (IGF-1)-expressing plasmid has demonstrated attenuation of hepatocellular apoptosis and liver injury in rats with BDL. IGF-1 promotes amelioration of cholestatic disease through activation of the phosphatidylinositol-3-kinase pathway, the inhibition of glycogen synthase kinase-3 beta, and the blockade of caspase-9 cleavage. Additionally, inactivation of hepatic stellate cells has been observed, which may explain the notable improvement in the degree of liver fibrosis [94].

3.1.2. Reduction of Mitochondrial Oxidative Stress

Reducing oxidative stress has been shown to be a therapeutic target for acquired liver cholestasis. For example, Adv-mediated mitochondrial superoxide dismutase (SOD) gene delivery leads to a reduction in liver injury by avoiding the formation of oxygen free radicals derived from the accumulation of hydrophobic BAs and preventing the release of proinflammatory cytokines, such as TNFα and TGF-β, in mice with BDL [95]. Similarly, administration of Adv vectors expressing an inhibitor gene of proinflammatory cytokine signaling like collagen triple helix repeat containing-1 (Cthrc-1) has shown a reduction of liver fibrosis in mice subjected to BDL and drug-mediated cholestasis through the inhibition of TGF-β signaling caused by the accelerating degradation of phospho-Smad3 [96].

3.1.3. Anti-Fibrotic Therapies

Anti-fibrotic therapies for cholestatic disorders via reducing pro-inflammatory factors tend to promote collagen degradation and thus reduce the degree of liver fibrosis. Adv vectors expressing the urokinase-plasminogen activator (uPA) gene resulted in a slight reduction of liver fibrosis, leading to a partial improvement of liver histology in rats with BDL associated with the activation of metalloproteinases that trigger collagen degradation [97,98]. Additionally, AAV vectors that allow hepatic expression of angiotensin-converting enzyme (ACE2) provided a sustained anti-fibrotic effect in different animal models of BDL and drug-induced cholestasis [99]. A different strategy to fight fibrosis is based on the gene delivery of human hepatocyte nuclear factor 4 alpha (HNF4A) via AAV vectors or mRNA containing LNP. This type of gene therapy was able to decrease the expression of genes involved in profibrogenic activity and revert fibrosis in several mouse models with induced or genetic cholestasis [100].

3.1.4. Amelioration of Bile Flow

Finally, Adv-mediated hepatic delivery of aquaporin-1 (AQP1) has shown an improvement in the bile flow of estrogen-induced cholestatic rats [101]. In fact, this approach resulted in a marked reduction of serum ALP, as well as serum and biliary concentrations of bile salts. Moreover, AQP1 gene transfer increased biliary output as mediated by a significant increase in BSEP transport activity [102].

Thus, gene therapy approaches may offer a new avenue for the development of novel treatments for acquired cholestatic disorders.

3.2. *Gene Therapy for Inherited Cholestasis*

Gene therapy for the treatment of inherited hepatic diseases has garnered a great deal of attention after demonstrating that AAV vectors expressing human coagulation factors IX and VIII in the livers of patients with hemophilia B and A, respectively, resulted in a sustained therapeutic effect for more than three years [103]. In fact, a large number of gene therapy products have demonstrated promising therapeutic effects in clinically relevant animal models, leading to clinical trials for inherited liver disorders, such as phenylketonuria, familial hypercholesterolemia, ornithine transcarbamylase deficiency, acute intermittent porphyria, methylmalonic acidemia, and Wilson's disease, among others [88]. In the next sections of the review, we will focus on the use of gene therapy for inherited cholestatic diseases, which include genetic disorders with associated cholestasis and the different forms of PFIC.

3.2.1. Gene Therapy of Genetic Disorders with Associated Cholestasis

Preclinical studies have shown promising results in animal models of Cerebrotendinous xanthomatosis (CTX) and Crigler-Najjar syndrome type 1. In the first case, the administration of an AAV8 vector expressing CYP27A was able to restore BA metabolism and normalize the concentration of most BAs in plasma in a mouse model of CTX [104]. Interestingly, this therapeutic effect was achieved with only 20% of transduced hepatocytes, which could greatly facilitate the clinical translation of this approach. Secondly, treatment of Crigler–Najjar syndrome type 1 with an AAV8 vector expressing UDP-glucuronosyltransferase family 1-member A1 (UGT1A) showed normalization of total serum bilirubin levels in two animal models of the disease, Gunn rats and *Ugt1a1*$^{-/-}$ mice [105]. In this last model, a therapeutic effect was also demonstrated in newborn mice, although high doses of vector were required to maintain the effect [106]. These preclinical results led to a phase I/II clinical trial sponsored by Genethon (Évry, France), which is currently ongoing (NCT03466463).

The results observed in preclinical studies of Crigler–Najjar syndrome showed that one of the main limitations for gene therapy of genetic cholestatic diseases could be related to the loss of viral genomes associated with hepatocyte proliferation occurring in young patients [107].

3.2.2. Gene Therapy for PFIC Diseases

Gene therapy approaches for PFIC can be based on gene supplementation or gene editing strategies to modify and repair the affected genes. The implementation of gene therapy for the different types of PFIC has some limitations. Firstly, in some types of PFIC in order to achieve stable and long-term therapeutic efficacy, it could be necessary to transduce most of the hepatocytes, which may require the use of high doses of the viral vector with the concomitant safety concerns [107,108]. Secondly, some types of PFIC have extrahepatic clinical manifestations hampering the liver-targeted treatment [109]. Finally, PFIC diseases requiring therapy are generally diagnosed in pediatric patients, and gene therapy based on non-integrative vectors, such as AAV, may be inefficient due to the loss of viral genomes associated with hepatocyte proliferation in a growing liver [107]. The decision to undergo gene therapy for PFIC, as well as the outcome of the therapy, will likely be influenced by the type of mutations present in the affected gene. For example, patients with missense mutations leading to decreased protein activity will probably respond better than those with a complete deficiency.

Although the loss of viral genomes could be a problem for most inherited cholestasis, ABCB4 deficiency, which causes PFIC3, has certain advantages over other PFIC types for liver gene therapy. For example, previous results using hepatocyte transplantation in a mouse model of PFIC3 showed that engraftment of 12% of healthy hepatocytes was enough to achieve therapeutic efficacy [110]. This evidence led to four preclinical studies examining the feasibility of gene therapy for PFIC3 in three different *Abcb4*$^{-/-}$ mouse models with a range of phenotypes depending on the mouse strain [111].

Gene Therapy for PFIC3 Based on ABCB4 Supplementation

The first study tested gene therapy in C57BL/6 *Abcb4*$^{-/-}$ mice that were challenged with a BA-enriched diet to increase liver toxicity due to their mild phenotype. Treatment with an AAV8 vector expressing ABCB4 demonstrated long-term efficacy by preventing the increase of serum transaminases and the loss of biliary PC levels after BA challenge [112]. In a second study, performed by our group, we evaluated PFIC3 AAV-based gene therapy in FVB *Abcb4*$^{-/-}$ mice, which have a clinically relevant phenotype characterized by high serum levels of bile salts and transaminases, hepatosplenomegaly, and liver fibrosis [113]. In this model, we demonstrated that an AAV8 vector containing a codon-optimized *ABCB4* sequence downstream of the liver specific alpha-1 antitrypsin (AAT) promoter resulted in stable and long-term correction of PFIC3 by improving all disease markers. Interestingly, this therapy was not only able to prevent disease progression in young mice (two-week-old), in which symptoms had not yet developed, but also in older mice with an established phenotype (five-week-old and sixteen-week-old mice). The therapeutic effect was dose dependent, and it was observed that restoration of biliary PC levels above 12–13% (over 4000 μM) of wild-type levels was enough to have a curative effect. This indicates that

PFIC3 could be treated even if only a small fraction of hepatocytes were transduced, in this way resembling gene therapy of other diseases like hemophilia B, in which therapeutic effects can be obtained with a small percentage of transduced hepatocytes. In our study, the therapeutic threshold was achieved with as little as 2–3% of wild-type ABCB4 expression levels [113]. Interestingly, this therapy was more efficacious in male mice compared to females, although a sustained therapeutic effect could be obtained in females by the administration of a second vector dose [113].

Recently, a preclinical study based on LNP-encapsulated mRNA therapy was able to transiently reverse the disease phenotype in BALB/c *Abcb4*$^{-/-}$ mice [114]. BALB/c *Abcb4*$^{-/-}$ show similar levels of serum biomarkers as the FVB *Abcb4*$^{-/-}$ mice, but with a faster progression of liver fibrosis, leading to early development of primary liver cancers as well as an earlier onset of other complications, such as portal hypertension [111]. Five repeat *ABCB4* mRNA-LNP injections were able to restore ABCB4 expression and biliary PC levels (~42% of wild-type levels), as well as improve serum biomarker levels, liver fibrosis, and hepatomegaly [114,115]. However, these previously described non-integrative vector-based gene therapy strategies may have important limitations, such as loss of transgene expression, either because of loss of viral genomes due to hepatocyte division or because the short half-life of mRNA requires periodic administration to maintain the therapeutic effect. An alternative strategy to solve this hurdle is gene delivery mediated by an integrative vector.

Using this type of approach, Siew et al. tested PFIC3 correction by the use of an integrative hybrid vector based on the expression of a piggyBac transposase and an AAV8 vector containing a piggyBac ABCB4 expression cassette in FVB *Abcb4*$^{-/-}$ mice. A single dose of the hybrid vector in neonates demonstrated the recovery of biliary PC levels and normalization of serum biomarkers. Additionally, the hybrid AAV-piggyBac treatment prevented biliary cirrhosis and reduced tumorigenesis [116]. However, the possibility of this vector integrating into oncogenic sites represents a high risk for clinical application. Results from these preclinical studies have led to orphan drug designation of an AAV vector harboring a codon optimized version of ABCB4 (VTX-803) developed by Vivet Therapeutics (Paris, France), opening a promising pathway for the treatment of patients with this cholestatic disorder (Table 2).

Gene Therapy for PFIC3 Targeting Mechanisms of Disease

Although gene supplementation or correction of the affected gene is the most straightforward gene therapy strategy for PFIC3, several studies have shown that it is also possible to treat this disease by altering the expression of other genes that are involved in this pathology. One example is the delivery of vectors that express genes that contribute to the attenuation of liver fibrosis, such as ACE2 and HNF4A, as described in Section 3.1.3. In this sense, an AAV8 vector expressing ACE2 was able to reduce liver fibrosis in early- and late-stage FVB *Abcb4*$^{-/-}$ mice [117]. Moreover, hepatocyte-targeted administration of *HNF4A* mRNA encapsulated with a biodegradable lipid restored the metabolic activity of hepatocytes in FVB *Abcb4*$^{-/-}$ mice, leading to a robust inhibition of fibrogenesis [100].

A novel approach that could be used to treat cholestatic diseases is based on the regulation of BA synthesis and homeostasis. It has recently been described that Limb expression 1-like protein (LIX1L) is increased in the liver of patients with cholestatic diseases and that the normalization of its expression alleviates cholestatic liver injury in different cholestatic mouse models, including FVB *Abcb4*$^{-/-}$ mice. LIX1L regulates the levels of miR-191-3p, a microRNA that downregulates transcription factor liver receptor homolog-1 (LRH-1), thereby inhibiting Cyp7a1 and Cyp8b1 expression, two enzymes required for BA synthesis. Based on these data, Li et al. [118], recently showed that an AAV vector overexpressing miR-191-3p was able to ameliorate cholestasis in FVB *Abcb4*$^{-/-}$ mice by direct repression of LRH-1 expression, thereby reducing de novo BA synthesis [118]. Another potential target for reducing liver fibrosis through gene therapy of cholestatic disorders is the suppression of the neurokinin 1 receptor (NK1R) axis as well as transforming growth factor-β1 (TGF-β1)/miR-31 signaling. In FVB *Abcb4*$^{-/-}$ mice, knock-out of NK1R has been shown to decrease the levels of miR-31 and of proinflammatory molecules such as TFG-β1, resulting in the reduction of liver inflammation and fibrosis [119]. These therapeutic approaches could be very useful for either acquired cholestatic disorders or PFIC.

Table 2. Gene therapy approaches for PFIC3.

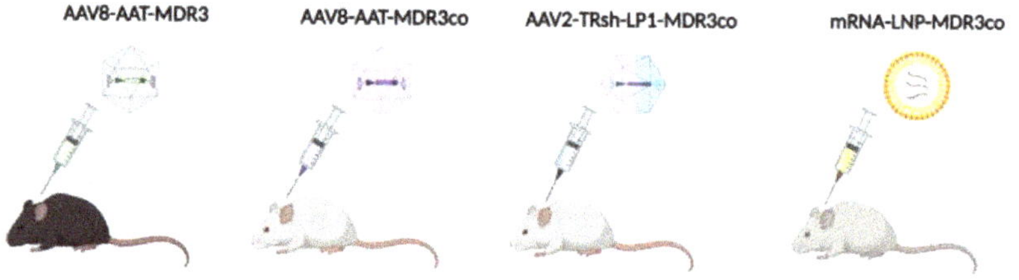

	Aronson et al. [112]	Weber et al. [113]	Siew et al. [116]	Wei et al. [114]
Strain Background	C57BL/6 *Abcb4*$^{-/-}$	FVB *Abcb4*$^{-/-}$	FVB *Abcb4*$^{-/-}$	BALB/c *Abcb4*$^{-/-}$
Phenotype	Mild (requiring cholate-enriched diet)	Severe (similar to patients)	Severe (similar to patients)	More severe
Vector	AAV8	AAV8	Hybrid AAV-piggyBac transposon	LNP
Dose	5×10^{13} vg/kg	1×10^{14} vg/kg	~2×10^{14} vg/kg	1.0 mg/kg
Age of treatment	10-week-old	2- or 5-week-old	Newborn	4-week-old
Outcomes	Increased biliary PC and cholesterol content. Rescue of serum ALT, ALP and bilirubin levels. Prevention of liver fibrosis.	Increased biliary PC. Rescue of serum transaminases, ALP and BA levels. Improvement of the degree of hepatosplenomegaly. Prevention and reversal of liver fibrosis.	Increased biliary PC. Decreased hepatomegaly and serum parameters (ALT, ALP, BAs). Reduced liver fibrosis and liver tumor incidence.	Increased biliary PC (10–25% WT) and %BW. Decreased hepatomegaly and serum parameters (ALT, ALP, BAs). Normalization of liver fibrosis and portal hypertension.
Advantages	Long-term correction. No risk of mutagenesis.	Granted orphan drug designation. Long-term prevention and correction at early and late stages of PFIC3, respectively. No risk of mutagenesis.	Long-term correction. Preventing genome loss by hepatocellular proliferation during liver growth.	No risk of mutagenesis. Less immune responses.
Disadvantages	Need for challenge with BA-enriched dietary supplementation (model). Need to evaluate efficacy in younger mice more representative of the age of patients. Risks of using a high viral dose.	Loss of long-term therapeutic effect in half of the females treated with a single dose. Need to address the immune response based on anti-AAV neutralizing antibody for repeated administrations of the vector. Risks of using a high viral dose.	Risk of mutagenesis. Transposase overexpression Lack of serotype that efficiently transduces human hepatocytes.	Less durable expression. Requires repeated parenteral dosing.

AAT, alpha-1 antitrypsin; AAV, adeno-associated vector; ALP, alkaline phosphatase; ALT, alanine aminotransferase; BW, body weight; LNP, lipid nanoparticles; LP1, liver-specific transcriptional control unit; PC, phosphatidylcholine; TRsh, short piggyBac terminal repeats; VG, viral genomes; WT, wild-type.

Gene Therapy for Other Types of PFIC

For other types of PFIC, although gene supplementation using vectors expressing the specific mutated gene is also an option, there are certain barriers that make the development of these treatments more challenging than for PFIC3. For example, patients with PFIC1, PFIC4, PFIC5, and PFIC6 have extrahepatic manifestations that cannot be rescued by liver-targeted gene therapy [109,120]. In addition, in contrast to gene therapy for PFIC3, where liver toxicity arises in the bile canaliculi and transgene delivery to a fraction of hepatocytes leads to sufficient ABCB4 protein to reverse toxicity, in other types of PFIC where toxicity occurs in hepatocytes, it is likely that correction of a high percentage of these cells will be required to achieve a therapeutic effect [110,121]. One additional problem to develop gene therapy strategies for some types of PFIC is the lack of suitable animal models that adequately recapitulate the phenotype of patients. Currently, there are no *TJP2*-deficient animal models available to test the feasibility of gene therapy for PFIC4 [121]. Likewise, the existing animal model for PFIC6 is not suitable, because it has a complete knock-out of the MYO5B protein, which is not an appropriate model for this cholestatic disease. For that, it is necessary to develop an animal model with missense mutations of the *MYO5B* gene that affect the motor domain but do not result in complete deficiency of the protein [122]. In the case of PFIC2, there are several animal models that show a varying degree of pathology depending on the genetic background. *Abcb11*$^{-/-}$ mice in a C57BL/6 background represent the closest model to the patient disease phenotype, showing a drastic decrease in bile salt content in the bile that leads to increased levels of serum transaminases, liver fibrosis, and hepatomegaly, with these changes being more severe in females than in males [123]. However, unlike PFIC2 patients, these mice only show a mild elevation of serum bile salts, which is one of the main biomarkers of the disease.

Finally, the loss of transgene expression by hepatocyte cell division is a drawback for the use of non-integrative vectors, such as AAV, in gene therapy of these inherited cholestatic disorders that need to be treated at very early ages, as only a few hepatocytes will maintain episomal AAV genomes [124]. Unlike PFIC3, for which partial gene therapy supplementation or correction of the affected gene is feasible, other types of PFIC may benefit from other gene therapy strategies aimed at reversing liver damage at several levels.

4. Future Directions

Due to the growing success of liver-targeted gene therapies and preclinical studies showing therapeutic efficacy against cholestatic diseases, such as PFIC3, the need to overcome challenges involved in taking these products from bench to bedside is even more critical.

One of the main challenges that gene therapy of cholestatic disorders faces is the potential loss of therapeutic effect in pediatric patients. This could be due to a decrease of viral genomes as a result of hepatocyte divisions in a growing liver in the case of AAV-based therapies, or to the transient expression of non-viral vector-mediated mRNA delivery [107,125]. Other challenges include immune responses to treatment (vector or transgene) and vector-mediated toxicities, particularly as a result of using very high vector doses. Strategies for addressing these challenges will guide the possible directions for present and future research.

First, the administration of repeated doses of the vector could allow the maintenance of the therapeutic effect. However, this is only straightforward for non-viral vectors, such as mRNA-loaded nanoparticles, although it will greatly increase the cost of this therapy [115,125]. For viral vectors, such as AAV, the induction of vector-neutralizing antibodies after the first dose prevents the use of the same vector for additional administrations. However, several strategies have been proposed to allow vector re-administrations, which include the use of alternative AAV serotypes without cross-reactivity [126], the elimination of neutralizing antibodies using IgG-degrading endopeptidases [127], and the prevention of humoral and cellular responses against the virus via co-administration of the vector with rapamycin encapsulated in LNPs [128].

Second, the combination of gene therapy vectors with pharmacological therapies, such as UDCA, could provide synergistic therapeutic effects, especially in PFIC3 patients with more severe pathology who do not respond to UDCA treatment [19]. The use of pharmacological therapies in some pediatric patients could lead to a healthier liver status, improving the vector transduction efficiency and/or allowing the administration of the gene therapy product at an older age, at which vector genomes could be maintained for longer periods of time.

Third, the sequential therapy of non-viral vectors such as mRNA-loaded nanoparticles in pediatric patients with growing livers followed by the administration of a viral vector that allows safe and stable long-term expression of the transgene at an older age, or the combination of vectors that, after reducing liver injury, facilitate the long-term efficacy of gene therapy could be of interest.

Fourth, the improvement of gene therapy vectors by codon optimization or incorporating promoters that allow a more potent expression of the transgene with the aim of reducing the viral dose required to achieve a therapeutic effect could function to reduce the risk of toxicity from high doses [129,130]. Alternatively, inducible promoters could allow a safe, precise, and controlled expression of the transgene with physiological transgene regulation [131,132], thus avoiding unwanted effects of transgene overexpression, such as silencing, exacerbated immune responses, or cytotoxicity that could result in the elimination of the transduced hepatocytes [133,134]. The modification of the transgene via codon optimization with a reduced number of CpG motifs may also mitigate the risk of activating the Toll-like receptor 9 pathway [135], which has been theorized to result in loss of transduced hepatocytes [136].

And finally, for those cholestatic disorders in which correction of the majority of hepatocytes for a long-term therapeutic effect is likely necessary, as in the case of some PFIC subtypes [108,109], a promising alternative is the use of CRISPR/Cas9 to achieve specific gene correction by non-homologous end-joining, base editing, or prime editing. The high efficiency of liver-targeted gene delivery makes it an ideal organ for the application of gene editing strategies in animal models of PFIC [88]. However, there are still many barriers hampering the use of gene editing techniques in humans, such as reduced specificity of targeted integration leading to safety concerns, as well as the low efficacy of non-homologous end-joining [137]. However, for most patients with more severe extrahepatic pathologies, liver-targeted gene therapy by itself will not be sufficient [109,122]. In this sense, the combination of gene therapy products targeting the liver with other therapies that allow the alleviation of extrahepatic damage could show a beneficial effect in these patients.

5. Conclusions

Although pharmacological therapies can be used to treat cholestatic diseases with milder phenotypes, they are less efficient in patients with a more severe pathology. As addressed in this review, alternative approaches, such as gene therapy, could represent a promising novel approach. To date, many preclinical studies using liver-directed gene therapy in clinically relevant animal models of both inherited and induced cholestasis have shown promising results. Although there are still many challenges for the implementation of these emerging treatments in the clinic, it is likely that some of these therapies will be approved in the near future, giving new hope for many cholestatic patients.

Author Contributions: J.M.-G., N.D.W. and C.S., writing—original draft preparation; J.M.-G., A.M., G.G.-A., N.D.W. and C.S., writing—review and editing. All authors have read and agreed to the published version of the manuscript.

Funding: This work was supported by the following grant: Instituto Salud Carlos III financed with Feder Funds PI20/00415 ("A way to make Europe").

Conflicts of Interest: N.D.W. and G.G.-A. are Vivet Therapeutics employees and hold stock in the company.

References

1. Zollner, G.; Trauner, M. Mechanisms of Cholestasis. *Clin. Liver Dis.* **2008**, *12*, 1–26. [CrossRef]
2. Lee, J.; Boyer, J.L. Molecular Alterations in Hepatocyte Transport Mechanisms in Acquired Cholestatic Liver Disorders. *Semin. Liver Dis.* **2000**, *20*, 373–384. [CrossRef] [PubMed]
3. Yokoda, R.T.; Rodriguez, E.A. Review: Pathogenesis of Cholestatic Liver Diseases. *World J. Hepatol.* **2020**, *12*, 423–435. [CrossRef] [PubMed]
4. Kaplan, M.M.; Gershwin, M.E. Primary Biliary Cirrhosis. *N. Engl. J. Med.* **2005**, *353*, 1261–1273. [CrossRef] [PubMed]
5. Gulamhusein, A.F.; Hirschfield, G.M. Primary Biliary Cholangitis: Pathogenesis and Therapeutic Opportunities. *Nat. Rev. Gastroenterol. Hepatol.* **2020**, *17*, 93–110. [CrossRef] [PubMed]
6. Dyson, J.K.; Beuers, U.; Jones, D.E.J.; Lohse, A.W.; Hudson, M. Primary Sclerosing Cholangitis. *Lancet* **2018**, *391*, 2547–2559. [CrossRef]
7. Reyes, H.; Sjövall, J. Bile Acids and Progesterone Metabolites Intrahepatic Cholestasis of Pregnancy. *Ann. Med.* **2000**, *32*, 94–106. [CrossRef]
8. Pang, S.-Y.; Dai, Y.-M.; Zhang, R.-Z.; Chen, Y.-H.; Peng, X.-F.; Fu, J.; Chen, Z.-R.; Liu, Y.-F.; Yang, L.-Y.; Wen, Z.; et al. Autoimmune Liver Disease-Related Autoantibodies in Patients with Biliary Atresia. *World J. Gastroenterol.* **2018**, *24*, 387–396. [CrossRef]
9. Abbey, P.; Kandasamy, D.; Naranje, P. Neonatal Jaundice. *Indian J. Pediatr.* **2019**, *86*, 830–841. [CrossRef]
10. Visentin, M.; Lenggenhager, D.; Gai, Z.; Kullak-Ublick, G.A. Drug-Induced Bile Duct Injury. *Biochim. Biophys. Acta-Mol. Basis Dis.* **2018**, *1864*, 1498–1506. [CrossRef]
11. Jacquemin, E. Progressive Familial Intrahepatic Cholestasis. *Clin. Res. Hepatol. Gastroenterol.* **2012**, *36*, S26–S35. [CrossRef]
12. Srivastava, A. Progressive Familial Intrahepatic Cholestasis. *J. Clin. Exp. Hepatol.* **2014**, *4*, 25–36. [CrossRef] [PubMed]
13. Amirneni, S.; Haep, N.; Gad, M.A.; Soto-Gutierrez, A.; Squires, J.E.; Florentino, R.M. Molecular Overview of Progressive Familial Intrahepatic Cholestasis. *World J. Gastroenterol.* **2020**, *26*, 7470–7484. [CrossRef]
14. Imagawa, K.; Hayashi, H.; Sabu, Y.; Tanikawa, K.; Fujishiro, J.; Kajikawa, D.; Wada, H.; Kudo, T.; Kage, M.; Kusuhara, H.; et al. Clinical Phenotype and Molecular Analysis of a Homozygous ABCB11 Mutation Responsible for Progressive Infantile Cholestasis. *J. Hum. Genet.* **2018**, *63*, 569–577. [CrossRef] [PubMed]
15. Gomez-Ospina, N.; Potter, C.J.; Xiao, R.; Manickam, K.; Kim, M.-S.; Kim, K.H.; Shneider, B.L.; Picarsic, J.L.; Jacobson, T.A.; Zhang, J.; et al. Mutations in the Nuclear Bile Acid Receptor FXR Cause Progressive Familial Intrahepatic Cholestasis. *Nat. Commun.* **2016**, *7*, 10713. [CrossRef] [PubMed]
16. Gonzales, E.; Taylor, S.A.; Davit-Spraul, A.; Thébaut, A.; Thomassin, N.; Guettier, C.; Whitington, P.F.; Jacquemin, E. MYO5B Mutations Cause Cholestasis with Normal Serum Gamma-glutamyl Transferase Activity in Children without Microvillous Inclusion Disease. *Hepatology* **2017**, *65*, 164–173. [CrossRef]
17. Luketic, V.A.; Shiffman, M.L. Benign Recurrent Intrahepatic Cholestasis. *Clin. Liver Dis.* **2004**, *8*, 133–149. [CrossRef]
18. Lam, P.; Soroka, C.; Boyer, J. The Bile Salt Export Pump: Clinical and Experimental Aspects of Genetic and Acquired Cholestatic Liver Disease. *Semin. Liver Dis.* **2010**, *30*, 125–133. [CrossRef]
19. Sticova, E.; Jirsa, M. ABCB4 Disease: Many Faces of One Gene Deficiency. *Ann. Hepatol.* **2020**, *19*, 126–133. [CrossRef]
20. Feranchak, A.P.; Sokol, R.J. Cholangiocyte Biology and Cystic Fibrosis Liver Disease. *Semin. Liver Dis.* **2001**, *21*, 471–488. [CrossRef]
21. Mitchell, E.; Gilbert, M.; Loomes, K.M. Alagille Syndrome. *Clin. Liver Dis.* **2018**, *22*, 625–641. [CrossRef] [PubMed]
22. Zhang, P.; Zhao, J.; Peng, X.-M.; Qian, Y.-Y.; Zhao, X.-M.; Zhou, W.-H.; Wang, J.-S.; Wu, B.-B.; Wang, H.-J. Cholestasis as a Dominating Symptom of Patients with CYP27A1 Mutations: An Analysis of 17 Chinese Infants. *J. Clin. Lipidol.* **2021**, *15*, 116–123. [CrossRef] [PubMed]
23. Sokal, E.M. Liver Transplantation for Inborn Errors of Liver Metabolism. *J. Inherit. Metab. Dis.* **2006**, *29*, 426–430. [CrossRef] [PubMed]
24. Nevens, F. PBC-Transplantation and Disease Recurrence. *Best Pract. Res. Clin. Gastroenterol.* **2018**, *34–35*, 107–111. [CrossRef]
25. Jadlowiec, C.C. Liver Transplantation: Current Status and Challenges. *World J. Gastroenterol.* **2016**, *22*, 4438. [CrossRef]
26. Liu, Y.; Sun, L.-Y.; Zhu, Z.-J.; Wei, L.; Qu, W.; Zeng, Z.-G. Liver Transplantation for Progressive Familial Intrahepatic Cholestasis. *Ann. Transplant.* **2018**, *23*, 666–673. [CrossRef]
27. Kubitz, R.; Dröge, C.; Kluge, S.; Stross, C.; Walter, N.; Keitel, V.; Häussinger, D.; Stindt, J. Autoimmune BSEP Disease: Disease Recurrence After Liver Transplantation for Progressive Familial Intrahepatic Cholestasis. *Clin. Rev. Allergy Immunol.* **2015**, *48*, 273–284. [CrossRef]
28. Stindt, J.; Kluge, S.; Dröge, C.; Keitel, V.; Stross, C.; Baumann, U.; Brinkert, F.; Dhawan, A.; Engelmann, G.; Ganschow, R.; et al. Bile Salt Export Pump-Reactive Antibodies Form a Polyclonal, Multi-Inhibitory Response in Antibody-Induced Bile Salt Export Pump Deficiency. *Hepatology* **2016**, *63*, 524–537. [CrossRef]
29. Bull, L.N.; Pawlikowska, L.; Strautnieks, S.; Jankowska, I.; Czubkowski, P.; Dodge, J.L.; Emerick, K.; Wanty, C.; Wali, S.; Blanchard, S.; et al. Outcomes of Surgical Management of Familial Intrahepatic Cholestasis 1 and Bile Salt Export Protein Deficiencies. *Hepatol. Commun.* **2018**, *2*, 515–528. [CrossRef]
30. Bjørnland, K.; Hukkinen, M.; Gatzinsky, V.; Arnell, H.; Pakarinen, M.P.; Almaas, R.; Svensson, J.F. Partial Biliary Diversion May Promote Long-Term Relief of Pruritus and Native Liver Survival in Children with Cholestatic Liver Diseases. *Eur. J. Pediatr. Surg.* **2021**, *31*, 341–346. [CrossRef]

31. Cielecka-Kuszyk, J.; Lipiński, P.; Szymańska, S.; Ismail, H.; Jankowska, I. Long-Term Follow-up in Children with Progressive Familial Intrahepatic Cholestasis Type 2 after Partial External Biliary Diversion with Focus on Histopathological Features. *Pol. J. Pathol.* **2019**, *70*, 79–83. [CrossRef] [PubMed]
32. Lemoine, C.; Bhardwaj, T.; Bass, L.M.; Superina, R.A. Outcomes Following Partial External Biliary Diversion in Patients with Progressive Familial Intrahepatic Cholestasis. *J. Pediatr. Surg.* **2017**, *52*, 268–272. [CrossRef] [PubMed]
33. Alam, S.; Lal, B.B. Recent Updates on Progressive Familial Intrahepatic Cholestasis Types 1, 2 and 3: Outcome and Therapeutic Strategies. *World J. Hepatol.* **2022**, *14*, 98–118. [CrossRef] [PubMed]
34. Abbas, N.; Quraishi, M.N.; Trivedi, P. Emerging Drugs for the Treatment of Primary Sclerosing Cholangitis. *Curr. Opin. Pharmacol.* **2022**, *62*, 23–35. [CrossRef] [PubMed]
35. Cabrera, D.; Arab, J.P.; Arrese, M. UDCA, NorUDCA, and TUDCA in Liver Diseases: A Review of Their Mechanisms of Action and Clinical Applications. In *Bile Acids and Their Receptors*; Handbook of Experimental Pharmacology; Springer: Cham, Switzerland, 2019; pp. 237–264.
36. Manna, L.B.; Papacleovoulou, G.; Flaviani, F.; Pataia, V.; Qadri, A.; Abu-Hayyeh, S.; McIlvride, S.; Jansen, E.; Dixon, P.; Chambers, J.; et al. Ursodeoxycholic Acid Improves Feto-Placental and Offspring Metabolic Outcomes in Hypercholanemic Pregnancy. *Sci. Rep.* **2020**, *10*, 10361. [CrossRef]
37. Carey, E.J.; Ali, A.H.; Lindor, K.D. Primary Biliary Cirrhosis. *Lancet* **2015**, *386*, 1565–1575. [CrossRef]
38. Gordo-Gilart, R.; Andueza, S.; Hierro, L.; Martínez-Fernández, P.; D'Agostino, D.; Jara, P.; Alvarez, L. Functional Analysis of ABCB4 Mutations Relates Clinical Outcomes of Progressive Familial Intrahepatic Cholestasis Type 3 to the Degree of MDR3 Floppase Activity. *Gut* **2015**, *64*, 147–155. [CrossRef]
39. Ghonem, N.S.; Assis, D.N.; Boyer, J.L. Fibrates and Cholestasis. *Hepatology* **2015**, *62*, 635–643. [CrossRef]
40. Stapelbroek, J.M.; van Erpecum, K.J.; Klomp, L.W.J.; Houwen, R.H.J. Liver Disease Associated with Canalicular Transport Defects: Current and Future Therapies. *J. Hepatol.* **2010**, *52*, 258–271. [CrossRef]
41. Fickert, P.; Hirschfield, G.M.; Denk, G.; Marschall, H.-U.; Altorjay, I.; Färkkilä, M.; Schramm, C.; Spengler, U.; Chapman, R.; Bergquist, A.; et al. NorUrsodeoxycholic Acid Improves Cholestasis in Primary Sclerosing Cholangitis. *J. Hepatol.* **2017**, *67*, 549–558. [CrossRef]
42. Chazouillères, O. 24-Norursodeoxycholic Acid in Patients with Primary Sclerosing Cholangitis: A New "Urso Saga" on the Horizon? *J. Hepatol.* **2017**, *67*, 446–447. [CrossRef] [PubMed]
43. Ma, H.; Zeng, M.; Han, Y.; Yan, H.; Tang, H.; Sheng, J.; Hu, H.; Cheng, L.; Xie, Q.; Zhu, Y.; et al. A Multicenter, Randomized, Double-Blind Trial Comparing the Efficacy and Safety of TUDCA and UDCA in Chinese Patients with Primary Biliary Cholangitis. *Medicine* **2016**, *95*, e5391. [CrossRef] [PubMed]
44. Trauner, M.; Nevens, F.; Shiffman, M.L.; Drenth, J.P.H.; Bowlus, C.L.; Vargas, V.; Andreone, P.; Hirschfield, G.M.; Pencek, R.; Malecha, E.S.; et al. Long-Term Efficacy and Safety of Obeticholic Acid for Patients with Primary Biliary Cholangitis: 3-Year Results of an International Open-Label Extension Study. *Lancet Gastroenterol. Hepatol.* **2019**, *4*, 445–453. [CrossRef]
45. Kowdley, K.V.; Vuppalanchi, R.; Levy, C.; Floreani, A.; Andreone, P.; LaRusso, N.F.; Shrestha, R.; Trotter, J.; Goldberg, D.; Rushbrook, S.; et al. A Randomized, Placebo-Controlled, Phase II Study of Obeticholic Acid for Primary Sclerosing Cholangitis. *J. Hepatol.* **2020**, *73*, 94–101. [CrossRef] [PubMed]
46. D'Amato, D.; de Vincentis, A.; Malinverno, F.; Viganò, M.; Alvaro, D.; Pompili, M.; Picciotto, A.; Palitti, V.P.; Russello, M.; Storato, S.; et al. Real-World Experience with Obeticholic Acid in Patients with Primary Biliary Cholangitis. *JHEP Rep.* **2021**, *3*, 100248. [CrossRef] [PubMed]
47. Wang, L.; Luo, Q.; Zeng, S.; Lou, Y.; Li, X.; Hu, M.; Lu, L.; Liu, Z. Disordered Farnesoid X Receptor Signaling Is Associated with Liver Carcinogenesis in *Abcb11* -deficient Mice. *J. Pathol.* **2021**, *255*, 412–424. [CrossRef]
48. Fiorucci, S.; Di Giorgio, C.; Distrutti, E. Obeticholic Acid: An Update of Its Pharmacological Activities in Liver Disorders. In *Bile Acids and Their Receptors*; Handbook of Experimental Pharmacology; Springer: Cham, Switzerland, 2019; pp. 283–295.
49. Trauner, M.; Gulamhusein, A.; Hameed, B.; Caldwell, S.; Shiffman, M.L.; Landis, C.; Eksteen, B.; Agarwal, K.; Muir, A.; Rushbrook, S.; et al. The Nonsteroidal Farnesoid X Receptor Agonist Cilofexor (GS-9674) Improves Markers of Cholestasis and Liver Injury in Patients With Primary Sclerosing Cholangitis. *Hepatology* **2019**, *70*, 788–801. [CrossRef]
50. Jiang, L.; Liu, X.; Wei, H.; Dai, S.; Qu, L.; Chen, X.; Guo, M.; Chen, Y. Structural Insight into the Molecular Mechanism of Cilofexor Binding to the Farnesoid X Receptor. *Biochem. Biophys. Res. Commun.* **2022**, *595*, 1–6. [CrossRef]
51. Massafra, V.; Pellicciari, R.; Gioiello, A.; van Mil, S.W.C. Progress and Challenges of Selective Farnesoid X Receptor Modulation. *Pharmacol. Ther.* **2018**, *191*, 162–177. [CrossRef]
52. van de Wiel, S.M.W.; Bijsmans, I.T.G.W.; Van Mil, S.W.C.; van de Graaf, S.F.J. Identification of FDA-Approved Drugs Targeting the Farnesoid X Receptor. *Sci. Rep.* **2019**, *9*, 2193. [CrossRef]
53. Baghdasaryan, A.; Chiba, P.; Trauner, M. Clinical Application of Transcriptional Activators of Bile Salt Transporters. *Mol. Asp. Med.* **2014**, *37*, 57–76. [CrossRef] [PubMed]
54. Beaudoin, J.J.; Brouwer, K.L.R.; Malinen, M.M. Novel Insights into the Organic Solute Transporter Alpha/Beta, OSTα/β: From the Bench to the Bedside. *Pharmacol. Ther.* **2020**, *211*, 107542. [CrossRef]
55. Slijepcevic, D.; van de Graaf, S.F.J. Bile Acid Uptake Transporters as Targets for Therapy. *Dig. Dis.* **2017**, *35*, 251–258. [CrossRef] [PubMed]

56. Slijepcevic, D.; Roscam Abbing, R.L.P.; Fuchs, C.D.; Haazen, L.C.M.; Beuers, U.; Trauner, M.; Oude Elferink, R.P.J.; van de Graaf, S.F.J. Na^+-Taurocholate Cotransporting Polypeptide Inhibition Has Hepatoprotective Effects in Cholestasis in Mice. *Hepatology* **2018**, *68*, 1057–1069. [CrossRef]
57. Kamath, B.M.; Stein, P.; Houwen, R.H.J.; Verkade, H.J. Potential of Ileal Bile Acid Transporter Inhibition as a Therapeutic Target in Alagille Syndrome and Progressive Familial Intrahepatic Cholestasis. *Liver Int.* **2020**, *40*, 1812–1822. [CrossRef] [PubMed]
58. Karpen, S.J.; Kelly, D.; Mack, C.; Stein, P. Ileal Bile Acid Transporter Inhibition as an Anticholestatic Therapeutic Target in Biliary Atresia and Other Cholestatic Disorders. *Hepatol. Int.* **2020**, *14*, 677–689. [CrossRef]
59. Deeks, E.D. Odevixibat: First Approval. *Drugs* **2021**, *81*, 1781–1786. [CrossRef]
60. Mayo, M.J.; Pockros, P.J.; Jones, D.; Bowlus, C.L.; Levy, C.; Patanwala, I.; Bacon, B.; Luketic, V.; Vuppalanchi, R.; Medendorp, S.; et al. A Randomized, Controlled, Phase 2 Study of Maralixibat in the Treatment of Itching Associated with Primary Biliary Cholangitis. *Hepatol. Commun.* **2019**, *3*, 365–381. [CrossRef]
61. Shirley, M. Maralixibat: First Approval. *Drugs* **2022**, *82*, 71–76. [CrossRef]
62. Gonzales, E.; Hardikar, W.; Stormon, M.; Baker, A.; Hierro, L.; Gliwicz, D.; Lacaille, F.; Lachaux, A.; Sturm, E.; Setchell, K.D.R.; et al. Efficacy and Safety of Maralixibat Treatment in Patients with Alagille Syndrome and Cholestatic Pruritus (ICONIC): A Randomised Phase 2 Study. *Lancet* **2021**, *398*, 1581–1592. [CrossRef]
63. Mazzetti, M.; Marconi, G.; Mancinelli, M.; Benedetti, A.; Marzioni, M.; Maroni, L. The Management of Cholestatic Liver Diseases: Current Therapies and Emerging New Possibilities. *J. Clin. Med.* **2021**, *10*, 1763. [CrossRef] [PubMed]
64. Kulkarni, S.R.; Soroka, C.J.; Hagey, L.R.; Boyer, J.L. Sirtuin 1 Activation Alleviates Cholestatic Liver Injury in a Cholic Acid-Fed Mouse Model of Cholestasis. *Hepatology* **2016**, *64*, 2151–2164. [CrossRef] [PubMed]
65. Claveria-Cabello, A.; Colyn, L.; Uriarte, I.; Latasa, M.U.; Arechederra, M.; Herranz, J.M.; Alvarez, L.; Urman, J.M.; Martinez-Chantar, M.L.; Banales, J.M.; et al. Dual Pharmacological Targeting of HDACs and PDE5 Inhibits Liver Disease Progression in a Mouse Model of Biliary Inflammation and Fibrosis. *Cancers* **2020**, *12*, 3748. [CrossRef]
66. Mareux, E.; Lapalus, M.; Amzal, R.; Almes, M.; Aït-Slimane, T.; Delaunay, J.; Adnot, P.; Collado-Hilly, M.; Davit-Spraul, A.; Falguières, T.; et al. Functional Rescue of an ABCB11 Mutant by Ivacaftor: A New Targeted Pharmacotherapy Approach in Bile Salt Export Pump Deficiency. *Liver Int.* **2020**, *40*, 1917–1925. [CrossRef]
67. Cançado, G.G.L.; Couto, C.A.; Guedes, L.V.; Braga, M.H.; Terrabuio, D.R.B.; Cançado, E.L.R.; Ferraz, M.L.G.; Villela-Nogueira, C.A.; Nardelli, M.J.; Faria, L.C.; et al. Fibrates for the Treatment of Primary Biliary Cholangitis Unresponsive to Ursodeoxycholic Acid: An Exploratory Study. *Front. Pharmacol.* **2022**, *12*, 818089. [CrossRef]
68. Joutsiniemi, T.; Timonen, S.; Leino, R.; Palo, P.; Ekblad, U. Ursodeoxycholic Acid in the Treatment of Intrahepatic Cholestasis of Pregnancy: A Randomized Controlled Trial. *Arch. Gynecol. Obstet.* **2014**, *289*, 541–547. [CrossRef]
69. Hopf, C.; Grieshaber, R.; Hartmann, H.; Hinrichsen, H.; Eisold, M.; Cordes, H.-J.; Greinwald, R.; Rust, C. Therapeutic Equivalence of Ursodeoxycholic Acid Tablets and Ursodeoxycholic Acid Capsules for the Treatment of Primary Biliary Cirrhosis. *Clin. Pharmacol. Drug Dev.* **2013**, *2*, 231–236. [CrossRef] [PubMed]
70. Poupon, R.E.; Eschwège, E.; Poupon, R.; Poupon, R.; Poupon, R.E.; Eschwège, E.; Attali, P.; Capron, J.P.; Erlinger, S.; Beaugrand, M.; et al. Ursodeoxycholic Acid for the Treatment of Primary Biliary Cirrhosis. *J. Hepatol.* **1990**, *11*, 16–21. [CrossRef]
71. Jacquemin, E.; Hermans, D.; Myara, A.; Habes, D.; Debray, D.; Hadchouel, M.; Sokal, E.M.; Bernard, O. Ursodeoxycholic Acid Therapy in Pediatric Patients with Progressive Familial Intrahepatic Cholestasis. *Hepatology* **1997**, *25*, 519–523. [CrossRef]
72. Nevens, F.; Andreone, P.; Mazzella, G.; Strasser, S.I.; Bowlus, C.; Invernizzi, P.; Drenth, J.P.H.; Pockros, P.J.; Regula, J.; Beuers, U.; et al. A Placebo-Controlled Trial of Obeticholic Acid in Primary Biliary Cholangitis. *N. Engl. J. Med.* **2016**, *375*, 631–643. [CrossRef]
73. Kowdley, K.V.; Luketic, V.; Chapman, R.; Hirschfield, G.M.; Poupon, R.; Schramm, C.; Vincent, C.; Rust, C.; Parés, A.; Mason, A.; et al. A Randomized Trial of Obeticholic Acid Monotherapy in Patients with Primary Biliary Cholangitis. *Hepatology* **2018**, *67*, 1890–1902. [CrossRef]
74. Schramm, C.; Hirschfield, G.; Mason, A.L.; Wedemeyer, H.; Klickstein, L.; Neelakantham, S.; Koo, P.; Sanni, J.; Badman, M.; Jones, D. Early Assessment of Safety and Efficacy of Tropifexor, a Potent Non Bile-Acid FXR Agonist, in Patients with Primary Biliary Cholangitis: An Interim Analysis of an Ongoing Phase 2 Study. *J. Hepatol.* **2018**, *68*, S103. [CrossRef]
75. Slavetinsky, C.; Sturm, E. Odevixibat and Partial External Biliary Diversion Showed Equal Improvement of Cholestasis in a Patient with Progressive Familial Intrahepatic Cholestasis. *BMJ Case Rep.* **2020**, *13*, e234185. [CrossRef]
76. Baumann, U.; Sturm, E.; Lacaille, F.; Gonzalès, E.; Arnell, H.; Fischler, B.; Jørgensen, M.H.; Thompson, R.J.; Mattsson, J.P.; Ekelund, M.; et al. Effects of Odevixibat on Pruritus and Bile Acids in Children with Cholestatic Liver Disease: Phase 2 Study. *Clin. Res. Hepatol. Gastroenterol.* **2021**, *45*, 101751. [CrossRef]
77. Hegade, V.S.; Kendrick, S.F.W.; Dobbins, R.L.; Miller, S.R.; Thompson, D.; Richards, D.; Storey, J.; Dukes, G.E.; Corrigan, M.; Oude Elferink, R.P.J.; et al. Effect of Ileal Bile Acid Transporter Inhibitor GSK2330672 on Pruritus in Primary Biliary Cholangitis: A Double-Blind, Randomised, Placebo-Controlled, Crossover, Phase 2a Study. *Lancet* **2017**, *389*, 1114–1123. [CrossRef]
78. Cholangitis, H. GLIMMER Trial-A Randomized, Double-Blind, Placebo-Controlled Study of Linerixibat, an Inhibitor of the Ileal Bile Acid Transporter, in the Treatment of Cholestatic Pruritus in Primary Biliary Cholangitis. *Gastroenterol. Hepatol.* **2021**, *17*, 11–12.
79. Sanyal, A.J.; Ling, L.; Beuers, U.; DePaoli, A.M.; Lieu, H.D.; Harrison, S.A.; Hirschfield, G.M. Potent Suppression of Hydrophobic Bile Acids by Aldafermin, an FGF19 Analogue, across Metabolic and Cholestatic Liver Diseases. *JHEP Rep.* **2021**, *3*, 100255. [CrossRef] [PubMed]

80. Corpechot, C.; Chazouillères, O.; Rousseau, A.; Le Gruyer, A.; Habersetzer, F.; Mathurin, P.; Goria, O.; Potier, P.; Minello, A.; Silvain, C.; et al. A Placebo-Controlled Trial of Bezafibrate in Primary Biliary Cholangitis. *N. Engl. J. Med.* **2018**, *378*, 2171–2181. [CrossRef]
81. Schattenberg, J.M.; Pares, A.; Kowdley, K.V.; Heneghan, M.A.; Caldwell, S.; Pratt, D.; Bonder, A.; Hirschfield, G.M.; Levy, C.; Vierling, J.; et al. A Randomized Placebo-Controlled Trial of Elafibranor in Patients with Primary Biliary Cholangitis and Incomplete Response to UDCA. *J. Hepatol.* **2021**, *74*, 1344–1354. [CrossRef]
82. Kremer, A.E.; Mayo, M.J.; Hirschfield, G.; Levy, C.; Bowlus, C.L.; Jones, D.E.; Steinberg, A.; McWherter, C.A.; Choi, Y. Seladelpar Improved Measures of Pruritus, Sleep, and Fatigue and Decreased Serum Bile Acids in Patients with Primary Biliary Cholangitis. *Liver Int.* **2022**, *42*, 112–123. [CrossRef]
83. High, K.A.; Roncarolo, M.G. Gene Therapy. *N. Engl. J. Med.* **2019**, *381*, 455–464. [CrossRef] [PubMed]
84. Szabó, G.T.; Mahiny, A.J.; Vlatkovic, I. COVID-19 mRNA vaccines: Platforms and current developments. *Mol. Ther.* **2022**, *30*, 1850–1868. [CrossRef] [PubMed]
85. Dunbar, C.E.; High, K.A.; Joung, J.K.; Kohn, D.B.; Ozawa, K.; Sadelain, M. Gene Therapy Comes of Age. *Science* **2018**, *359*, eaan4672. [CrossRef] [PubMed]
86. Baruteau, J.; Waddington, S.N.; Alexander, I.E.; Gissen, P. Gene Therapy for Monogenic Liver Diseases: Clinical Successes, Current Challenges and Future Prospects. *J. Inherit. Metab. Dis.* **2017**, *40*, 497–517. [CrossRef]
87. van der Laan, L.J.; Wang, Y.; Tilanus, H.W.; Janssen, H.L.; Pan, Q. AAV-Mediated Gene Therapy for Liver Diseases: The Prime Candidate for Clinical Application? *Expert Opin. Biol. Ther.* **2011**, *11*, 315–327. [CrossRef]
88. Maestro, S.; Weber, N.D.; Zabaleta, N.; Aldabe, R.; Gonzalez-Aseguinolaza, G. Novel Vectors and Approaches for Gene Therapy in Liver Diseases. *JHEP Rep.* **2021**, *3*, 100300. [CrossRef]
89. Mendell, J.R.; Al-Zaidy, S.A.; Rodino-Klapac, L.R.; Goodspeed, K.; Gray, S.J.; Kay, C.N.; Boye, S.L.; Boye, S.E.; George, L.A.; Salabarria, S.; et al. Current Clinical Applications of In Vivo Gene Therapy with AAVs. *Mol. Ther.* **2021**, *29*, 464–488. [CrossRef]
90. Russell, S.; Bennett, J.; Wellman, J.A.; Chung, D.C.; Yu, Z.-F.; Tillman, A.; Wittes, J.; Pappas, J.; Elci, O.; McCague, S.; et al. Efficacy and Safety of Voretigene Neparvovec (AAV2-HRPE65v2) in Patients with RPE65 -Mediated Inherited Retinal Dystrophy: A Randomised, Controlled, Open-Label, Phase 3 Trial. *Lancet* **2017**, *390*, 849–860. [CrossRef]
91. Mendell, J.R.; Al-Zaidy, S.; Shell, R.; Arnold, W.D.; Rodino-Klapac, L.R.; Prior, T.W.; Lowes, L.; Alfano, L.; Berry, K.; Church, K.; et al. Single-Dose Gene-Replacement Therapy for Spinal Muscular Atrophy. *N. Engl. J. Med.* **2017**, *377*, 1713–1722. [CrossRef]
92. Mariotti, V.; Strazzabosco, M.; Fabris, L.; Calvisi, D.F. Animal Models of Biliary Injury and Altered Bile Acid Metabolism. *Biochim. Biophys. Acta-Mol. Basis Dis.* **2018**, *1864*, 1254–1261. [CrossRef]
93. Fernández-Ramos, D.; Fernández-Tussy, P.; Lopitz-Otsoa, F.; Gutiérrez-de-Juan, V.; Navasa, N.; Barbier-Torres, L.; Zubiete-Franco, I.; Simón, J.; Fernández, A.F.; Arbelaiz, A.; et al. MiR-873-5p Acts as an Epigenetic Regulator in Early Stages of Liver Fibrosis and Cirrhosis. *Cell Death Dis.* **2018**, *9*, 958. [CrossRef] [PubMed]
94. Wang, K.P.-C.; Lee, L.-M.; Lin, T.-J.; Sheen-Chen, S.-M.; Lin, J.-W.; Chiu, W.-T.; Wang, C.-C.; Hung, K.-S. Gene Transfer of IGF1 Attenuates Hepatocellular Apoptosis After Bile Duct Ligation. *J. Surg. Res.* **2011**, *167*, 237–244. [CrossRef] [PubMed]
95. Zhong, Z.; Froh, M.; Wheeler, M.; Smutney, O.; Lehmann, T.; Thurman, R. Viral Gene Delivery of Superoxide Dismutase Attenuates Experimental Cholestasis-Induced Liver Fibrosis in the Rat. *Gene Ther.* **2002**, *9*, 183–191. [CrossRef] [PubMed]
96. Bian, Z.; Miao, Q.; Zhong, W.; Zhang, H.; Wang, Q.; Peng, Y.; Chen, X.; Guo, C.; Shen, L.; Yang, F.; et al. Treatment of Cholestatic Fibrosis by Altering Gene Expression of Cthrc1: Implications for Autoimmune and Non-Autoimmune Liver Disease. *J. Autoimmun.* **2015**, *63*, 76–87. [CrossRef]
97. Miranda-Díaz, A.; Rincón, A.R.; Salgado, S.; Vera-Cruz, J.; Gálvez, J.; Islas, M.C.; Berumen, J.; Aguilar Cordova, E.; Armendáriz-Borunda, J. Improved Effects of Viral Gene Delivery of Human UPA plus Biliodigestive Anastomosis Induce Recovery from Experimental Biliary Cirrhosis. *Mol. Ther.* **2004**, *9*, 30–37. [CrossRef]
98. Salgado, S.; Garcia, J.; Vera, J.; Siller, F.; Bueno, M.; Miranda, A.; Segura, A.; Grijalva, G.; Segura, J.; Orozco, H.; et al. Liver Cirrhosis Is Reverted by Urokinase-Type Plasminogen Activator Gene Therapy. *Mol. Ther.* **2000**, *2*, 545–551. [CrossRef]
99. Mak, K.Y.; Chin, R.; Cunningham, S.C.; Habib, M.R.; Torresi, J.; Sharland, A.F.; Alexander, I.E.; Angus, P.W.; Herath, C.B. ACE2 Therapy Using Adeno-Associated Viral Vector Inhibits Liver Fibrosis in Mice. *Mol. Ther.* **2015**, *23*, 1434–1443. [CrossRef]
100. Yang, T.; Poenisch, M.; Khanal, R.; Hu, Q.; Dai, Z.; Li, R.; Song, G.; Yuan, Q.; Yao, Q.; Shen, X.; et al. Therapeutic HNF4A MRNA Attenuates Liver Fibrosis in a Preclinical Model. *J. Hepatol.* **2021**, *75*, 1420–1433. [CrossRef]
101. Marrone, J.; Lehmann, G.L.; Soria, L.R.; Pellegrino, J.M.; Molinas, S.; Marinelli, R.A. Adenoviral Transfer of Human Aquaporin-1 Gene to Rat Liver Improves Bile Flow in Estrogen-Induced Cholestasis. *Gene Ther.* **2014**, *21*, 1058–1064. [CrossRef]
102. Marrone, J.; Soria, L.R.; Danielli, M.; Lehmann, G.L.; Larocca, M.C.; Marinelli, R.A. Hepatic Gene Transfer of Human Aquaporin-1 Improves Bile Salt Secretory Failure in Rats with Estrogen-induced Cholestasis. *Hepatology* **2016**, *64*, 535–548. [CrossRef]
103. Nathwani, A.C.; Tuddenham, E.G.D.; Rangarajan, S.; Rosales, C.; McIntosh, J.; Linch, D.C.; Chowdary, P.; Riddell, A.; Pie, A.J.; Harrington, C.; et al. Adenovirus-Associated Virus Vector–Mediated Gene Transfer in Hemophilia B. *N. Engl. J. Med.* **2011**, *365*, 2357–2365. [CrossRef] [PubMed]
104. Lumbreras, S.; Ricobaraza, A.; Baila-Rueda, L.; Gonzalez-Aparicio, M.; Mora-Jimenez, L.; Uriarte, I.; Bunuales, M.; Avila, M.A.; Monte, M.J.; Marin, J.J.G.; et al. Gene Supplementation of CYP27A1 in the Liver Restores Bile Acid Metabolism in a Mouse Model of Cerebrotendinous Xanthomatosis. *Mol. Ther.-Methods Clin. Dev.* **2021**, *22*, 210–221. [CrossRef] [PubMed]

105. Collaud, F.; Bortolussi, G.; Guianvarc'h, L.; Aronson, S.J.; Bordet, T.; Veron, P.; Charles, S.; Vidal, P.; Sola, M.S.; Rundwasser, S.; et al. Preclinical Development of an AAV8-HUGT1A1 Vector for the Treatment of Crigler-Najjar Syndrome. *Mol. Ther.-Methods Clin. Dev.* **2019**, *12*, 157–174. [CrossRef] [PubMed]
106. Ronzitti, G.; Bortolussi, G.; van Dijk, R.; Collaud, F.; Charles, S.; Leborgne, C.; Vidal, P.; Martin, S.; Gjata, B.; Sola, M.S.; et al. A Translationally Optimized AAV-UGT1A1 Vector Drives Safe and Long-Lasting Correction of Crigler-Najjar Syndrome. *Mol. Ther.-Methods Clin. Dev.* **2016**, *3*, 16049. [CrossRef]
107. Ginocchio, V.M.; Ferla, R.; Auricchio, A.; Brunetti-Pierri, N. Current Status on Clinical Development of Adeno-Associated Virus-Mediated Liver-Directed Gene Therapy for Inborn Errors of Metabolism. *Hum. Gene Ther.* **2019**, *30*, 1204–1210. [CrossRef] [PubMed]
108. Bull, L.N.; Thompson, R.J. Progressive Familial Intrahepatic Cholestasis. *Clin. Liver Dis.* **2018**, *22*, 657–669. [CrossRef]
109. Bosma, P.J.; Wits, M.; Oude-Elferink, R.P.J. Gene Therapy for Progressive Familial Intrahepatic Cholestasis: Current Progress and Future Prospects. *Int. J. Mol. Sci.* **2020**, *22*, 273. [CrossRef]
110. de Vree, J.M.L.; Ottenhoff, R.; Bosma, P.J.; Smith, A.J.; Aten, J.; Oude Elferink, R.P.J. Correction of Liver Disease by Hepatocyte Transplantation in a Mouse Model of Progressive Familial Intrahepatic Cholestasis. *Gastroenterology* **2000**, *119*, 1720–1730. [CrossRef]
111. Ikenaga, N.; Liu, S.B.; Sverdlov, D.Y.; Yoshida, S.; Nasser, I.; Ke, Q.; Kang, P.M.; Popov, Y. A New Mdr2$^{-/-}$ Mouse Model of Sclerosing Cholangitis with Rapid Fibrosis Progression, Early-Onset Portal Hypertension, and Liver Cancer. *Am. J. Pathol.* **2015**, *185*, 325–334. [CrossRef]
112. Aronson, S.J.; Bakker, R.S.; Shi, X.; Duijst, S.; Bloemendaal, L.T.; de Waart, D.R.; Verheij, J.; Ronzitti, G.; Elferink, R.P.O.; Beuers, U.; et al. Liver-Directed Gene Therapy Results in Long-Term Correction of Progressive Familial Intrahepatic Cholestasis Type 3 in Mice. *J. Hepatol.* **2019**, *71*, 153–162. [CrossRef]
113. Weber, N.D.; Odriozola, L.; Martínez-García, J.; Ferrer, V.; Douar, A.; Bénichou, B.; González-Aseguinolaza, G.; Smerdou, C. Gene Therapy for Progressive Familial Intrahepatic Cholestasis Type 3 in a Clinically Relevant Mouse Model. *Nat. Commun.* **2019**, *10*, 5694. [CrossRef] [PubMed]
114. Wei, G.; Cao, J.; Huang, P.; An, P.; Badlani, D.; Vaid, K.A.; Zhao, S.; Wang, D.Q.-H.; Zhuo, J.; Yin, L.; et al. Synthetic Human ABCB4 MRNA Therapy Rescues Severe Liver Disease Phenotype in a BALB/c.Abcb4 Mouse Model of PFIC3. *J. Hepatol.* **2021**, *74*, 1416–1428. [CrossRef] [PubMed]
115. Weber, N.D.; Martínez-García, J.; González-Aseguinolaza, G. Comment on "Synthetic Human ABCB4 MRNA Therapy Rescues Severe Liver Disease Phenotype in a BALB/c.Abcb4 Mouse Model of PFIC3". *J. Hepatol.* **2022**, *76*, 749–751. [CrossRef] [PubMed]
116. Siew, S.M.; Cunningham, S.C.; Zhu, E.; Tay, S.S.; Venuti, E.; Bolitho, C.; Alexander, I.E. Prevention of Cholestatic Liver Disease and Reduced Tumorigenicity in a Murine Model of PFIC Type 3 Using Hybrid AAV-PiggyBac Gene Therapy. *Hepatology* **2019**, *70*, 2047–2061. [CrossRef] [PubMed]
117. Rajapaksha, I.G.; Angus, P.W.; Herath, C.B. Current Therapies and Novel Approaches for Biliary Diseases. *World J. Gastrointest. Pathophysiol.* **2019**, *10*, 1–10. [CrossRef]
118. Li, J.; Zhu, X.; Zhang, M.; Zhang, Y.; Ye, S.; Leng, Y.; Yang, T.; Kong, L.; Zhang, H. Limb Expression 1-like (LIX1L) Protein Promotes Cholestatic Liver Injury by Regulating Bile Acid Metabolism. *J. Hepatol.* **2021**, *75*, 400–413. [CrossRef]
119. Ceci, L.; Francis, H.; Zhou, T.; Giang, T.; Yang, Z.; Meng, F.; Wu, N.; Kennedy, L.; Kyritsi, K.; Meadows, V.; et al. Knockout of the Tachykinin Receptor 1 in the Mdr2$^{-/-}$ (Abcb4$^{-/-}$) Mouse Model of Primary Sclerosing Cholangitis Reduces Biliary Damage and Liver Fibrosis. *Am. J. Pathol.* **2020**, *190*, 2251–2266. [CrossRef]
120. Giang, S.; Gordon, R.L.; Haas, K.B. A Diagnostic Quagmire: PFIC5 Presenting as a Rare Cause of Neonatal Cholestasis. *ACG Case Rep. J.* **2021**, *8*, e00558. [CrossRef]
121. Sambrotta, M.; Strautnieks, S.; Papouli, E.; Rushton, P.; Clark, B.E.; Parry, D.A.; Logan, C.V.; Newbury, L.J.; Kamath, B.M.; Ling, S.; et al. Mutations in TJP2 Cause Progressive Cholestatic Liver Disease. *Nat. Genet.* **2014**, *46*, 326–328. [CrossRef]
122. Overeem, A.W.; Li, Q.; Qiu, Y.; Cartón-García, F.; Leng, C.; Klappe, K.; Dronkers, J.; Hsiao, N.; Wang, J.; Arango, D.; et al. A Molecular Mechanism Underlying Genotype-Specific Intrahepatic Cholestasis Resulting From MYO5B Mutations. *Hepatology* **2020**, *72*, 213–229. [CrossRef]
123. Zhang, Y.; Li, F.; Patterson, A.D.; Wang, Y.; Krausz, K.W.; Neale, G.; Thomas, S.; Nachagari, D.; Vogel, P.; Vore, M.; et al. Abcb11 Deficiency Induces Cholestasis Coupled to Impaired β-Fatty Acid Oxidation in Mice. *J. Biol. Chem.* **2012**, *287*, 24784–24794. [CrossRef] [PubMed]
124. Hu, C.; Busuttil, R.W.; Lipshutz, G.S. RH10 Provides Superior Transgene Expression in Mice When Compared with Natural AAV Serotypes for Neonatal Gene Therapy. *J. Gene Med.* **2010**, *12*, 766–778. [CrossRef] [PubMed]
125. Kowalski, P.S.; Rudra, A.; Miao, L.; Anderson, D.G. Delivering the Messenger: Advances in Technologies for Therapeutic MRNA Delivery. *Mol. Ther.* **2019**, *27*, 710–728. [CrossRef] [PubMed]
126. Rivière, C.; Danos, O.; Douar, A.M. Long-Term Expression and Repeated Administration of AAV Type 1, 2 and 5 Vectors in Skeletal Muscle of Immunocompetent Adult Mice. *Gene Ther.* **2006**, *13*, 1300–1308. [CrossRef]
127. Ros-Gañán, I.; Hommel, M.; Trigueros-Motos, L.; Tamarit, B.; Rodríguez-García, E.; Salas, D.; Pérez, G.; Douar, A.; Combal, J.P.; Benichou, B.; et al. Optimising the IgG-degrading Enzyme Treatment Regimen for Enhanced Adeno-associated Virus Transduction in the Presence of Neutralising Antibodies. *Clin. Transl. Immunol.* **2022**, *11*, e1375. [CrossRef]

128. Meliani, A.; Boisgerault, F.; Hardet, R.; Marmier, S.; Collaud, F.; Ronzitti, G.; Leborgne, C.; Verdera, H.C.; Sola, M.S.; Charles, S.; et al. Antigen-Selective Modulation of AAV Immunogenicity with Tolerogenic Rapamycin Nanoparticles Enables Successful Vector Re-Administration. *Nat. Commun.* **2018**, *9*, 4098. [CrossRef]
129. Buscara, L.; Gross, D.-A.; Daniele, N. Of RAAV and Men: From Genetic Neuromuscular Disorder Efficacy and Toxicity Preclinical Studies to Clinical Trials and Back. *J. Pers. Med.* **2020**, *10*, 258. [CrossRef]
130. Chand, D.; Mohr, F.; McMillan, H.; Tukov, F.F.; Montgomery, K.; Kleyn, A.; Sun, R.; Tauscher-Wisniewski, S.; Kaufmann, P.; Kullak-Ublick, G. Hepatotoxicity Following Administration of Onasemnogene Abeparvovec (AVXS-101) for the Treatment of Spinal Muscular Atrophy. *J. Hepatol.* **2021**, *74*, 560–566. [CrossRef]
131. Suzuki, M.; Singh, R.N.; Crystal, R.G. Regulatable Promoters for Use in Gene Therapy Applications: Modification of the 5′-Flanking Region of the CFTR Gene with Multiple CAMP Response Elements to Support Basal, Low-Level Gene Expression That Can Be Upregulated by Exogenous Agents That Raise Int. *Hum. Gene Ther.* **1996**, *7*, 1883–1893. [CrossRef]
132. Martínez-García, J.; Molina, M.; Odriozola, L.; Molina, A.; González-Aseguinolaza, G.; Weber, N.D.; Smerdou, C. A Minimal Bile Salt Excretory Pump Promoter Allows Bile Acid-Driven Physiological Regulation of Transgene Expression from a Gene Therapy Vector. *Cell Biosci.* **2022**, *12*. [CrossRef]
133. Chen, S.-J.; Johnston, J.; Sandhu, A.; Bish, L.T.; Hovhannisyan, R.; Jno-Charles, O.; Sweeney, H.L.; Wilson, J.M. Enhancing the Utility of Adeno-Associated Virus Gene Transfer through Inducible Tissue-Specific Expression. *Hum. Gene Ther. Methods* **2013**, *24*, 270–278. [CrossRef] [PubMed]
134. Toscano, M.G.; Romero, Z.; Muñoz, P.; Cobo, M.; Benabdellah, K.; Martin, F. Physiological and Tissue-Specific Vectors for Treatment of Inherited Diseases. *Gene Ther.* **2011**, *18*, 117–127. [CrossRef] [PubMed]
135. Konkle, B.A.; Walsh, C.E.; Escobar, M.A.; Josephson, N.C.; Young, G.; von Drygalski, A.; McPhee, S.W.J.; Samulski, R.J.; Bilic, I.; de la Rosa, M.; et al. BAX 335 Hemophilia B Gene Therapy Clinical Trial Results: Potential Impact of CpG Sequences on Gene Expression. *Blood* **2021**, *137*, 763–774. [CrossRef] [PubMed]
136. Wright, J.F. Codon Modification and PAMPs in Clinical AAV Vectors: The Tortoise or the Hare? *Mol. Ther.* **2020**, *28*, 701–703. [CrossRef] [PubMed]
137. Suzuki, K.; Tsunekawa, Y.; Hernandez-Benitez, R.; Wu, J.; Zhu, J.; Kim, E.J.; Hatanaka, F.; Yamamoto, M.; Araoka, T.; Li, Z.; et al. In Vivo Genome Editing via CRISPR/Cas9 Mediated Homology-Independent Targeted Integration. *Nature* **2016**, *540*, 144–149. [CrossRef] [PubMed]

biomedicines

Review

Update on the Pharmacological Treatment of Primary Biliary Cholangitis

Annarosa Floreani [1,2], Daniela Gabbia [3] and Sara De Martin [3,*]

[1] Department of Surgery, Oncology and Gastroenterology, University of Padova, 35131 Padova, Italy
[2] IRCCS Negrar, 37024 Verona, Italy
[3] Department of Pharmaceutical and Pharmacological Sciences, University of Padova, 35131 Padova, Italy
* Correspondence: sara.demartin@unipd.it

Abstract: Ursodeoxycholic acid (UDCA) is the first-line therapy used for the treatment of PBC. In recent years, new pharmacological agents have been proposed for PBC therapy to cure UDCA-non-responders. Obeticholic acid (OCA) is registered in many countries for PBC, and fibrates also seem to be effective in ameliorating biochemistry alteration and symptoms typical of PBC. Moreover, a variety of new agents, acting with different mechanisms of action, are under clinical evaluation for PBC treatment, including PPAR agonists, anti-NOX agents, immunomodulators, and mesenchymal stem cell transplantation. Since an insufficient amount of data is currently available about the effect of these novel approaches on robust clinical endpoints, such as transplant-free survival, their clinical approval needs to be supported by the consistent improvement of these parameters. The intensive research in this field will hopefully lead to a novel treatment landscape for PBC in the near future, with innovative therapies based on the combination of multiple agents acting on different pathogenetic mechanisms.

Keywords: PBC; ursodeoxycholic acid (UDCA); obeticholic acid (OCA); fibrates; FXR agonists; PPAR agonists; budesonide

Citation: Floreani, A.; Gabbia, D.; De Martin, S. Update on the Pharmacological Treatment of Primary Biliary Cholangitis. *Biomedicines* **2022**, *10*, 2033. https://doi.org/10.3390/biomedicines10082033

Academic Editor: Jinghua Wang

Received: 22 July 2022
Accepted: 18 August 2022
Published: 20 August 2022

1. Introduction

Primary biliary cholangitis (PBC) is a chronic liver disease characterized by autoimmune responses, in which the small interlobular bile ducts are progressively disrupted, causing cholestasis. As in other chronic liver diseases, PBC can evolve into hepatic fibrosis and cirrhosis, causing the need for liver transplantation to prevent liver failure and death [1]. In regard to its geographical distribution, the highest number of patients is diagnosed in Northern Europe and North America, even though this disease is also quite common in Europe (mainly in the Southern countries), Asia, and Australia. Its global prevalence is 14.6 per 100.000, and the global incidence is 1.76 per 100,000 per year [2,3]. A gender difference can be observed in PBC patients, with a female predominancy. A F/M ratio of 9:1 was reported in a cohort series analyzing epidemiology, natural history, and clinical characteristics of PBC patients [1].

The clinical features and natural evolution of PBC may vary greatly between patients, who can experience either asymptomatic, slowly progressive, symptomatic, or rapidly evolving disease. Over the last 30 years, a modification of PBC symptoms was observed, which has changed from a disease with evident clinical manifestations, such as portal hypertension, to a milder condition, characterized by a long outcome [4]. The etiology of PBC is complex, and some mechanistic issues remain to be solved. Nevertheless, there is a general consensus indicating a predisposing genetic background that could lead to the onset of the disease in combination with infective, immunological, and/or environmental triggers [5–7]. The therapeutic management of PBC is a fascinating challenge, and several drugs with different mechanisms of action are either approved or under development (Figure 1).

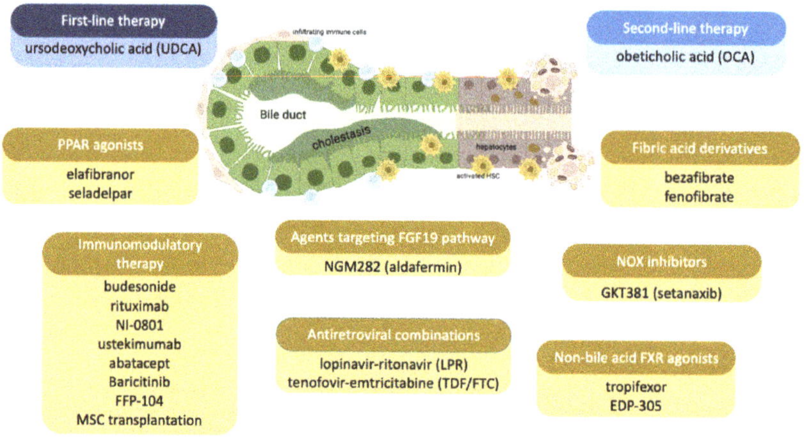

Figure 1. Drugs approved (in blue) or under evaluation (in yellow) for the treatment of PBC.

2. Ursodeoxycholic Acid (UDCA) as First-Line PBC Therapy

The standard therapy for PBC is currently ursodeoxycholic acid (UDCA), a natural hydrophilic tertiary bile acid with choleretic properties, used in clinical practice at the dose of 13–15 mg/Kg per day, according to the European guidelines. The mechanism of action of UDCA is complex and involves several molecular pathways, which have been extensively studied in preclinical settings. There is a general consensus that its therapeutic effect on PBC is mainly due to: (1) the stimulation of hepatocellular secretion and (2) the stimulation of cholangiocellular secretion, both resulting in a choleretic effect; (3) anti-apoptotic effects on hepatocytes; (4) the reduction of bile acid toxicity. UDCA exerts its mechanisms of action by interacting with a panel nuclear receptors, i.e., retinoid X receptor (RXR), peroxisome proliferator-activated receptor α (PPARα), and pregnane X receptor (PXR), all of which transcriptionally modulate the synthesis and homeostasis of bile components [8]. The drug is given as a single dose, or divided into multiple doses, due to tolerability issues [9]. Observational studies evaluating PBC patients treated with UDCA helped to define an achievement of biochemical response in therapy-responding patients, evaluating also the prolongation of liver transplant (LT)-free survival, with respect to non-responders. Altogether, the data collected with these clinical studies helped to define a population of PBC patients in which UCDA therapy is beneficial [10–15]. A multicentric study evaluating PBC patients treated with UDCA or placebo demonstrated that plasma bilirubin values below the current upper limits of normal (ULN) are predictive of survival, and a threshold of 0.6 x ULN was selected for assessing the increased risk of LT or death [16]. Furthermore, a study observed that a relevant proportion of PBC patients has an incomplete biochemical response to UDCA therapy, according to the Paris II criteria, and the presence of cirrhosis, elevated GGT, and alkaline phosphatase (ALP) at diagnosis could represent predictive factors for an incomplete UDCA response [17]. However, UDCA therapy has been demonstrated to improve LT-free survival in all PBC patients, irrespective of diseases severity and whether or not they meet the accepted criteria for the definition of a UDCA responder [18]. Thus, these observations are likely to prove that the improvement of cholestatic biochemical parameters in PBC patients, even of modest entity, can generate long-term benefits. However, despite all these efforts, the correlation between the lack of UDCA efficacy and survival in PBC patients still needs to be defined in detail. Two groups, i.e., the Global PBC Study Group and the United Kingdom (UK)-PBC Consortium, have been created with the aim of setting up a prognostic model for disease progression in UDCA-treated patients. These two groups independently developed and evaluated the risk of PBC progression. In 2015, the first score, called the GLOBE score, was introduced to assess PBC risk progression. The setting up of this score accounted for a wide derivation cohort (accounting for 2488 patients) and a validation cohort accounting for 1634 UDCA-treated patients. In the same years, another score was proposed by the United Kingdom (UK)-PBC Consortium, called the UK-PBC risk score (www.uk.pbc.com (accessed on 15 July 2022)), based on a nation-wide cohort of 1916 patients and validated in a cohort of 1249 UDCA-treated patients. These two predictive models have also been validated in PBC subjects not treated with UDCA, providing indications of disease activity and stage, based on biochemical liver function markers. The two main differences between the two models rely on the different endpoints used for calculating the scores. First, the GLOBE-PBC score takes into account all-cause mortality, in addition to LT-related mortality, whereas the UK-PBC score considers only liver-related death. Interestingly, in the study population of the Obeticholic Acid International Study of Efficacy (PBC POISE), both models demonstrated a potential usefulness in individualizing risk prediction, both in clinical practice and therapeutic trials for PBC [19]. It should be noted that the UDCA non-responder patients are around 30–40% of all UDCA-treated patients. Since they have a poorer prognosis due to a higher risk of disease progression, and the plausibility to require liver transplantation, as well as a greater mortality risk [20], the identification of novel effective treatments still represents an urgent medical need.

3. Other Therapeutic Agents for PBC

To overcome the problem of the incomplete response to UDCA and/or toxicity issues, several alternative therapeutic approaches have been proposed, and many clinical trials are currently ongoing to assess the possibility of repositioning approved drugs after the demonstration of their efficacy in PBC patients. Furthermore, a variety of candidate drugs are under evaluation in clinical trials for PBC patients because of their promising mechanisms of action, i.e., bile acid modulation, immunomodulation, and antifibrotic and anti-inflammatory effects. Table 1 summarizes the ongoing clinical trials.

Table 1. Ongoing controlled trials with experimental agents in PBC.

Agent	Study Design	Aim/Outcome	Nr. pts	Phase	Duration	NCT nr.
PPAR agonists						
BEZA	RCT	Utility of BEZA as add-on therapy/complete biochemical response	34	3	12 m	NCT02937012
FENO	RCT	Clinical efficacy of FENO + UDCA/amelioration of ALP	72	1–2	12 m	NCT02965911
FENO	OL	Utility of FENO + UDCA/complete biochemical response	200	3	44 w	NCT02823353
Seladelpar	OL	Long-term safety and tolerability of seladelpar/measures of adverse events, death	500	3	60 m	NCT03301506
Seladelpar	RCT	Safety and effect of 2 seladelpar regimens on cholestasis/percentage of participants to composite endpoint	240	3	52 w	NCT03602560
BEZA	observational	Influence of BEZA on macrophage activation markers and fibrosis/sCD163 levels	100	3	36 m	NCT04514965
Seladelpar	RCT	Effect of seladelpar on cholestasis/composite endpoint of ALP and total bilirubin	180	3	12 m	NCT04620733
Seladelpar	OL	Effect of hepatic impairment on the pharmacokinetics of seladelpar/pharmacokinetic measures	24	1	17 w	NCT04950764

Table 1. *Cont.*

Agent	Study Design	Aim/Outcome	Nr. pts	Phase	Duration	NCT nr.
Saroglitazar Mg	RCT	Safety, tolerability, and efficacy of saroglitazar/improvement in ALP levels	36	2	16 w	NCT03112681
Saroglitazar Mg (EPICS-III)	RCT	Efficacy and safety of saroglitazas/ biochemical response on the composite endpoint of ALP and total bilirubin	192	2 b–3	52 w	NCT05133336
FXR agonists + PPAR agonists						
OCA + BEZA	RCT	Effect of OCA + BEZA/change in ALP	75	2	12 w	NCT04594694
OCA + BEZA	RCT	Effect of BEZA alone or in combination with OCA/change in ALP	60	2	12 w	NCT05239468
FXR Agonists						
EDP-305	RCT	Safety, tolerability, and efficacy of EDP-305/percentage of participants with at least 20% reduction in ALP	119	2	12 w	NCT03394924
Cilofexor	RCT	Safety and tolerability of cilofexor/percentage of adverse events	71	2	12 w + 30 d	NCT02943447
Immunomodulants						
Baricitinib	RCT	Safety and efficacy of baricitinib/change in ALP	52	2	12 w	NCT03742973
MSCs transplantation	RCT	Safety and efficacy of MSC/change in ALP	14	1–2	12 m	NCT03668145
MSCs transplantation	RCT	Safety and efficacy of UC-MSC/change in ALP	100	1–2	12 w	NCT01662973
CNP-104 nanoparticle Incapsulating PDC-E2	RCT	Safety, tolerability, pharmacodynamics of CNP-104 nanoparticle/frequency of adverse events, changes in ALP	40	2	12 d + 20 m	NCT05104853
Antiretroviral therapy						
Tenofovir, raltegravir	RCT	Efficacy of antiretroviral therapy/change in ALP	60	2	24 m	NCT03954327

Abbreviations: OCA = obeticholic acid; OL = open label; RCT = randomized controlled trial; MSCs = mesenchymal stem cells; N/A = not available.

3.1. Obeticholic Acid

The only second-line drug approved for the treatment of PBC is obeticholic acid (OCA), which is indicated for patients who are non-tolerant or non-responding to UDCA after 12 months of treatment. OCA is a chemically modified derivative of BA chenodeoxycholic acid. Its mechanism relies on an agonistic activity on the farnesoid X receptor (FXR). Thanks to its affinity to FXR, OCA regulates the synthesis and export of bile acids (BAs), thereby preventing hepatic toxicity due to their toxic accumulation [21]. Beside the regulation of BA homeostasis, its complex and multifaced mechanism of action comprises anti-inflammatory and antifibrotic effects, as demonstrated by preclinical and clinical studies [21,22], thereby targeting a panel of pathological processes involved in PBC development.

The first clinical indication for the use of OCA in monotherapy came from an international randomized, double blind, placebo-controlled phase 2 study investigating the benefit of treating PBC patients with OCA in monotherapy [23]. In this study, patients were randomized into three groups, i.e., 23 PBC patients treated with placebo, 20 with

OCA (10 mg dose), and 16 patients with OCA (50 mg dose) for 3 months. As a primary endpoint, the ALP percentage change from baseline was considered. OCA significantly reduced ALP levels in patients treated at both dosage with respect to placebo. This study also reported an improvement in many biochemical parameters, among which were GGT, alanine aminotransferase, conjugated bilirubin, and immunoglobulins. The most common adverse drug reactions (ADRs) observed after OCA therapy was pruritus, which was reported in this study in patients treated with both OCA 10 mg (15%) and 50 mg (38%).

The FDA approved OCA in 2016 after the results of the phase 3 international trial POISE, with a multicentric randomized controlled design, enrolling more than 200 PBC patients [24]. Interestingly, it should be emphasized that more than 50% of UDCA-non-responders had a beneficial effect by receiving the combination therapy of OCA plus UDCA for 12 months, as indicated by the achievement of the clinical endpoint, which was an ALP level lower than 1.67 times ULN, reduced by at least 15% from baseline. After 12 months, all patients received OCA therapy in the extension phase [25]. In the following 3-year interim analysis, OCA obtained good results on both efficacy and safety, demonstrating a stable therapeutic performance, even associated with a significant reduction in total and direct bilirubin, more evident in patients with high baseline direct bilirubin [26], and good tolerability. The most common adverse drug reactions (ADRs) reported in the POISE trial were pruritus and fatigue, which were experienced by 77% and 33% of OCA-treated patients, respectively [26]. Pruritus received the score "mild-to-moderate" by the visual analogue scale (VAS), and 8% of patients (n = 16) had to withdraw due to this ADR. However, most patients experiencing severe pruritus have been treated with specific drugs. The histological analysis of a subgroup of 17 patients recruited in the POISE trial who underwent liver biopsy at the time of enrollment and after 3 years of treatment, showed that the chronic therapy with OCA led to an improvement or at least a stabilization of the histology of PBC patients, assessed by evaluating ductular injury, fibrosis, and collagen morphometry [27]. Another sub-analysis of patients enrolled in the POISE trial investigated the beneficial effects of OCA on AST to platelet ratio (APRI) and transient elastography (TE), which are both non-invasive markers of liver fibrosis [28]. A significant APRI reduction from the baseline could be observed in OCA-treated patients and during the open-label extension phase with respect to placebo-treated group. Furthermore, the treatment with OCA 10 mg caused a decreasing tendency toward liver stiffness, while both patients treated with lower dosages of OCA or placebo showed a mean increase in liver stiffness [28]. Despite the small sample size, this study can be considered as a milestone in PBC therapy, since it demonstrated that most patients who respond inadequately to UDCA ameliorated or stabilized multiple histological PBC features when treated with OCA.

The decision to implement PBC pharmacological therapy with OCA deserves consideration if at least one of the following conditions is met: (i) ALP $\geq$ 1.67 x ULN (in Italy, the ALP threshold is 1.5 ULN); (ii) total bilirubin > ULN, but < 2 x ULN.

Three clinical studies analyzing real-world cohorts of OCA patients have been published so far, all reporting results for 12 months of OCA treatment [29–31]. The first real-world analysis on the effectiveness of OCA treatment was conducted on 64 Canadian PBC patients experiencing incomplete UDCA response, or who were intolerant to UDCA [29]. Among the 44 patients meeting the inclusion criteria of POISE, 39% (n = 17) underwent a 1-year biochemical evaluation. While only 18% of these patients (3 out of 17) reached the POISE primary endpoint after 12 months of treatment, 43% of patients (9 out of 21) achieved this target after a 19-month observation period. Overall, a significant ALP, GGT, transaminases, and IgM reduction was reported in the whole cohort. As regarding pruritus, either new onset or exacerbation was reported in 26 patients (41%), and 5 of them had to discontinue the drug for this reason. Other reasons for therapy discontinuation reported in this cohort were skin rash (n = 2), liver toxicity (n = 2), and incomplete response after 12 months of treatment (n = 2). In the Iberian cohort [30], 120 patients were enrolled (21.7% of them had cirrhosis and 26.7% received or were taking concomitant treatment with fibrates). A total of 78 patients completed at least 1 year of treatment. The GLOBE-PBC score significantly decreased to 0.17 ($p = 0.005$), whereas the UK-PBC score decreased to 0.17, without reaching any significant difference ($p = 0.11$). According to the POISE criteria, 29.5% of patients achieved a response. In the Italian cohort recruited into the Italian PBC registry, 191 patients were analyzed [31], and 43% of them responded to OCA, according to the POISE criteria. Patients with cirrhosis showed lower efficacy (29.5%). Patients with AIH/PBC overlap syndrome showed a comparable efficacy to classical PBC, with a higher ALT reduction at 6 months. A further analysis was conducted in 100 cirrhotic patients from the Italian cohort (De Vincentis A, unpublished). The response to treatment, according to the POISE criteria, was obtained in 41% of cases, also confirming the efficacy of the drug in cirrhotic stage. Of note, by applying the normal range criteria, 11.5% of the cirrhotic patients reached the endpoint. A total of 22 patients (22%) discontinued the treatment due to severe side effects (5 patients with jaundice and/or ascitic decompensation and 4 with upper digestive bleeding. One patient died after TIPS placement).

3.2. Non-Bile Acid FXR Agonists

Three compounds without the classical bile acid structure, but able to bind and activate FXR, have been proposed to treat PBC patients, i.e., tropifexor, cilofexor, and EDP-305.

Tropifexor is a highly potent FXR agonist with a positive effect in treating both cholestasis and steatosis in animal models, mainly by reducing fibrosis [32]. A phase 2 study investigated tropifexor efficacy in PBC patients characterized by an inadequate UDCA response. Patients were randomized in arms, receiving once daily doses of 30 µg, 60 µg, or 90 µg of tropifexor or placebo for 4 weeks [33]. Moreover, an interim analysis was conducted in the cohort of patients treated with 90 µg. In this group of patients, a rapid decrease in the levels of GGT (72% reduction), ALP, ALT, and AST could be observed at day 28, as well as a good tolerability of tropifexor. HDL was reduced by 33% and 26% at the doses of 60 and 90 µg, respectively, and restored to physiological levels by the end of the study. No increase was observed in total or LDL cholesterol. The results of this trial suggested that this FXR agonist is a candidate drug for PBC therapy [33].

Another non-steroidal FXR agonist, called cilofexor, was tested in a trial (NCT02943447) enrolling 71 UDCA non-responders with PBC. They were randomized into three groups treated with 30 or 100 mg cilofexor or placebo once a day for 12 weeks. Patients treated with 100 mg cilofexor achieved a significant median reduction in GGT (8–47.7%, $p < 0.001$), ALT (8–13.8%, $p = 0.05$), C-reactive protein (8–33.6%, $p = 0.03$), and primary bile acids (−30.5%, $p = 0.008$). The reduction in ALP was greater than 25% in 17% of the patients treated with the dose of 100 mg and in 18% of those treated with 30 mg cilofexor, in comparison with 0% obtained in the placebo group. The major ADR observed after cilofexor treatment was pruritus, particularly common in patients treated with the higher dose. Moreover, promising results were obtained from a phase 3 trial in patients with PSC, thus suggesting the potential benefit of using this new non-bile acid FXR agonist [34].

EDP-305 is a potent FXR agonist with a "mixed" structure, containing steroid and non-steroid moieties, without the classical carboxylic acid group of the other FXR agonists or natural bile acids. The INTREPID study (NCT03394924) evaluated its safety, tolerability, and efficacy in PBC patients with inadequate response to UDCA. A total of 68 subjects were randomized to receive either EDP-305 2.5 mg, 1 mg, or placebo for 42 weeks [35]. The primary endpoint was the proportion of patients with at least 20% ALP reduction from the pre-treatment value, or normalization of ALP at week 12. The intention-to-treat analysis showed that EDP-305 resulted in ALP reduction of 45% and 46% in the 1 mg and 2.5 mg treatment groups, respectively, whereas this reduction was only 11% in the placebo group. Five patients treated with 2.5 mg EDP-305 had severe pruritus. Pruritus was present in 51% of the 2.5 mg-treated patients, whereas less than 10% of patients treated with 1 mg experienced it. In general, the other most common ADRs were gastrointestinal-related symptoms, e.g., nausea, vomiting, diarrhea, or headache, and dizziness.

3.3. PPAR Agonists: Fibrates

Fibric acid derivatives, also called fibrates, are an old class of lipid-lowering agents proposed as a second-line PBC therapy in the late 1990s. The first drug belonging to this class was clofibrate, discovered in 1962 [36]. These drugs attracted great attention for treating PBC patients because they showed efficacy against cholestasis, inflammation, and fibrosis. Their mechanism of action relies on their agonist effect on peroxisome proliferator-activated receptors (PPARs), a family of nuclear receptors (NRs). Three main isoforms of PPARs have been described, i.e., α, β/δ, and γ, each encoded by distinct genes and characterized by a peculiar tissue distribution. Each fibric acid derivate displays a peculiar pattern of affinity towards these three PPAR isoforms, thus differently modulating PPAR-related pathways. Fenofibrate, by binding to PPARα, stimulates the transcription of the multidrug resistance protein 3 (MDR3) transporter, increasing the biliary secretion of phosphatidylcholine and improving cholestasis biomarkers [37]. At variance, bezafibrate, beside binding to PPARα and γ, is also an agonist of pregnane X receptor (PXR) [38], another transcription factor implicated in cholestatic liver disease [39]. The first placebo-controlled trial investigating the efficacy of fibrates in PBC treatment was the BEZURSO trial, a phase 3 study proposing a combination therapy with bezafibrate (BEZA) and UDCA. This study demonstrated that the addition of BEZA to the previous monotherapy of UDCA induced a significantly higher biochemical response with respect to patients of the placebo/UDCA arm [40]. This result was also associated with an improvement in PBC symptoms and surrogate markers of fibrosis. The main ADRs associated with the use of fibrates were linked to creatinine and transaminase increase and heartburn. In addition, gallstone formation, perhaps as consequence of the reduction in BA synthesis, and a paradoxical increase in cholesterol, have also been reported in PBC patients treated with clofibrate, even though the same ADRs have not been observed in patients treated with fenofibrate (FENO) or bezafibrate [41].

To compare the efficacy of OCA and fibrates as second-line therapies, a multicentric retrospective study including PBC patients from 30 centers has been undertaken in Spain [42]. A total of 86 patients receiving OCA (5 mg), 250 patients receiving fibrates (81% BEZA 400 mg, 19% FENO 200 mg), and 15 receiving OCA plus fibrates were enrolled. Both treatments decreased GGT and transaminases and improved the GLOBE score. ALP decrease was higher in patients treated with fibrates, whereas alanine aminotransferase was lower in OCA-treated patients. Discontinuation was more frequent in fenofibrate treatment due to low tolerability or the onset of ADRs. In summary, neither OCA nor fibrates emerged as a significantly better second-line treatment for PBC. Caution should be recommended, in any case.

At the AASLD meeting in Boston in 2019 [43], the results of another trial assessing the comparative efficacy of BEZA or OCA in 59 patients was presented. This study did not reveal significant differences in the incidence of severe hepatic impairment manifestations, such as varices, variceal bleeding, ascites, and LT list insertion between patients treated with OCA or bezafibrate. However, ALP reduction was more evident in bezafibrate-treated patients with respect to those treated with OCA ($p < 0.001$). A higher percentage of BEZA-treated patients experienced an elevation of bilirubin. These two studies offer great insight by presenting real-world data regarding the use of OCA and fibrates in PBC patients, paving the way for the design of future trials.

The additive effects of the combination of fibrates and OCA were investigated in a multicenter retrospective cohort of 58 patients with PBC [44]. A total of 50 of them were treated with a combination of OCA (5–10 mg/day), fibrates (BEZA 400 mg/day or FENO 200 mg/day), and UDCA (13–15 mg/day). Triple therapy was associated with a significant decrease in ALP levels with respect to dual therapy, and with an odds ratio for ALP normalization of 5.5 (95% CI: 1.8–17.1, $p = 0.003$).

Regarding the effect of fibrates on pruritus, this deserves a separate discussion. The benefit of fibrates in improving this symptom is well documented. The Fibrates for Cholestatic Itch (FITCH) trial was designed to investigate the effects of BEZA on pruritus in 70 patients with PBC, primary sclerosing cholangitis (PSC), or secondary sclerosing cholangitis who reported pruritus scored as "moderate to severe" [45]. The primary endpoint of this trial was the achievement of a reduction of more than 50% of VAS-assessed pruritus. BEZA (400 mg/day) led to this achievement in 45% of patients (41% PSC, 55% PBC), whereas only 11% reached the primary endpoint in the placebo group ($p = 0.003$). This effect in relieving cholestasis-associated pruritus occurs via an autotaxin-independent mechanism [46]. This improving effect on pruritus ensures that fibrates should be employed as a second-line option for PBC therapy in patients experiencing moderate to severe pruritus.

Since fibric acid derivates reduce cholesterol levels, they should be considered for the treatment of PBC patients with hypercholesterolemia associated with low levels of high-density lipoprotein [HDL], in whom these agents are protective against cardiovascular events.

3.4. Other PPAR Agonists

The efficacy of elafibranor (ELA), an agonist of PPAR α and δ, has been recently investigated in PBC patients enrolled in a phase 2, double-blind, placebo-controlled study [47]. A total of 45 PBC patients with inadequate UDCA response were randomized into three groups, receiving either ELA 80 mg or ELA 120 mg four times a day, or placebo four times a day for 12 weeks (NCT03124108). ELA significantly decreased mean ALP at week 12 in both groups (−48% in 80 mg-treated group and −40.6% in 120 mg-treated group, $p < 0.001$). The endpoint (ALP < 1.67 x ULN, ALP decrease >15%, and total bilirubin < ULN) was reached in most (67% and 79%) patients treated with the 80 or 120 mg doses, respectively. Moreover, in ELA caused an improvement in lipid and inflammatory markers (IgM, CRP, haptoglobin, fibrinogen) and a decrease in 7α-hydroxy-4-cholesten-3-one, or C4, an intermediate of bile acid synthesis. ELA at both dosages was well tolerated and did not cause induction or exacerbation of pruritus. In general, all these effects suggest that ELA is a promising drug candidate for PBC.

A 12-week double-blind, randomized, placebo-controlled phase 2 trial investigated the effect of seladelpar, a selective PPAR-δ agonist [48]. A total of 70 PBC patients with inadequate response or intolerance to UDCA were randomly divided into 3 experimental groups treated with 50 or 200 mg/day of seladelpar or placebo. Since 3 patients treated with seladelpar developed a grade 3 increase in ALT, even if fully reversible and asymptomatic, the study was terminated early. Despite these results, the safety and tolerability of seladelpar have been tested in a 52-week, phase 2, open-label uncontrolled dose-finding study [49,50]. This trial enrolled 120 patients who were treated for 12 weeks: 53 patients were treated with seladelpar 5 mg/day, 55 with seladelpar 10 mg/day, and 11 were assigned to the 2 mg/day group (United Kingdom sites after interim analysis), after which the dose could be increased to 10 mg/day. One year of observations indicated that seladelpar appeared to be safe and well-tolerated, while not inducing pruritus. A total of 4 patients discontinued seladelpar due to ADRs, 2 of which have been correlated to the drug treatment (grade 1 heartburn and grade 2 transaminase elevation). The composite endpoint (ALP < 1.67 x ULN, −15% reduction in ALP, total bilirubin < ULN) was met in 64% and 67% of seladelpar-treated patients. ALP normalization rates were 9%, 13%, and 33% in the 2 mg-, 5 mg-, and 10 mg-treated groups, respectively. After one year of treatment with seladelpar, 101 patients included in this trial self-reported using the pruritus VAS, the 5D-itch scale, and the PBC-40 questionnaire (evaluating itch and fatigue domains) [51]. Seladelpar led to consistent improvement in both pruritus and fatigue, along with a reduction in serum bile acid profiles. A phase 3, international, randomized, placebo-controlled study (ENHANCE) further assessed the safety and efficacy of seladelpar in PBC patients not responding to first-line treatment [52]. Enrolled participants were randomized into three groups of 80 patients: seladelpar 10 mg/day, seladelpar 5 mg/day, or placebo. After a first analysis after 26 weeks, patients were treated for an additional 26 weeks with either 5 mg or 10 mg of seladelpar. The primary endpoint was a composite response at month 3, which included an ALP of less than 1.67 times the ULN, a ≥15% ALP reduction, and total bilirubin at or below the ULN. After one year of treatment, this study demonstrated a mean ALP decrease of 40% in the 5/10-mg group and of 45% in the 10-mg group. In addition, in the 5-mg group uptitrated to 10 mg, 53% of the patients reached the composite endpoint, as well as 69% of patients in the 10 mg group. However, this trial was terminated early due to an unexpected histological finding of non-alcoholic steatohepatitis, even though the causality assessment with seladelpar treatment was not demonstrated. These results suggest that seladelpar is a drug candidate for the second-line therapy of PBC, although further evidence about its tolerability should be obtained.

3.5. Agents Targeting the FGF19 Pathway

Fibroblast growth factor 19 (FGF19) is a hormone encoded by the *FGF19* gene, directly reducing the gene expression of CYP7A1, a key enzyme catalyzing the first rate-limiting step of bile acid synthesis [53]. Since the suppression of hepatocyte bile acid synthesis is a rational mechanism for the improvement of bile acid homeostasis and the management of cholestasis, some attempts to find novel agents acting via the FGF19 axis have been made.

An engineered analogue of FGF19, NGM282 (aldafermin), was tested in a multicentric, randomized, double-blind phase 2 trial [54]. A total of 45 PBC patients with inadequate UDCA responses were randomly assigned to three groups: one received subcutaneous daily administration of NGM282 at a 0.3 mg dose (n = 14), another received 3 mg (n = 16), and the latter received the placebo (n = 15). NGM282 treatment significantly reduced ALP (primary endpoint) at both doses compared to placebo at the end of the treatment. Moreover, 50% of the patients receiving 0.3 mg and 46% of those receiving 3 mg were shown to have an ALP reduction higher than 15% from baseline compared to 7% in the placebo group. Most ADRs were gastrointestinal disorders of grade 1 and 2. Overall, the tolerability profile of NGM282 was acceptable. However, further studies are encouraged to ascertain whether the biochemical response is durable and related to a real improvement of robust clinical outcomes, rather than to a decrease in decompensation or death.

3.6. Agents Targeting the NADPH Oxidase (NOX) Enzymes

Besides their physiological functions, NADPH oxidases (NOXs), enzymes devoted to the production of reactive oxygen species [55], play a role in multiple pathological processes characterized by excessive oxidative stress. The NOX inhibitor GKT831 (setanaxib) was investigated in a phase 2 trial including 111 patients with PBC divided into 3 arms, one receiving 400 mg of GKT831 once daily (n = 38), another twice daily (n = 36), and the latter receiving placebo (n = 37) [56]. The primary endpoint was the change in GGT vs. baseline, and the secondary endpoints were the modification in ALP, liver stiffness evaluated by means of FibroScan, and overall quality of life after 24 weeks. GKT831 led to a reduction in cholestatic markers. Particularly, a greater GGT reduction was observed in patients with higher baseline values, thus suggesting that this NOX inhibitor may be useful in patients with more advanced disease. Moreover, GKT831 was shown to be well-tolerated, with no reported treatment discontinuation or interruption due to pruritus or fatigue. Due to the positive results obtained in this trial, a phase 3 trial in PBC patients is planned.

3.7. Agents with Immunomodulatory Properties

In recent years, many studies have pointed out that immunomodulators, such for example anti-IL antibodies, Janus kinase (JAK) 1/2 inhibitors and sphingosine-1-phosphate receptor agonists, may have a potential efficacy in the treatment of PBC, since the dysregulation of innate immune system plays a fundamental role in its pathogenesis. To date, some agents with immunomodulatory properties are in early-stage preclinical and/or clinical development for PBC treatment.

Budesonide, a synthetic corticosteroid displaying a high first-pass metabolism, has been evaluated in a placebo-controlled, double-blind trial in 62 non-responder patients to UDCA [57]. Participants were randomly assigned 2:10 to receive budesonide (9 mg/day) or placebo once daily for 36 months while maintaining UDCA treatment. The primary endpoint was the improvement of liver histology with respect to inflammation and no progression of fibrosis. Comparing patients with paired liver biopsies (n = 43) the histologic endpoint was not met; moreover, serious adverse events occurred in 10 patients receiving budesonide and 7 receiving placebo. Improvements in biochemical markers of disease activity were obtained with budesonide.

Recently budesonide has been recommended for patients diagnosed with AIH/PBC overlap syndrome [58]. This treatment can improve liver function tests and is relatively safe, although the risk of portal vein thrombosis remains a concern [59].

The efficacy of rituximab, an anti-CD20 chimeric monoclonal antibody, was evaluated in two open-label studies enrolling PBC patients with incomplete UDCA response. The results of both studies suggested a limited efficacy of rituximab in PBC patients, even though an impressive reduction in ALP levels was observed [60,61] in a limited number of patients. Moreover, the treatment with rituximab was demonstrated to be ineffective in reducing fatigue in a phase 2 trial in PBC patients [62].

Since PBC hepatic histology shows a lymphocytic infiltration in portal tracts and segmental inflammatory destruction of intrahepatic bile ducts, some studies have investigated the potential effects of antibodies directed against chemokine (C-X-C motif) ligand 10 (CXCL10) in PBC patients. CXCL10 is a chemokine secreted in response to interferon-γ-stimulation by several cell types, e.g., monocytes, endothelial cells, fibroblasts, cholangiocytes, and hepatocytes, and is implicated in the hepatic recruitment of inflammatory T cells. This effect is elicited through its binding to chemokine (C-X-C motif) receptor 3 (CXCR3), expressed on effector T cells [63]. Moreover, both CXCL10 and CXRC3 have been demonstrated to be upregulated in the serum and livers of PBC patients [64]. In particular, CXCR3+ cells have been found in the hepatic tissue of PBC patients [65]. Interestingly, in situ hybridization of PBC liver samples demonstrated the presence of the CXCL10 messenger in hepatocytes surrounded by infiltrating monocytes. The anti-CXCL10 monoclonal antibody NI-0801 was evaluated in a phase 2 study enrolling 29 UDCA-non-responder patients with PBC [66]. Each patient received an intravenous infusion of NI-0801 (10 mg/Kg, 6 doses) every 2 weeks. A 3-month follow-up was performed after the last infusion. No serious ADRs have been reported after treatment, and the most common ADRs were headaches (52%), pruritus (34%), fatigue (24%), and diarrhea (21%). However, the trial was terminated due to no significant therapeutic benefits obtained, despite the good pharmacological response observed in the blood, since the high rate of CXCL10 production makes it difficult to reach drug levels leading to an effective sustained neutralization of this chemokine [66].

Ustekimumab, a monoclonal antibody specifically binding the two interleukins IL-12 and IL-23, has been investigated in a multicentric, open-label study including PBC patients with an inadequate response to UDCA. Unfortunately, the results of this study failed to demonstrate the efficacy of this antibody in achieving a decrease, even moderate, in ALP levels [67].

Another open-label trial investigating abatacept, a fusion protein formed by the extracellular domain of the CTL4 and Fc region of the immunoglobulin IgG1, has demonstrated the inefficacy of this protein in achieving the required clinical outcomes [68].

Baricitinib is a JAK inhibitor, selective for the two subtypes JAK1 and JAK2, already approved in the US and Europe for the treatment of other autoimmune diseases, e.g., rheumatoid arthritis, and alopecia areata. JAK is a family of intracellular tyrosine kinases transducing cytokine-mediated signals. A randomized, double-blinded placebo-controlled trial in patients with PBC and inadequate response or intolerance to UDCA was performed [69]. Endpoints included change in ALP, itch numeric rating score, and fatigue scoring at 12 weeks post-baseline. Only two patients were enrolled and completed the trial (one received baricitinib and the other placebo). The patient treated with baricitinib demonstrated a 30% decrease in ALP and a 7-point improvement in itch scoring, but a 2-point increase in fatigue scoring.

FFP-104, an anti-CD40 monoclonal antibody, is a novel agent proposed for the treatment of PBC, since CD40 promotes the efficient T cell activation caused by the paracrine communications of antigen presenting cells, fibroblasts, and other non-lymphoid cells. As a consequence, its blockade could be exploited to counteract PBC autoimmune activation. A phase 2 trial including PBC patients is currently ongoing to determine the initial safety, tolerability, and pharmacodynamics of this antibody in PBC patients (NCT02193360). Interestingly, in a murine model of autoimmune cholangitis, administration of the anti-CD40 ligand reduced liver inflammation and lowered the levels of AMA, but these reductions were not sustained [70].

Mesenchymal stem cells (MSCs) transplantation has been studied as alternative to liver transplantation for patients with end-stage PBC [71]. MSCs are able to modulate and repair the injured tissue by affecting immune response by different mechanisms, such as cell-to-cell interactions and the production of useful paracrine factors [72]. The first clinical trial evaluating MSCs for PBC treatment was conducted in China (NCT01662973). This pilot study enrolled a small number of patients (n = 7) with an incomplete response to assess the safety and efficacy of umbilical cord-derived mesenchymal stem cells (UC-MSCs) [73]. All patients received 3 infusions of UC-MSCs every 4 weeks. After 48 weeks of follow-up, the treatment was well tolerated, and no relevant ADRs occurred. UC-MSCs significantly decreased serum levels of ALP and GGT. After these encouraging results, a second study was performed by the same research group testing MSCs derived from allogenic donors of the patients' family members [74]. Their efficacy was evaluated using a 1-year of follow-up. Although transaminases, GGT, and IgM were significantly improved, the histological analyses evaluating the presence and severity of fibrosis were stabilized by the treatment. Overall, further studies seem to be necessary to discriminate the real efficacy of the use of MSC therapy in PBC. A new study is currently ongoing (NCT03668145).

3.8. *Antiretroviral Therapy*

After the proposal of a Canadian research group of a viral involvement in the pathogenesis of PBC, a multicentric trial was designed to investigate the efficacy of antiretroviral therapy in PBC patients (NCT01614405) in a limited number of patients (n = 13), since most enrolled patients were intolerant to the lopinavir-ritonavir (LPRr) combination. Patients were randomized and received a combination of tenofovir-emtricitabine (TDF/FTC 300/200 mg), LPRr (800/200 mg), or placebo for 6 months [75]. A significant 25% reduction in ALP was observed after antiretroviral therapy ($p < 0.05$). However, an important limitation to the use of the antiviral combination was represented by the frequency of ADRs, which were much higher than those reported in HIV patients receiving the same therapy. A new trial investigating better-tolerated combination regimens is ongoing (NCT03954327). Another antiretroviral therapy with tenofovir/emtricitabine-based regimens in combination with lopinavir or raltegravir in recurrent PBC following liver transplantation improved hepatic biochemistry, but the antiretroviral therapy was associated with side-effects [76].

4. Agents for the Treatment of Specific Symptoms of PBC

4.1. *Agents Targeting Pruritus*

Pruritus represents a frequent and troublesome symptom, reported in 60–70% of patients [77,78]. Its pathogenesis is complex, and the results regarding therapy with UDCA showed that it was mostly ineffective in improving this symptom. Since the principal guideline-approved anti-pruritic agents, e.g., cholestyramine, rifampicin, naltrexone, and sertraline, are often ineffective to improve PBC-related pruritus, novel agents targeting this symptom have been developed and are under evaluation.

Ileal Bile Acid Transporter (IBAT) Inhibitors

The use of ileal bile acid transporter inhibitors has been suggested for the treatment of PBC-related pruritus due to their ability of decrease retained circulating BAs. IBATs is physiologically devoted to BA reabsorption from the ileum, thus maintaining their enterohepatic circulation. Since in many cholestatic liver diseases, ileal BA absorption is increased, several compounds capable of altering the ileal reabsorption of bile acids have been proposed and are discussed below.

Maralixibat, a selective, sodium-dependent, ileal apical, BA transport inhibitor was tested in a phase 2 trail in which its efficacy and safety were assessed in PBC patients with pruritus (CLARITY study [79]). Patients were divided into arms and treated for 13 weeks with either maralixibat (10 or 20 mg/day) or placebo, in addition to the standard UDCA therapy, when tolerated. The primary endpoint was defined as "adult itch reported outcome average sum score" from baseline to the end of the study. The main ADRs were gastrointestinal disorders, which were common in treated (78.6%) but also placebo (50%) patients. Despite an improvement of baseline risk scores, maralixibat caused no significant improvement of pruritus with respect to placebo.

The IBAT inhibitor GSK2330672, also called linerixibat, was evaluated in a phase 2 trial enrolling 21 patients [80] to assess the safety and tolerability of GSK2330672. The secondary endpoints were changes in patient-reported pruritus scores, assessed by means of different scales, namely a 0 to 10 numerical rating scale, PBC-40 itch domain score, 5-D itch scale, and changes in circulating bile acid levels (NCT01899703). Linerixibat was well tolerated, and diarrhea was the most experienced ADR. The percentage decrease in itch scores was −57% in the numerical rating scale, −31% in the PBC-40 itch domain, and −35% in the 5-D itch scale in linerixibat-treated patients, and these differences were statistically significant with respect to the placebo-treated group. A larger phase 2 study enrolling 147 patients is still ongoing to confirm these beneficial effects on PBS-related pruritus and to further assess the drug tolerability (NCT02966834).

The last proposed IBAT inhibitor, A4250 (odevixibat), was tested in an open-label phase 2 study that aimed to assess drug tolerability and efficacy in improving pruritus in 9 PBC patients (NCT02360852) [81]. Patients were treated with odevixibat at a dose of 0.75 mg (n = 4) or 1.5 mg (n = 5) for 4 weeks. A remarkable improvement in pruritus was observed in all 9 odevixibat-treated patients assessed by VAS, the 5-D itch scale, and the pruritus domain of the PBC-40 questionnaire [82]. Unfortunately, tolerability was low because of gastrointestinal symptoms. Odevixibat received its first approval in the EU in July 2021 for the treatment of progressive familial intrahepatic cholestasis (PFIC) in patients aged $\geq$ 6 months, followed by its approval in the US for pruritus in patients with PFIC aged $\geq$ 3 months [83].

4.2. Agents Targeting Fatigue

Another frequently reported PBC manifestation is fatigue, a complex syndrome characterized by feelings of discomfort, exhaustion, and lethargy that could significantly reduce the quality of life. The probability of improving fatigue after LT in advanced PBC is roughly 50% [84]. Currently, no pharmacological treatment is approved for PBC-related fatigue. The only prescribed suggestion is an exercise increase, even though this kind of prescription needs further evaluation. The results of a pilot study showed an improvement in muscle pH in PBC patients, and an amelioration of fatigue, social, and emotional symptoms in patients following an exercise program [85].

The first phase 2 randomized controlled trial of treatment of PBS-associated fatigue and daytime somnolence (NCT2376335, [62]) was performed in 57 PBC patients with moderate to severe fatigue. Patients were randomized to receive two doses of rituximab (1000 mg) or placebo. The primary outcome was assessed by measuring fatigue severity using a questionnaire at 3 months. The rationale of the use of rituximab was an improvement in the fatigue associated with a variety of other autoimmune diseases, e.g., Sjogren's syndrome, which has been also association with PBC. Rituximab, however, failed to show an improvement in fatigue in PBC patients.

Modafinil, an agent acting on the central nervous system and used for the treatment of daytime somnolence in narcoleptic patients, was tested in an open study enrolling 21 patients with PBC experiencing daytime somnolence and fatigue [86]. The starting dose of modafinil was 100 mg/day, which was titrated according to patient's tolerability and response. Unfortunately, only 14 patients could tolerate the full 2-month treatment, although in those patients, an improvement of excessive daytime somnolence and associated fatigue was observed. The suggestion from these data was to improve the design of the study with a placebo-controlled trial, to confirm modafinil's efficacy against fatigue.

A preclinical study on an animal model of hepatic cholestasis induced by the ligation of the bile duct demonstrated that early OCA administration was able to improve cognitive impairment [87]. Otherwise, these preclinical observations need to be validated in further studies.

A systematic meta-analysis of 16 studies evaluating UDCA, liver transplantation, serotonin reuptake inhibitors, colchicine, methotrexate, cyclosporine, modafinil, and OCA found some improvement in fatigue with liver transplantation, but a lack of high-quality evidence supporting the efficacy of any other intervention in the treatment of PBC-related fatigue [88].

5. Conclusions

In recent years, new candidate drugs have undergone or completed phase 2 and 3 clinical trials on PBC patients who did not respond to the first line therapy with UDCA. OCA represents the most promising drug and is approved in many countries for this indication. Fibrates seem to effectively ameliorate biochemistry alteration and symptoms typical of PBC. Moreover, a variety of new agents, acting with different mechanisms of action, are under clinical evaluations for PBC treatment, e.g., PPAR agonists, NOX inhibitors, immunomodulators, and mesenchymal stem cells transplantation. Even though most of these approaches seem to have beneficial effects on biochemical endpoints, no data are currently available regarding robust endpoints, such as transplant-free survival; thus, their clinical use needs to be supported by the consistent improvement of these parameters. In general, data on the efficacy of the new therapeutic agents are still undergoing investigation in clinical trials and are too premature to provide practical information to physicians. The crucial point when designing clinical trials is the choice of a combination treatment with nuclear receptor ligands and other agents with different mechanism and therapeutic effects [89]. This huge armamentarium of new therapeutic options will likely lead to a novel treatment landscape for PBC in the near future, with novel therapies based on the combinations of multiple agents acting on different pathogenetic mechanisms [90]. Another crucial point is that the ideal therapy for PBC would achieve a complete biochemical remission, namely normalization of serum ALP and bilirubin, and would be well tolerated. Furthermore, the ideal therapy must be safe for patients with advanced or decompensated disease and should aim to reduce the need for liver transplantation [91].

Author Contributions: Conceptualization, A.F. and S.D.M.; writing—original draft preparation, A.F. and D.G.; writing—review and editing, S.D.M. All authors have read and agreed to the published version of the manuscript.

Funding: This research received no external funding.

Institutional Review Board Statement: Not applicable.

Informed Consent Statement: Not applicable.

Conflicts of Interest: A.F. has received consultancy fees during the last two years from Intercept.

References

1. Gulamhusein, A.F.; Hirschfield, G.M. Primary biliary cholangitis: Pathogenesis and therapeutic opportunities. *Nat. Rev. Gastroenterol. Hepatol.* **2020**, *17*, 93–110. [CrossRef] [PubMed]
2. Lv, T.; Chen, S.; Li, M.; Zhang, D.; Kong, Y.; Jia, J. Regional variation and temporal trend of primary biliary cholangitis epidemiology: A systematic review and meta-analysis. *J. Gastroenterol. Hepatol.* **2021**, *36*, 1423–1434. [CrossRef] [PubMed]
3. Baldursdottir, T.R.; Bergmann, O.M.; Jonasson, J.G.; Ludviksson, B.R.; Axelsson, T.A.; Björnsson, E.S. The epidemiology and natural history of primary biliary cirrhosis. *Eur. J. Gastroenterol. Hepatol.* **2012**, *24*, 824–830. [CrossRef]

4. Perez, C.F.M.; Goet, J.C.; Lammers, W.J.; Gulamhusein, A.; van Buuren, H.R.; Ponsioen, C.Y.; Carbone, M.; Mason, A.; Corpechot, C.; Invernizzi, P.; et al. Milder disease stage in patients with primary biliary cholangitis over a 44-year period: A changing natural history. *Hepatology* **2018**, *67*, 1920–1930. [CrossRef] [PubMed]
5. Juran, B.D.; Lazaridis, K.N. Environmental Factors in Primary Biliary Cirrhosis. *Semin. Liver Dis.* **2014**, *34*, 265–272. [CrossRef] [PubMed]
6. Webb, G.; Hirschfield, G. Using GWAS to identify genetic predisposition in hepatic autoimmunity. *J. Autoimmun.* **2016**, *66*, 25–39. [CrossRef] [PubMed]
7. Bianchi, I.; Carbone, M.; Lleo, A.; Invernizzi, P. Genetics and Epigenetics of Primary Biliary Cirrhosis. *Semin. Liver Dis.* **2014**, *34*, 255–264. [CrossRef] [PubMed]
8. Beuers, U.; Trauner, M.; Jansen, P.; Poupon, R. New paradigms in the treatment of hepatic cholestasis: From UDCA to FXR, PXR and beyond. *J. Hepatol.* **2015**, *62*, S25–S37. [CrossRef]
9. Hirschfield, G.M.; Beuers, U.; Corpechot, C.; Invernizzi, P.; Jones, D.; Marzioni, M.; Schramm, C. EASL Clinical Practice Guidelines: The diagnosis and management of patients with primary biliary cholangitis. *J. Hepatol.* **2017**, *67*, 145–172. [CrossRef]
10. Parés, A.; Caballeria, L.; Rodés, J. Excellent Long-Term Survival in Patients with Primary Biliary Cirrhosis and Biochemical Response to Ursodeoxycholic Acid. *Gastroenterology* **2006**, *130*, 715–720. [CrossRef]
11. Corpechot, C.; Abenavoli, L.; Rabahi, N.; Chrétien, Y.; Andréani, T.; Johanet, C.; Chazouillères, O.; Poupon, R. Biochemical response to ursodeoxycholic acid and long-term prognosis in primary biliary cirrhosis. *Hepatology* **2008**, *48*, 871–877. [CrossRef] [PubMed]
12. Kuiper, E.M.M.; Hansen, B.E.; de Vries, R.A.; den Ouden–Muller, J.W.; van Ditzhuijsen, T.J.M.; Haagsma, E.B.; Houben, M.H.M.G.; Witteman, B.J.M.; van Erpecum, K.J.; van Buuren, H.R. Improved Prognosis of Patients with Primary Biliary Cirrhosis That Have a Biochemical Response to Ursodeoxycholic Acid. *Gastroenterology* **2009**, *136*, 1281–1287. [CrossRef] [PubMed]
13. Corpechot, C.; Chazouillères, O.; Poupon, R. Early primary biliary cirrhosis: Biochemical response to treatment and prediction of long-term outcome. *J. Hepatol.* **2011**, *55*, 1361–1367. [CrossRef] [PubMed]
14. Lammers, W.J.; van Buuren, H.R.; Hirschfield, G.M.; Janssen, H.L.; Invernizzi, P.; Mason, A.L.; Ponsioen, C.Y.; Floreani, A.; Corpechot, C.; Mayo, M.J.; et al. Levels of Alkaline Phosphatase and Bilirubin Are Surrogate End Points of Outcomes of Patients with Primary Biliary Cirrhosis: An International Follow-up Study. *Gastroenterology* **2014**, *147*, 1338–1349.e5. [CrossRef] [PubMed]
15. Kumagi, T.; Guindi, M.; Fischer, S.E.; Arenovich, T.; Abdalian, R.; Coltescu, C.; Heathcote, J.E.; Hirschfield, G. Baseline Ductopenia and Treatment Response Predict Long-Term Histological Progression in Primary Biliary Cirrhosis. *Am. J. Gastroenterol.* **2010**, *105*, 2186–2194. [CrossRef]
16. Perez, C.F.M.; Harms, M.H.; Lindor, K.D.; van Buuren, H.R.; Hirschfield, G.M.; Corpechot, C.; van der Meer, A.J.; Feld, J.J.; Gulamhusein, A.; Lammers, W.J.; et al. Goals of Treatment for Improved Survival in Primary Biliary Cholangitis: Treatment Target Should Be Bilirubin within the Normal Range and Normalization of Alkaline Phosphatase. *Am. J. Gastroenterol.* **2020**, *115*, 1066–1074. [CrossRef]
17. Cortez-Pinto, H.; Liberal, R.; Lopes, S.; Machado, M.V.; Carvalho, J.; Dias, T.; Santos, A.; Agostinho, C.; Figueiredo, P.; Loureiro, R.; et al. Predictors for incomplete response to ursodeoxycholic acid in primary biliary cholangitis. Data from a national registry of liver disease. *United Eur. Gastroenterol. J.* **2021**, *9*, 699–706. [CrossRef]
18. Harms, M.H.; van Buuren, H.R.; Corpechot, C.; Thorburn, D.; Janssen, H.L.; Lindor, K.D.; Hirschfield, G.M.; Parés, A.; Floreani, A.; Mayo, M.J.; et al. Ursodeoxycholic acid therapy and liver transplant-free survival in patients with primary biliary cholangitis. *J. Hepatol.* **2019**, *71*, 357–365. [CrossRef]
19. Carbone, M.; Harms, M.H.; Lammers, W.; Marmon, T.; Pencek, R.; MacConell, L.; Shapiro, D.; Jones, D.E.; Mells, G.F.; Hansen, B.E. Clinical application of the GLOBE and United Kingdom-primary biliary cholangitis risk scores in a trial cohort of patients with primary biliary cholangitis. *Hepatol. Commun.* **2018**, *2*, 683–692. [CrossRef]
20. Selmi, C.; Bowlus, C.L.; Gershwin, M.E.; Coppel, R.L. Primary biliary cirrhosis. *Lancet* **2011**, *377*, 1600–1609. [CrossRef]
21. Gerussi, A.; Lucà, M.; Cristoferi, L.; Ronca, V.; Mancuso, C.; Milani, C.; D'Amato, D.; O'Donnell, S.E.; Carbone, M.; Invernizzi, P. New Therapeutic Targets in Autoimmune Cholangiopathies. *Front. Med.* **2020**, *7*, 117. [CrossRef] [PubMed]
22. Modica, S.; Petruzzelli, M.; Bellafante, E.; Murzilli, S.; Salvatore, L.; Celli, N.; Di Tullio, G.; Palasciano, G.; Moustafa, T.; Halilbasic, E.; et al. Selective Activation of Nuclear Bile Acid Receptor FXR in the Intestine Protects Mice Against Cholestasis. *Gastroenterology* **2012**, *142*, 355–365.e4. [CrossRef]
23. Kowdley, K.V.; Luketic, V.; Chapman, R.; Hirschfield, G.M.; Poupon, R.; Schramm, C.; Vincent, C.; Rust, C.; Parés, A.; Mason, A.; et al. A randomized trial of obeticholic acid monotherapy in patients with primary biliary cholangitis. *Hepatology* **2018**, *67*, 1890–1902. [CrossRef] [PubMed]
24. Nevens, F.; Andreone, P.; Mazzella, G.; Strasser, S.I.; Bowlus, C.; Invernizzi, P.; Drenth, J.P.; Pockros, P.J.; Regula, J.; Beuers, U.; et al. A Placebo-Controlled Trial of Obeticholic Acid in Primary Biliary Cholangitis. *N. Engl. J. Med.* **2016**, *375*, 631–643. [CrossRef] [PubMed]
25. Trauner, M.; Nevens, F.; Shiffman, M.L.; Drenth, J.P.H.; Bowlus, C.L.; Vargas, V.; Andreone, P.; Hirschfield, G.M.; Pencek, R.; Malecha, E.S.; et al. Long-term efficacy and safety of obeticholic acid for patients with primary biliary cholangitis: 3-year results of an international open-label extension study. *Lancet Gastroenterol. Hepatol.* **2019**, *4*, 445–453. [CrossRef]

26. Parés, A.; Shiffman, M.; Vargas, V.; Invernizzi, P.; Malecha, E.S.; Liberman, A.; MacConell, L.; Hirschfield, G. Reduction and stabilization of bilirubin with obeticholic acid treatment in patients with primary biliary cholangitis. *Liver Int.* **2020**, *40*, 1121–1129. [CrossRef]
27. Bowlus, C.L.; Pockros, P.J.; Kremer, A.E.; Parés, A.; Forman, L.M.; Drenth, J.P.; Ryder, S.D.; Terracciano, L.; Jin, Y.; Liberman, A.; et al. Long-Term Obeticholic Acid Therapy Improves Histological Endpoints in Patients With Primary Biliary Cholangitis. *Clin. Gastroenterol. Hepatol.* **2020**, *18*, 1170–1178.e6. [CrossRef]
28. Hirschfield, G.M.; Floreani, A.; Trivedi, P.J.; Pencek, R.; Liberman, A.; Marmon, T.; MacConell, L. PTU-097 Long-term effect of obeticholic acid on transient elastography and ast to platelet ratio index in patients with pbc. *BMJ Gut* **2017**, *66*, A98–A99. [CrossRef]
29. Roberts, S.B.; Ismail, M.; Kanagalingam, G.; Mason, A.L.; Swain, M.G.; Vincent, C.; Yoshida, E.M.; Tsien, C.; Flemming, J.A.; Janssen, H.L.; et al. Real-World Effectiveness of Obeticholic Acid in Patients with Primary Biliary Cholangitis. *Hepatol. Commun.* **2020**, *4*, 1332–1345. [CrossRef]
30. Gomez, L.E.; Garcia Buey, E.; Molina, M.; Casado, I.; Conde, M.; Berenguer, F.; Jorquera, M.-A.; Simón, A.; Olveira, M.; Hernández-Guerra, M.; et al. Effectiveness and safety of obeticholic acid in a Southern European multicentre cohort of patients with primary biliary cholangitis and suboptimal response to ursodeoxycholic acid. *Aliment. Pharm. Ther.* **2021**, *53*, 519–530. [CrossRef]
31. D'Amato, D.; De Vincentis, A.; Malinverno, F.; Viganò, M.; Alvaro, D.; Pompili, M.; Picciotto, A.; Palitti, V.P.; Russello, M.; Storato, S.; et al. Real-world experience with obeticholic acid in patients with primary biliary cholangitis. *JHEP Rep.* **2021**, *3*, 100248. [CrossRef] [PubMed]
32. Tully, D.C.; Rucker, P.V.; Chianelli, D.; Williams, J.; Vidal, A.; Alper, P.B.; Mutnick, D.; Bursulaya, B.; Schmeits, J.; Wu, X.; et al. Discovery of Tropifexor (LJN452), a Highly Potent Non-bile Acid FXR Agonist for the Treatment of Cholestatic Liver Diseases and Nonalcoholic Steatohepatitis (NASH). *J. Med. Chem.* **2017**, *60*, 9960–9973. [CrossRef] [PubMed]
33. Schramm, C.; Hirschfield, G.; Mason, A.; Wedemeyer, H.; Klickstein, L.; Neelakantham, S.; Koo, P.; Sanni, J.; Badman, M.; Jones, D. Early assessment of safety and efficacy of tropifexor, a potent non bile-acid FXR agonist, in patients with primary biliary cholangitis: An interim analysis of an ongoing phase 2 study. *J. Hepatol.* **2018**, *68*, S103. [CrossRef]
34. Trauner, M.; Gulamhusein, A.; Hameed, B.; Caldwell, S.; Shiffman, M.L.; Landis, C.; Eksteen, B.; Agarwal, K.; Muir, A.; Rushbrook, S.; et al. The Nonsteroidal Farnesoid X Receptor Agonist Cilofexor (GS-9674) Improves Markers of Cholestasis and Liver Injury in Patients with Primary Sclerosing Cholangitis. *Hepatology* **2019**, *70*, 788–801. [CrossRef] [PubMed]
35. Kowdley, K.V.; Bonder, A.; Heneghan, M.A.; Hodge, A.D.; Ryder, S.D.; Sanchez, A.J.; Vargas, V.; Zeuzem, S.; Ahmad, A.; Larson, K.; et al. Final data of the phase 2a INTREPID study with EDP-305, a non-bile acid farnesoid X receptor (FXR) agonist. *Hepatology* **2020**, *72*, 131–1159. [CrossRef]
36. Corpechot, C. The Role of Fibrates in Primary Biliary Cholangitis. *Curr. Hepatol. Rep.* **2019**, *18*, 107–114. [CrossRef]
37. Ghonem, N.S.; Ananthanarayanan, M.; Soroka, C.J.; Boyer, J.L. Peroxisome proliferator-activated receptor α activates human multidrug resistance transporter 3/ATP-binding cassette protein subfamily B4 transcription and increases rat biliary phosphatidylcholine secretion. *Hepatology* **2014**, *59*, 1030–1042. [CrossRef]
38. Honda, A.; Ikegami, T.; Nakamuta, M.; Miyazaki, T.; Iwamoto, J.; Hirayama, T.; Saito, Y.; Takikawa, H.; Imawari, M.; Matsuzaki, Y. Anticholestatic effects of bezafibrate in patients with primary biliary cirrhosis treated with ursodeoxycholic acid. *Hepatology* **2013**, *57*, 1931–1941. [CrossRef]
39. Gabbia, D.; Dalla Pozza, A.; Albertoni, L.; Lazzari, R.; Zigiotto, G.; Carrara, M.; Baldo, V.; Baldovin, T.; Floreani, A.; De Martin, S. Pregnane X receptor and constitutive androstane receptor modulate differently CYP3A-mediated metabolism in early- and late-stage cholestasis. *World J. Gastroenterol.* **2017**, *23*, 7519–7530. [CrossRef]
40. Corpechot, C.; Chazouillères, O.; Rousseau, A.; Le Gruyer, A.; Habersetzer, F.; Mathurin, P.; Goria, O.; Potier, P.; Minello, A.; Silvain, C.; et al. A Placebo-Controlled Trial of Bezafibrate in Primary Biliary Cholangitis. *N. Engl. J. Med.* **2018**, *378*, 2171–2181. [CrossRef]
41. Summerfield, J.; Elias, E.; Sherlock, S. Effects of Clofibrate in Primary Biliary Cirrhosis Hypercholesterolemia and Gallstones. *Gastroenterology* **1975**, *69*, 998–1000. [CrossRef]
42. Reig, A.; Álvarez-Navascués, C.; Gómez, M.V.; Domińguez, E.G.; Moya, A.G.; Pérez-Medrano, I.; Fábrega, E.; Guerra, M.H.; Haym, M.B.; Estevez, P.; et al. Comparative effects of second-line therapy with obeticholic acid or fibrates in primary biliary cholangitis patients. *J. Hepatol.* **2020**, *73*, S460–S461. [CrossRef]
43. Culver, E.; Hayden, J.; Thornburn, D.; Marshall, A. Obeticholic acid and bezafibrate in primary biliary cholangitis: A comparative evaluation of efficacy through real world clinical practice. *Hepatology* **2019**, *70* (Suppl. S1), 770A.
44. D'Amato, D.; O'Donnell, S.; Cazzagon, N.; Marconi, G.; Gerussi, A.; Cristoferi, L.; Malinverno, F.; Mancuso, C.; Milani, C.; Marzioni, M.; et al. Additive beneficial effects of Fibrates combined with Obeticholic acid in the treatment of patients with Primary Biliary Cholangitis and inadequate response to second-line therapy: Data from the Italian PBC Study Group. *Dig. Liver Dis.* **2020**, *52*, e32. [CrossRef]
45. de Vries, E.; Bolier, R.; Goet, J.; Parés, A.; Verbeek, J.; de Vree, M.; Drenth, J.; van Erpecum, K.; van Nieuwkerk, K.; van der Heide, F.; et al. Fibrates for Itch (FITCH) in Fibrosing Cholangiopathies: A Double-Blind, Randomized, Placebo-Controlled Trial. *Gastroenterology* **2021**, *160*, 734–743.e6. [CrossRef] [PubMed]
46. Floreani, A.; De Martin, S. Treatment of primary sclerosing cholangitis. *Dig. Liver Dis.* **2021**, *53*, 1531–1538. [CrossRef]

47. Schattenberg, J.M.; Pares, A.; Kowdley, K.V.; Heneghan, M.A.; Caldwell, S.; Pratt, D.; Bonder, A.; Hirschfield, G.M.; Levy, C.; Vierling, J.; et al. A randomized placebo-controlled trial of elafibranor in patients with primary biliary cholangitis and incomplete response to UDCA. *J. Hepatol.* **2021**, *74*, 1344–1354. [CrossRef]
48. Jones, D.; Boudes, P.F.; Swain, M.G.; Bowlus, C.L.; Galambos, M.R.; Bacon, B.R.; Doerffel, Y.; Gitlin, N.; Gordon, S.C.; Odin, J.A.; et al. (Sasha) Steinberg, FRI133-Durability of treatment response after 1 year of therapy with seladelpar in patients with prima-ry biliary cholangitis (PBC): Final results of an international phase 2 study. *J. Hepatol.* **2020**, *73*, S464–S465.
49. Levy, C.; Bowlus, C.; Neff, G.; Swain, M.G.; Michael, G.; Mayo, M.J.; Goel, A.; Trivedi, P.; Hirschfield, G.; Aspinall, R.; et al. (Sasha) Steinberg, FRI133 - Durability of treatment response after 1 year of therapy with seladelpar in patients with primary biliary cholangitis (PBC): Final results of an international phase 2 study. *J. Hepatol.* **2020**, *73*, S464–S465. [CrossRef]
50. Bowlus, C.L.; Galambos, M.R.; Aspinall, R.J.; Hirschfield, G.M.; Jones, D.E.; Dörffel, Y.; Gordon, S.C.; Harrison, S.A.; Kremer, A.E.; Mayo, M.J.; et al. A phase II, randomized, open-label, 52-week study of seladelpar in patients with primary biliary cholangitis. *J. Hepatol.* **2022**, *77*, 353–364. [CrossRef]
51. Kremer, A.E.; Mayo, M.J.; Hirschfield, G.; Levy, C.; Bowlus, C.L.; Jones, D.E.; Steinberg, A.; McWherter, C.A.; Choi, Y. Seladelpar improved measures of pruritus, sleep, and fatigue and decreased serum bile acids in patients with primary biliary cholangitis. *Liver Int.* **2022**, *42*, 112–123. [CrossRef] [PubMed]
52. ENHANCE: Safety and Efficacy of Seladelpar in Patients With Primary Biliary Cholangitis-A Phase 3, International, Randomized, Placebo-Controlled Study. *Gastroenterol. Hepatol.* **2021**, *17*, 5–6.
53. Russell, D.W. Fifty years of advances in bile acid synthesis and metabolism. *J. Lipid Res.* **2009**, *50*, S120–S125. [CrossRef] [PubMed]
54. Mayo, M.J.; Wigg, A.J.; Leggett, B.; Arnold, H.; Thompson, A.J.; Weltman, M.; Carey, E.J.; Muir, A.J.; Ling, L.; Rossi, S.J.; et al. NGM 282 for Treatment of Patients With Primary Biliary Cholangitis: A Multicenter, Randomized, Double-Blind, Placebo-Controlled Trial. *Hepatol. Commun.* **2018**, *2*, 1037–1050. [CrossRef]
55. Gabbia, D.; Cannella, L.; De Martin, S. The Role of Oxidative Stress in NAFLD–NASH–HCC Transition—Focus on NADPH Oxidases. *Biomedicines* **2021**, *9*, 687. [CrossRef]
56. Dalekos, G.; Invernizzi, P.; Nevens, F.; Hans, V.V.; Zigmond, E.; Andrade, R.J.; Ben Ari, Z.; Heneghan, M.; Huang, J.; Harrison, S.; et al. GS-02-Efficacy of GKT831 in patients with primary biliary cholangitis and inadequate response to ursodeoxy-cholic acid: Interim efficacy results of a phase 2 clinical trial. *J. Hepatol.* **2019**, *70*, e1–e2. [CrossRef]
57. Hirschfield, G.M.; Beuers, U.; Kupcinskas, L.; Ott, P.; Bergquist, A.; Färkkilä, M.; Manns, M.P.; Parés, A.; Spengler, U.; Stiess, M.; et al. A placebo-controlled randomised trial of budesonide for PBC following an insufficient response to UDCA. *J. Hepatol.* **2021**, *74*, 321–329. [CrossRef]
58. Guo, C.; Zhang, H.; Yang, J.; Zhu, R.; Zheng, Y.; Dai, W.; Wang, F.; Chen, K.; Li, J.; Wang, C.; et al. Combination therapy of ursodeoxycholic acid and budesonide for PBC–AIH overlap syndrome: A meta-analysis. *Drug Des. Dev. Ther.* **2015**, *9*, 567–574. [CrossRef]
59. Hempfling, W.; Grunhage, F.; Dilger, K.; Reichel, C.; Sauerbruch, T. Pharmacokinetics and pharmacodynamic action of budesonide in early- and late-stage primary biliary cirrhosis. *Hepatology* **2003**, *38*, 196–202. [CrossRef]
60. Tsuda, M.; Moritoki, Y.; Lian, Z.-X.; Zhang, W.; Yoshida, K.; Wakabayashi, K.; Yang, G.-X.; Nakatani, T.; Vierling, J.; Lindor, K.; et al. Biochemical and immunologic effects of rituximab in patients with primary biliary cirrhosis and an incomplete response to ursodeoxycholic acid. *Hepatology* **2012**, *55*, 512–521. [CrossRef]
61. Myers, R.P.; Swain, M.G.; Lee, S.S.; Shaheen, A.A.M.; Burak, K.W. B-Cell Depletion with Rituximab in Patients with Primary Biliary Cirrhosis Refractory to Ursodeoxycholic Acid. *Am. J. Gastroenterol.* **2013**, *108*, 933–941. [CrossRef] [PubMed]
62. Khanna, A.; Jopson, L.; Howel, D.; Bryant, A.; Blamire, A.; Newton, J.L.; Jones, D.E. Rituximab Is Ineffective for Treatment of Fatigue in Primary Biliary Cholangitis: A Phase 2 Randomized Controlled Trial. *Hepatology* **2019**, *70*, 1646–1657. [CrossRef] [PubMed]
63. Groom, J.R.; Luster, A.D. CXCR3 ligands: Redundant, collaborative and antagonistic functions. *Immunol. Cell Biol.* **2011**, *89*, 207–215. [CrossRef] [PubMed]
64. Lleo, A.; Zhang, W.; Zhao, M.; Tan, Y.; Bernuzzi, F.; Zhu, B.; Liu, Q.; Tan, Q.; Malinverno, F.; Valenti, L.; et al. DNA methylation profiling of the X chromosome reveals an aberrant demethylation on CXCR3 promoter in primary biliary cirrhosis. *Clin. Epigenetics* **2015**, *7*, 61. [CrossRef] [PubMed]
65. Chuang, Y.-H.; Lian, Z.-X.; Cheng, C.-M.; Lan, R.Y.; Yang, G.-X.; Moritoki, Y.; Chiang, B.-L.; Ansari, A.A.; Tsuneyama, K.; Coppel, R.L.; et al. Increased levels of chemokine receptor CXCR3 and chemokines IP-10 and MIG in patients with primary biliary cirrhosis and their first degree relatives. *J. Autoimmun.* **2005**, *25*, 126–132. [CrossRef]
66. De Graaf, K.L.; Lapeyre, G.; Guilhot, F.; Ferlin, W.; Curbishley, S.M.; Carbone, M.; Richardson, P.; Moreea, S.; McCune, C.A.; Ryder, S.D.; et al. NI-0801, an anti-chemokine (C-X-C motif) ligand 10 antibody, in patients with primary biliary cholangitis and an incomplete response to ursodeoxycholic acid. *Hepatol. Commun.* **2018**, *2*, 492–503. [CrossRef] [PubMed]
67. Hirschfield, G.M.; Gershwin, M.E.; Strauss, R.; Mayo, M.J.; Levy, C.; Zou, B.; Johanns, J.; Nnane, I.P.; Dasgupta, B.; Li, K.; et al. Ustekinumab for patients with primary biliary cholangitis who have an inadequate response to ursodeoxycholic acid: A proof-of-concept study. *Hepatology* **2016**, *64*, 189–199. [CrossRef]
68. Bowlus, C.L.; Yang, G.-X.; Liu, C.H.; Johnson, C.R.; Dhaliwal, S.S.; Frank, D.; Levy, C.; Peters, M.G.; Vierling, J.M.; Gershwin, M.E. Therapeutic trials of biologics in primary biliary cholangitis: An open label study of abatacept and review of the literature. *J. Autoimmun.* **2019**, *101*, 26–34. [CrossRef]

69. Gordon, S.C.; Trudeau, S.; Regev, A.; Uhas, J.M.; Chakladar, S.; Pinto-Correia, A.; Gottlieb, K.; Schlichting, D. Baricitinib and primary biliary cholangitis. *J. Transl. Autoimmun.* **2021**, *4*, 100107. [CrossRef]
70. Tanaka, H.; Yang, G.; Iwakoshi, N.; Knechtle, S.J.; Kawata, K.; Tsuneyama, K.; Leung, P.; Coppel, R.L.; Ansari, A.A.; Joh, T.; et al. Anti-CD40 ligand monoclonal antibody delays the progression of murine autoimmune cholangitis. *Clin. Exp. Immunol.* **2013**, *174*, 364–371. [CrossRef]
71. Arsenijevic, A.; Harrell, C.R.; Fellabaum, C.; Volarevic, V. Mesenchymal Stem Cells as New Therapeutic Agents for the Treatment of Primary Biliary Cholangitis. *Anal. Cell. Pathol.* **2017**, *2017*, 7492836. [CrossRef] [PubMed]
72. Alfaifi, M.; Eom, Y.W.; Newsome, P.N.; Baik, S.K. Mesenchymal stromal cell therapy for liver diseases. *J. Hepatol.* **2018**, *68*, 1272–1285. [CrossRef] [PubMed]
73. Wang, L.; Li, J.; Liu, H.; Li, Y.; Fu, J.; Sun, Y.; Xu, R.; Lin, H.; Wang, S.; Lv, S.; et al. A pilot study of umbilical cord-derived mesenchymal stem cell transfusion in patients with primary biliary cirrhosis. *J. Gastroenterol. Hepatol.* **2013**, *28*, 85–92. [CrossRef] [PubMed]
74. Wang, L.; Han, Q.; Chen, H.; Wang, K.; Shan, G.-L.; Kong, F.; Yang, Y.-J.; Li, Y.-Z.; Zhang, X.; Dong, F.; et al. Allogeneic Bone Marrow Mesenchymal Stem Cell Transplantation in Patients with UDCA-Resistant Primary Biliary Cirrhosis. *Stem Cells Dev.* **2014**, *23*, 2482–2489. [CrossRef] [PubMed]
75. Lytvyak, E.; Hosamani, I.; Montano-Loza, A.J.; Saxinger, L.; Mason, A.L. Randomized clinical trial: Combination antiretroviral therapy with tenofovir-emtricitabine and lopinavir-ritonavir in patients with primary biliary cholangitis. *Can. Liver J.* **2019**, *2*, 31–44. [CrossRef]
76. Lytvyak, E.; Niazi, M.; Pai, R.; He, D.; Zhang, G.; Hübscher, S.G.; Mason, A.L. Combination antiretroviral therapy improves recurrent primary biliary cholangitis following liver transplantation. *Liver Int.* **2021**, *41*, 1879–1883. [CrossRef]
77. Talwalkar, J.A.; Souto, E.; Jorgensen, R.A.; Lindor, K.D. Natural history of pruritus in primary biliary cirrhosis. *Clin. Gastroenterol. Hepatol.* **2003**, *1*, 297–302. [CrossRef]
78. Hegade, V.; Mells, G.; Lammert, C.; Juran, B.; Lleo, A.; Carbone, M.; Lazaridis, K.; Invernizzi, P.; Kendrick, S.; Sandford, R.; et al. P1152: A Comparative study of pruritus in PBC cohorts from UK, USA and Italy. *J. Hepatol.* **2015**, *62*, S785. [CrossRef]
79. Mayo, M.J.; Pockros, P.J.; Jones, D.; Bowlus, C.L.; Levy, C.; Patanwala, I.; Bacon, B.; Luketic, V.; Vuppalanchi, R.; Medendorp, S.; et al. A Randomized, Controlled, Phase 2 Study of Maralixibat in the Treatment of Itching Associated with Primary Biliary Cholangitis. *Hepatol. Commun.* **2019**, *3*, 365–381. [CrossRef]
80. Hegade, V.S.; Kendrick, S.; Dobbins, R.L.; Miller, S.R.; Thompson, D.; Richards, D.; Storey, J.; Dukes, G.E.; Corrigan, M.; Elferink, R.P.J.O.; et al. Effect of ileal bile acid transporter inhibitor GSK2330672 on pruritus in primary biliary cholangitis: A double-blind, randomised, placebo-controlled, crossover, phase 2a study. *Lancet* **2017**, *389*, 1114–1123. [CrossRef]
81. Al-Dury, S.; Wahlström, A.; Wahlin, S.; Langedijk, J.; Elferink, R.O.; Ståhlman, M.; Marschall, H.-U. Pilot study with IBAT inhibitor A4250 for the treatment of cholestatic pruritus in primary biliary cholangitis. *Sci. Rep.* **2018**, *8*, 6658. [CrossRef] [PubMed]
82. Jacoby, A. Development, validation, and evaluation of the PBC-40, a disease specific health related quality of life measure for primary biliary cirrhosis. *Gut* **2005**, *54*, 1622–1629. [CrossRef] [PubMed]
83. Deeks, E.D. Odevixibat: First Approval. *Drugs* **2021**, *81*, 1781–1786. [CrossRef] [PubMed]
84. Zenouzi, R.; Weiler-Normann, C.; Lohse, A.W. Is fatigue in primary biliary cirrhosis cured by transplantation? *J. Hepatol.* **2013**, *59*, 418–419. [CrossRef]
85. Hollingsworth, K.G.; Newton, J.L.; Taylor, R.; McDonald, C.; Palmer, J.M.; Blamire, A.M.; Jones, D.E. Pilot Study of Peripheral Muscle Function in Primary Biliary Cirrhosis: Potential Implications for Fatigue Pathogenesis. *Clin. Gastroenterol. Hepatol.* **2008**, *6*, 1041–1048. [CrossRef]
86. Jones, D.E.J.; Newton, J.L. An open study of modafinil for the treatment of daytime somnolence and fatigue in primary biliary cirrhosis. *Aliment. Pharmacol. Ther.* **2007**, *25*, 471–476. [CrossRef]
87. Millar, B.; Richardson, C.; McKay, K.; Pechlivanis, A.; Innes, B.; Kirby, J.; Jones, D.; Holmes, E.; Oakley, F. Obeticholic acid therapy improves cognitive decline in cholestatic liver disease. *J. Hepatol.* **2017**, *66*, S364–S365. [CrossRef]
88. Lee, J.Y.; Danford, C.J.; Trivedi, H.D.; Tapper, E.B.; Patwardhan, V.R.; Bonder, A. Treatment of Fatigue in Primary Biliary Cholangitis: A Systematic Review and Meta-Analysis. *Am. J. Dig. Dis.* **2019**, *64*, 2338–2350. [CrossRef]
89. Bertolini, A.; Fiorotto, R.; Strazzabosco, M. Bile acids and their receptors: Modulators and therapeutic targets in liver inflammation. *Semin. Immunopathol.* **2022**, *44*, 547–564. [CrossRef]
90. Mayo, M.J. Mechanisms and molecules: What are the treatment targets for primary biliary cholangitis? *Hepatology* **2022**, *76*, 518–531. [CrossRef]
91. Gochanour, E.M.; Kowdley, K.V. Investigational drugs in early phase development for primary biliary cholangitis. *Expert Opin. Investig. Drugs* **2021**, *30*, 131–141. [CrossRef] [PubMed]

biomedicines

Review

Obeticholic Acid for Primary Biliary Cholangitis

Annarosa Floreani [1,2,*], Daniela Gabbia [3] and Sara De Martin [3]

1 Department of Surgery, Oncology and Gastroenterology, University of Padova, 35131 Padova, Italy
2 Scientific Institute for Research, Hospitalization and Healthcare, 37024 Verona, Italy
3 Department of Pharmaceutical and Pharmacological Sciences, University of Padova, 35131 Padova, Italy
* Correspondence: annarosa.floreani@unipd.it; Tel.: +39-3899-4188-41

Abstract: Primary biliary cholangitis (PBC) is a rare autoimmune cholestatic liver disease that may progress to fibrosis and/or cirrhosis. Treatment options are currently limited. The first-line therapy for this disease is the drug ursodeoxycholic acid (UDCA), which has been proven to normalize serum markers of liver dysfunction, halt histologic disease progression, and lead to a prolongation of transplant-free survival. However, 30–40% of patients unfortunately do not respond to this first-line therapy. Obeticholic acid (OCA) is the only registered agent for second-line treatment in UDCA-non responders. In this review, we focus on the pharmacological features of OCA, describing its mechanism of action of and its tolerability and efficacy in PBC patients. We also highlight current perspectives on future therapies for this condition.

Keywords: primary biliary cholangitis; obeticholic acid; ursodeoxycholic acid; farnesoid X receptor

Citation: Floreani, A.; Gabbia, D.; De Martin, S. Obeticholic Acid for Primary Biliary Cholangitis. *Biomedicines* **2022**, *10*, 2464. https://doi.org/10.3390/biomedicines10102464

Academic Editors: Giovanni Squadrito and Francesco Vasuri

Received: 23 July 2022
Accepted: 28 September 2022
Published: 2 October 2022

1. Introduction

Primary biliary cholangitis (PBC) is a chronic disease characterized by the accumulation of bile acids in the liver, potentially progressing to cirrhosis, end-stage liver disease, hepatocellular carcinoma, and even death [1]. The existence of gender differences in PBC development has been widely reported. Indeed, PBC develops more frequently in females than males [1]. In the global population, a prevalence of 14.6 cases per 100,000 people has been observed, with a female:male ratio of 9:1, and 1.76 new cases diagnosed per 100,000 people each year [2]. Due to more careful routine testing and/or incompletely understood changes in environmental factors, the definition and outcome of PBC have been reconsidered over the last 30 years, from a severe symptomatic disease characterized by symptoms of portal hypertension to a milder disease with a long natural history [3]. As a consequence, many patients are asymptomatic, and most new diagnoses (up to 60%) are made after the discovery of increased serum biochemical markers of liver function during check-ups performed for unrelated purposes [4,5]. This autoimmune cholestatic disease is characterized by increased plasma levels of alkaline phosphatase (ALP) and the presence of a high titer of antimitochondrial antibodies (AMAs) in over 90% of patients, as well as a PBC-specific anti-nuclear antibody (ANA). The current EASL guidelines suggest that a diagnosis of PBC can be determined in adult patients in the presence of cholestasis and the absence of other systemic diseases, when the ALP value is elevated and AMAs are present with a titer >1:40 [6].

Ursodeoxycholic acid (UDCA) represents the gold standard for PBC therapy, and it is generally administered as a daily oral treatment (recommended dose: 13–15 mg/kg) [6]. UDCA therapy improves liver transplantation (LT)-free survival in PBC patients, including those with early and advanced disease, and also in patients who did not meet the accepted criteria for UDCA response [7]. Even though the improvement of biochemical parameters after UDCA treatment is modest, patients experience a long-term benefit in terms of improved survival. Regardless, non-responders represent 30–40% of all UDCA-treated patients, and globally have a higher risk of PBC progression and a greater need for transplant than responder patients, as well as a higher mortality [8]. A young age at diagnosis and male sex have been associated with a reduced chance of biochemical response to UDCA therapy in a large cohort study from the UK-PBC study group [9]. Accordingly, another large, multicenter long-term follow-up study (n = 4355) found that young PBC patients (aged <45) had significantly lower response rates to UDCA than their older counterparts (aged >65) [10]. However, the biological mechanisms underpinning this clinical observation in non-responders to UDCA are far from completely understood.

Therefore, the proposal of a second-line therapy devoted to UDCA non-responders provides the rationale to overcome the observed limitations of drug efficacy. To date, obeticholic acid (OCA) represents the only second-line treatment recommended for non-responder PBC patients, which are intolerant to UDCA therapy or in whom a 12 month-treatment haven't produced benefit. As demonstrated by clinical trials, including the phase III POISE study described in detail below, OCA is effective in improving the serum and histological endpoints of PBC patients in monotherapy. In this review, we focus on the mechanism of action of OCA and its tolerability and efficacy in PBC, and offer a perspective on the future treatment of this condition.

2. Pharmacological Actions of OCA

OCA, a synthetic derivative of the bile acid (BA) chenodeoxycholic acid, is an agonist of the farnesoid X receptor (FXR) [11], a key nuclear receptor mainly expressed in the liver and gut, which orchestrates complex signaling pathways related to the homeostasis of bile acids (BAs) (Figure 1). In vitro pharmacological studies have demonstrated that OCA is an FXR agonist with a potency 100 times higher than endogenous BAs [12]. BA synthesis occurs in the liver starting from hepatic cholesterol. After their synthesis, BAs are secreted into the gut to help digestion and consequently the absorption of nutrients, in particular lipids and liposoluble vitamins, by virtue of their emulsifying ability [13]. After their secretion, about 95% of BAs are reabsorbed from the terminal ileum, thus entering into the enterohepatic circulation. As FXR agonists, BAs themselves participate in the finely tuned regulation of their own synthesis and secretion through the modulation of FXR activation. In PBC-related cholestasis, the enterohepatic circulation of BAs is impaired, leading to hepatic inflammation and damage.

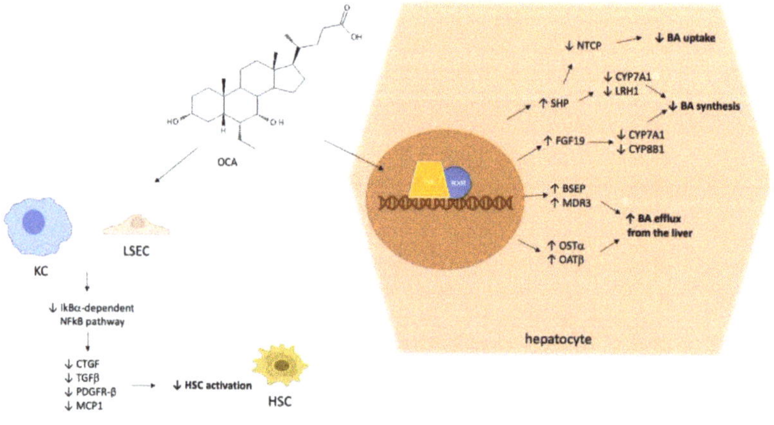

Figure 1. Molecular mechanism of hepatic OCA pharmacodynamics. OCA activates FXR, thereby triggering cellular pathways leading to a reduction in the synthesis and hepatic uptake of BAs, and an increase in their efflux from the liver. Furthermore, OCA acts on LSEC and KC, exerting anti-inflammatory and antifibrotic effects by reducing the production of proinflammatory cytokines

and HSC activation, respectively. Abbreviations: farnesoid X receptor (FXR), retinoid X receptor (RXR), bile acid (BA), Kupffer cell (KC), liver sinusoidal endothelial cell (LSEC), hepatic stellate cell (HSC), small heterodimer partner (SHP), liver receptor homolog 1 (LRH-1), fibroblast growth factor-19 (FGF-19), sodium taurocholate co-transporting polypeptide (NTCP), bile salt export pump (BSEP), multidrug resistance protein-3 (MDR3), organic solute transporters (OST), transforming growth-factor β (TGFβ), connective tissue growth factor (CTGF), platelet-derived growth factor β-receptor (PDGFR-β), monocyte chemo-attractant protein-1 (MCP1), nuclear factor kappa-light-chain-enhancer of activated B cells (NF-κB), inhibitor of kB (IκB).

Similar to other nuclear receptors [14,15], upon activation, FXR binds to the retinoid X receptor (RXR). The binding of the FXR–RXR heterodimer to DNA responsive elements results in the induction of the small heterodimer partner (SHP) gene, finally causing the transcriptional repression of rate-limiting enzymes in BA synthesis, such as cytochrome P450 (CYP)7A1 and liver receptor homolog 1 (LRH-1) [16]. LRH-1 is a transcription factor with a key role in the regulation of BA and cholesterol homeostasis, and also in coordinating a panel of other hepatic metabolic processes [17]. In addition, FXR stimulates the synthesis of fibroblast growth factor-19 (FGF-19), which in turn participates in the inhibition of CYP7A1 and CYP8B1 expression through the fibroblast growth factor receptor-4 (FGFR4) pathway in hepatocytes [18]. As a result, the above-described FXR/SHP and FXR/FGF19/FGFR4 pathways are major negative regulators of BA synthesis. Furthermore, FXR inhibits the sodium taurocholate co-transporting polypeptide (NTCP) via SHP, thereby repressing hepatic BA uptake [19]. FXR activation also increases the efflux of BAs from the liver to the canalicular lumen by targeting the transporter bile salt export pump (BSEP) and multidrug resistance protein-3 (MDR3), triggering another mechanism responsible for the anticholestatic effects of FXR agonists [20]. FXR activation also leads to an increase in the expression of the organic solute transporters OSTα and β, which also enhance BA efflux from the liver to the portal vein [21]. Besides its pivotal activity as a BA-responsive transcription regulator of BA synthesis and metabolism, as described in detail above, it has been demonstrated that FXR-mediated signaling plays a role in hepatic fibrogenesis, although controversial results have been obtained regarding this function. Hence, it has been observed that FXR knock-out mice develop hepatic inflammation, fibrosis, and liver tumors over time [22] and, accordingly, it has been demonstrated that OCA-induced FXR activation reduced liver fibrosis in two different experimental in vivo models of liver fibrosis [23]. Other authors have suggested that FXR in liver fibrosis models can be either detrimental or irrelevant, depending on the type of damage [24]. Notably, no direct effects of FXR agonists could be observed on the activation of cultured hepatic stellate cells (HSCs) [25,26], which are the main cell types triggering the fibrogenesis process [27].

OCA exerted both anti-inflammatory and ant-fibrotic effects by targeting the activation of both liver sinusoidal endothelial cells (LSECs) and Kupffer cells [26]. In particular, OCA reduces the production of inflammatory cytokines and chemokines (transforming growth-factor β, connective tissue growth factor, platelet-derived growth factor β-receptor, monocyte chemo-attractant protein-1) by these two types of sinusoidal cells, which in turn activate HSCs [28]. Hence, the mechanism of the anti-inflammatory effect relies on the inhibition of the NF-κB signaling pathway via the up-regulation of its inhibitor IκBα. In summary, OCA acts by a complex mechanism, comprising several actions: (a) the regulation of bile acid transport; (b) the reduction in inflammation; (c) the modulation of cellular pathways triggering fibrogenesis [29]. Due to the induction of a signaling pathway which modulates the activity of fibroblast growth factor-19 (FGF-19), OCA exerts greater hepatoprotection than UDCA. OCA also induces the expression and secretion of gut-derived hormones, e.g., FGF-19 [30]. This hormone is absorbed and secreted by enterocytes into the portal blood, thereby reaching the liver through the portal venous system. In the liver, FGF-19 is involved in the anticholestatic mechanisms described above.

3. Pre-Registration Studies

OCA has been evaluated in monotherapy in a phase II study in which PBC patients were enrolled with the aim of assessing its benefit in the absence of UDCA treatment [31]. After randomization, patients were treated with a placebo (23 patients), or two doses of OCA (10 mg in 20 patients and 50 mg in 16 patients) for 3 months, and followed up by a 6-year open-label extension. The ALP reduction, measured as the percentage difference from the baseline, was evaluated as the primary endpoint of this study. The treatment with both dosages induced a significant ALP reduction compared to the placebo. Accordingly, other plasma parameters were reduced in OCA-treated patients, e.g., conjugated bilirubin, GGT, AST, and immunoglobulins. In this study, the most common adverse effect reported after OCA treatment was pruritus, having been experienced by 15% of the 10 mg-treated patients and 38% of the 50 mg-treated patients.

The first approval of OCA was obtained following the results of a phase III trial that enrolled 216 patients [32], and demonstrated that about 59% of UDCA-non-responders benefitted from a one-year treatment with a combination of OCA and UDCA. These patients reached the clinical endpoint, set as an ALP level of less than 1.67 times the upper limit of the normal range, with a reduction of at least 15% from the baseline). Thereafter, the study underwent an open-label extension phase in which 193 enrolled patients were switched to OCA treatment [33]. The results of the following 3-year interim analysis showed that OCA therapy was well tolerated and could be demonstrated to maintain its performance over time. Additionally, a post-hoc analysis revealed that OCA induced a significant bilirubin reduction (both total and direct) that was particularly evident in those patients with a high baseline value of direct bilirubin [34]. This analysis thus confirmed the beneficial effects of OCA therapy in high-risk patients. Furthermore, the histological analysis of liver biopsies at baseline and after a 3-year treatment with OCA in a subgroup of patients (n = 17) revealed the improvement or stabilization of a panel of histologic disease features, e.g., ductular injury, fibrosis, and collagen morphometry [35]. This analysis, despite the limited number of assessed liver biopsies, further demonstrated that OCA is effective in UDCA-non-responders. The most reported adverse effects related to OCA treatment were pruritus and fatigue, which were experienced by 77% and 33% of patients, respectively [34]. As regards pruritus, only 8% of the OCA-treated patients interrupted the treatment during the open-label extension phase and, in general, patients reported a mild-to-moderate pruritus, and those experiencing severe pruritus were treated with specific medication after a clinical consult. In general, the results of this clinical trial demonstrate that 3 years of OCA treatment were efficient in ameliorating or stabilizing multiple histological features of PBC in most patients with an inadequate UDCA response, and supported the approval of OCA from the FDA in 2016.

Another sub-analysis of the above-reported trial observed that OCA treatment induced a significant reduction in the AST to platelet ratio (APRI). This effect was observed after a 1-year treatment and in the open-label extension phase in the groups treated with 10 and 50 mg OCA with respect to the placebo [36]. Liver stiffness (LS) was evaluated in 39 patients randomized and dosed with the placebo, 35 patients dosed with OCA 5–10 mg, and 32 patients dosed with OCA 10 mg. LS at baseline was 12.7 $\pm$ 10.7, 10.7 $\pm$ 8.6, and 11.4 $\pm$ 8.2 kPa, respectively. During the double-blind and open-label phases, a decrease, while not significant, was only observed in the OCA 10 mg group, while both the OCA 5–10 mg and placebo groups displayed mean increases in liver stiffness [36]. In other words, a trend towards a reduction in LS was observed only in the arm treated with the highest dose of OCA. In another scenario, namely non-alcoholic steatohepatitis, patients enrolled in the phase III REGENERATE study with OCA showed a significant reduction in LS after 18 months in the OCA 25 mg group vs. the placebo [37]. Thus, the assessment of the antifibrotic activity of OCA in a clinical setting has several limitations, mainly considering that changes in LS occur during a median interval of 2 years.

The main pre-registration studies evaluating the efficacy and safety of OCA are reported in Table 1.

Table 1. Summary of the main pre-registration studies described in the text.

NCT Number [Ref]	Type of Study	Therapeutic Scheme	Population	Outcome	Adverse Events
NCT00570765 [31]	Phase II study, 3-month randomized, double-blind, placebo-controlled, parallel group phase, followed by a long-term safety extension (LTSE)	OCA monotherapy (10 or 50 mg)	60 PBC patients (18–70 years)	ALP reduction at both dosages after a 3-month treatment. Improvement of GGT, ALT, conjugated bilirubin, IgG	Pruritus (placebo 35%, OCA 10 70%, 94% OCA 50
NCT01473524 [32,33]	Phase III study, international 12-month randomized, double-blind (DB), placebo-controlled, parallel group phase, followed by a long-term safety extension (LTSE) phase of up to 5 years	OCA 5 mg (6 months) up to 10 mg or 10 mg vs. placebo	217 patients (≥18 years)	ALP reduction only after 12-month treatment with combination Reduction in total and direct bilirubin	Pruritus (56% in the 5–10% group and 68% in the 10 mg group vs. 38% placebo
NCT03253276 [38]	Early phase I, double-blind placebo-controlled crossover study	OCA vs. placebo	8 PBC patients	OCA reduced the time hepatocytes are exposed to potentially cytotoxic bile acids.	1 patient dropped for pruritus
NCT00550862 [39]	Phase II, randomized, double-blind study	OCA (10, 25, 50 mg) plus UDCA combination	165 patients (18–75 years)	Significant reduction in ALP, γ-GT, and ALT compared with placebo, in patients with PBC experiencing an inadequate response to UDCA	13% discontinuation for pruritus

4. Real-World Data on OCA

Currently, OCA is available as tablets containing 5 and 10 mg under the brand name Ocaliva. Typically, therapy for PBC patients is started with the administration of an initial dose of 5 mg once daily, which can be titrated to a maximum of 10 mg daily [40]. The general recommendation for patients with advanced cirrhosis (Child–Pugh B or C) is to start with a dose of 5 mg once weekly, which is then increased to a maximum of 10 mg twice weekly if the drug is well-tolerated.

The most significant ADRs caused by OCA therapy which have been reported in clinical trials are pruritus, fatigue, nausea, and headache. To a minor extent, hypersensitivity reactions and depression have also been observed [40]. As far as pruritus is concerned, it appears to be less severe if the patients are initially treated with a low dose, which can then be gradually increased. As a consequence of the alteration of lipid metabolism, which is due to other molecular signaling pathways triggered by FXR activation, an increase in total serum lipid levels and a small decrease in high-density lipoprotein (HDL) have also been reported in PBC patients treated with OCA, but to date these effects have not been correlated to a long-term increased cardiovascular risk [30].

Real-world data are crucial for understanding treatment effectiveness and safety in everyday clinical practice where: (i) patients' characteristics are more heterogeneous with respect to sub-phenotypes, e.g., cirrhosis and overlap syndrome between PBC and AIH; (ii) the treatment schedule may be less rigid and more "personalized" by each treating physician. A number of post-registration clinical trials are ongoing and recruiting patients (Table 2).

Table 2. Ongoing clinical trials recruiting patients for post-registration efficacy assessment.

NCT Number	Type of Study	Therapeutic Scheme	Estimated Enrollment	Primary Endpoints
NCT05450887	Randomized, double-blind, multicenter, placebo-controlled phase III clinical trial	OCA (5 mg titrated to 10 mg) ± UDCA vs. placebo ± UDCA (13~15 mg/kg/day)	156 PBC patients (18–75 years)	Percentage of PBC patients reaching ALP < 1.67× Upper Limit of Normal, and ALP decrease ≥ 15% from baseline, and total bilirubin ≤ ULN after 12-month treatment
NCT03703076	Post-authorization non-interventional observational, multi-site study	OCA (5 or 10 mg)	150 patients	Response to Ocaliva® after 12-month treatment (monotherapy or combination) assessed by Paris II response criteria
NCT05293938	Retrospective study	OCA (5 or 10 mg) and UDCA	2544 participants	Time to the first occurrence of the composite endpoint of all-cause death, liver transplant, or hospitalization for hepatic decompensation after 67 months
NCT05292872 (HEROES PBC)	Retrospective study	OCA (5 or 10 mg) and UDCA	3156 participants	Time to the first occurrence of all-cause death, liver transplant, or hospitalization for hepatic decompensation after 67 months
NCT05239468	Phase IIa, double-blind, randomized, active-controlled, parallel group study	Bezafibrate 100 or 200 mg, OCA 5 mg, Bezafibrate placebo, OCA placebo	60 patients	ALP change after 12 weeks vs. baseline
NCT04594694	Phase II, double-blind, randomized, parallel group study	Bezafibrate 200 or 400 mg, OCA mg, Bezafibrate placebos, OCA placebo	75 patients	ALP change after 12 weeks vs. baseline
NCT04076527	Prospective, multicenter cohort study	OCA vs. UDCA	1200 patients	Construction of a systematic registry to describe the characteristics and the recent state of usual clinical care of the respective population
NCT04956328	Multicenter, randomized, double-blind trial	OCA (5 to 10 mg) + UDCA, or placebo + UDCA	120 patients	Percentage of PBC patients reaching ALP < 1.67× ULN, and ALP decrease ≥ 15% from baseline, and total bilirubin ≤ ULN after 48week-treatment

Three real-world cohorts have been published thus far (Table 3), all reporting results for 12 months of OCA treatment [41–43]. Altogether, 375 patients treated with OCA were included in these three studies. The main characteristics of the three cohorts are respectively described in Table 3. The inclusion criteria were: hepatologist's discretion for the Canadian cohort, lack of response to Paris II criteria [44] for the Iberian cohort and ALP >1.5 times the normal according to the Italian Medicines Agency (AIFA) for the Italian cohort. The percentages of patients with cirrhosis were 6.3, 10, and 15%. The percentages of response at 12 months according to the POISE criteria were respectively 18, 29.5, and 51.9%. Due to the retrospective design of these studies, a comparable evaluation of the response to OCA is impossible. However, it has to be pointed out that in the Italian cohort, with one third of cirrhotic patients, the response rate was lower due to the higher drop-out and higher levels of bilirubin at baseline in cirrhotic patients. Within the Canadian cohort, 11 patients (17%) had a permanent discontinuation of treatment (2 of them with Child–Pugh A and B respectively) for suspected hepatotoxicity. The first case was a 67-year-old female who discontinued OCA due to an increase in ALP. The second patient was a 54-year-old female who developed severe cholestatic cirrhosis, who was transplanted for severe complications. Within the Iberian cohort, a total of 14 patients (11.67%) discontinued the treatment due to severe adverse events or decompensation of cirrhosis. Within the Italian cohort, 33 patients (17%) discontinued OCA for pruritus or other side-effects. In the same cohort, factors associated with a lack of response at 12 months were: previous treatment with fibrates, high levels of ALP at baseline, and high levels of bilirubin at baseline [43].

Table 3. Real-world data in three cohorts of patients with PBC.

Author	Country	N. of Patients	Inclusion Criteria	% of Cirrhosis	% of pts with AIH/PBC Overlap	% of Response According to POISE
Roberts	Canada	64	Hepatologist's discretion	23.7	6.3	18
Gomez	Spain/Portugal	120	Lack of response to Paris II criteria	21.7	10	29.5
D'Amato	Italy	191	ALP > 1.5 UNL	32	15	51.9

A further analysis was performed in 100 cirrhotic patients of the Italian cohort [45]. The response to treatment was obtained in 41% of cases, according to the POISE criteria, confirming OCA efficacy at this stage as well. In this case, the use of the normal range criteria means that the endpoint was reached by only 11.5% of the cirrhotic patients. Regarding the reported severe adverse effects, 22% of patients discontinued OCA therapy: 5 patients due to jaundice and/or ascitic decompensation, 4 due to upper digestive bleeding, and 1 subject died after the substitution of a transjugular intrahepatic portosystemic shunt.

A sub-analysis from the Italian and Iberian cohorts found that patients with PBC/AIH overlap syndrome had a similar response after OCA treatment [42,43].

Two further real-world studies were presented at an AASLD virtual meeting in 2020. The first study, derived from the GLOBAL PBC group, enrolled 290 patients in 11 centers located between Europe, North America, and Israel [46]. Among them, 215 patients met the POISE criteria for eligibility, 60 patients possessed available biochemical data for a period of 12 months, and 35% of patients reached the pre-defined POISE primary endpoint after 1 year of treatment. The second study was conducted on 319 patients that received OCA therapy between May 2016 and September 2019, and were considered eligible for OCA according to laboratory databases and American administrative claims [47]. According to the Toronto criteria, the proportion of patients achieving a biochemical response to the treatment was 48% after 1 year, 58% after 2 years, and 55% after 3 years which marked the end of the follow-up period [48]. More recently, a large nationwide experience of second-line therapy in PBC has been reported [49]. The study was conducted from August 2017 to June 2021 across 14 centers in the UK. A total of 457 PBC patients with an inadequate response to UDCA were recruited. Overall, 259 patients received OCA and 80 received fibrates (fibric acid derivatives) and completed 12 months of therapy, yielding a dropout rate of 25.7% and 25.9%, respectively. Treatment efficacy was quantified by the proportion of patients attaining a biochemical response according to propensity score matching. The 12-month biochemical response rates were 70.6% with OCA and 80% under fibric acid treatment, without reaching any statistical significance.

With the objective of evaluating the time to first occurrence of liver transplant or death, OCA-treated patients in the POISE trial and open-label extension were compared with non-OCA-treated external controls [50]. Propensity scores were generated for external control patients meeting POISE eligibility criteria from 1381 patients in the Global PBC registry study and 2135 in the UK PBC registry. Over the 6-year follow-up, patients treated with OCA had a significantly greater transplant-free survival than comparable external control patients.

5. Combined Therapy with OCA and Fibrates

Fibrates, well-known agents with anti-lipidemic properties, were proposed as a second-line treatment because their beneficial effects on inflammation, cholestasis, and fibrosis are documented, resulting from their activity as peroxisome proliferator-activated receptor (PPAR) agonists. Fibrates have different affinities to the three main PPAR isoforms, PPARα, PPARβ/δ, and PPARγ, and consequently can activate different signaling pathways. As an example, fenofibrate, a PPARα agonist, upon binding to its receptor, increases the expression of multidrug resistance protein 3 (MDR3) [51]. Furthermore, it increases biliary phosphatidylcholine secretion, thus ameliorating a recognized biomarker of cholestasis. Bezafibrate acts as a dual agonist of PPARα and PPARγ and is also a pregnane X receptor (PXR) agonist [52]. The BEZURSO trial is a Phase III study, employing bezafibrate in combination with UDCA, and was the first placebo-controlled trial evaluating the use of fibrates as a second-line treatment for PBC. In this study, the second-line combination therapy of bezafibrate and UDCA was effective in obtaining a complete biochemical response with a rate significantly higher than that observed in patients treated with a placebo and UDCA [53]. This regression was associated with a concurrent improvement of both symptoms and surrogate markers of liver fibrosis. The most frequently reported ADRs of fibrates include increased levels of creatinine and transaminases and heartburn. As a consequence of its main mechanism of action involving a reduction in BA synthesis, clofibrate treatment can lead to the formation of gallstones and hypercholesterolemia [54], two events which have not been observed during treatment with fenofibrate or bezafibrate.

A triple therapy with UDCA, OCA, and fibrates was studied in a multicenter retrospective cohort of patients with PBC [55]. Fifty-eight patients were treated with a combination of UDCA (13–15 mg/day), OCA (5–10 mg/day), and fibrates (fenofibrate 200 mg/day or bezafibrate 400 mg/day). This combination achieved a significant reduction in ALP level compared to dual therapy (odds ratio for ALP normalization of 5.5). The primary outcome (change in ALP) and the effect on pruritus are summarized in Table 4.

Table 4. Outcomes of triple therapy (UDCA + fibrates + OCA) [55].

Outcome	Baseline Dual	Baseline Triple	Last Follow-Up Triple
ALP (xULN)	2.5	1.8	1.1
Normal ALP (%)	0.7	10.3	47.4
Absence of pruritus	41.1	51.8	66.1

6. Conclusions

In May 2021, the Food and Drug Administration issued a new warning restricting the use of OCA in patients with advanced cirrhosis (https://www.fda.gov/drugs/drug-safety-and-availability/due-risk-serious-liver-injury-fda-restricts-use-ocaliva-obeticholic-acid-primary-biliary-cholangitis, accessed on 1 September 2022). Advanced cirrhosis was defined on the basis of current or prior evidence of liver decompensation (e.g., encephalopathy, coagulopathy) or portal hypertension (e.g., ascites, gastroesophageal varices, or persistent thrombocytopenia). A practical guidance statement was published thereafter by the AASLD [56]. In this statement, the AASLD reported the contraindication on cirrhosis announced by the FDA, namely decompensated cirrhosis, and further recommended the careful monitoring of any patient with cirrhosis, even if not advanced, receiving OCA. In eligible patients, the recommended starting dose of OCA is 5 mg, which can be titrated to 10 mg after 6 months if OCA is well-tolerated. It is also recommended by the AASLD to monitor liver function before and after the initiation of OCA therapy.

In conclusion, due to its complex and fascinating mechanism, OCA represents a complete intervention for the therapeutic management of those PBC patients who cannot be treated satisfactorily with UDCA for efficacy or safety reasons. However, more real-world data are needed to gain a full understanding of its pharmacological and toxicological features.

Author Contributions: Conceptualization, A.F.; writing—original draft preparation, A.F., D.G. and S.D.M.; writing—review and editing, A.F. and S.D.M. All authors have read and agreed to the published version of the manuscript.

Funding: This research received no external funding.

Institutional Review Board Statement: Not applicable.

Informed Consent Statement: Not applicable.

Conflicts of Interest: The authors declare no conflict of interest.

References

1. Gulamhusein, A.F.; Hirschfield, G.M. Primary Biliary Cholangitis: Pathogenesis and Therapeutic Opportunities. *Nat. Rev. Gastroenterol. Hepatol.* **2020**, *17*, 93–110. [CrossRef] [PubMed]
2. Lv, T.; Chen, S.; Li, M.; Zhang, D.; Kong, Y.; Jia, J. Regional Variation and Temporal Trend of Primary Biliary Cholangitis Epidemiology: A Systematic Review and Meta-analysis. *J. Gastroenterol. Hepatol.* **2021**, *36*, 1423–1434. [CrossRef] [PubMed]
3. Murillo Perez, C.F.; Goet, J.C.; Lammers, W.J.; Gulamhusein, A.; van Buuren, H.R.; Ponsioen, C.Y.; Carbone, M.; Mason, A.; Corpechot, C.; Invernizzi, P.; et al. Milder Disease Stage in Patients with Primary Biliary Cholangitis over a 44-year Period: A Changing Natural History. *Hepatology* **2018**, *67*, 1920–1930. [CrossRef] [PubMed]
4. Prince, M.I. Asymptomatic Primary Biliary Cirrhosis: Clinical Features, Prognosis, and Symptom Progression in a Large Population Based Cohort. *Gut* **2004**, *53*, 865–870. [CrossRef] [PubMed]
5. Invernizzi, P.; Lleo, A.; Podda, M. Interpreting Serological Tests in Diagnosing Autoimmune Liver Diseases. *Semin. Liver Dis.* **2007**, *27*, 161–172. [CrossRef] [PubMed]
6. European Association for the Study of the Liver; Hirschfield, G.M.; Beuers, U.; Corpechot, C.; Invernizzi, P.; Jones, D.; Marzioni, M.; Schramm, C. EASL Clinical Practice Guidelines: The Diagnosis and Management of Patients with Primary Biliary Cholangitis. *J. Hepatol.* **2017**, *67*, 145–172. [CrossRef] [PubMed]
7. Harms, M.H.; van Buuren, H.R.; Corpechot, C.; Thorburn, D.; Janssen, H.L.A.; Lindor, K.D.; Hirschfield, G.M.; Parés, A.; Floreani, A.; Mayo, M.J.; et al. Ursodeoxycholic Acid Therapy and Liver Transplant-Free Survival in Patients with Primary Biliary Cholangitis. *J. Hepatol.* **2019**, *71*, 357–365. [CrossRef]
8. Selmi, C.; Bowlus, C.L.; Gershwin, M.E.; Coppel, R.L. Primary Biliary Cirrhosis. *Lancet* **2011**, *377*, 1600–1609. [CrossRef]
9. Carbone, M.; Mells, G.F.; Pells, G.; Dawwas, M.F. Sex and age are determinants of the clinical phenotype of primary biliary cirrhosis and response to ursodeoxycholic acid. *Gastroenterology* **2013**, *144*, 560–569. [CrossRef]
10. Cheung, A.C.; Lammers, W.J.; Murillo Perez, C.F.; van Buuren, H.R.; Gulamhusein, A.; Trivedi, P.J.; Lazaridis, K.N. Effects of age and sex on response to ursodeoxycholic acid and transplant-free survival in patients with primary biliary cholangitis. *Clin. Gastreonetrol. Hepatol.* **2019**, *17*, 2076–2084. [CrossRef]
11. Beuers, U.; Trauner, M.; Jansen, P.; Poupon, R. New Paradigms in the Treatment of Hepatic Cholestasis: From UDCA to FXR, PXR and Beyond. *J. Hepatol.* **2015**, *62*, S25–S37. [CrossRef] [PubMed]
12. Pellicciari, R.; Costantino, G.; Camaioni, E.; Sadeghpour, B.M.; Entrena, A.; Willson, T.M.; Fiorucci, S.; Clerici, C.; Gioiello, A. Bile Acid Derivatives as Ligands of the Farnesoid X Receptor. Synthesis, Evaluation, and Structure-Activity Relationship of a Series of Body and Side Chain Modified Analogues of Chenodeoxycholic Acid. *J. Med. Chem.* **2004**, *47*, 4559–4569. [CrossRef] [PubMed]
13. Chiang, J.Y.L. Bile Acid Metabolism and Signaling in Liver Disease and Therapy. *Liver Res.* **2017**, *1*, 3–9. [CrossRef] [PubMed]
14. Sayaf, K.; Zanotto, I.; Russo, F.P.; Gabbia, D.; De Martin, S. The Nuclear Receptor PXR in Chronic Liver Disease. *Cells* **2021**, *11*, 61. [CrossRef]
15. Gabbia, D.; Dalla Pozza, A.; Albertoni, L.; Lazzari, R.; Zigiotto, G.; Carrara, M.; Baldo, V.; Baldovin, T.; Floreani, A.; De Martin, S. Pregnane X Receptor and Constitutive Androstane Receptor Modulate Differently CYP3A-Mediated Metabolism in Early- and Late-Stage Cholestasis. *World J. Gastroenterol.* **2017**, *23*, 7519–7530. [CrossRef]
16. Goodwin, B.; Jones, S.A.; Price, R.R.; Watson, M.A.; McKee, D.D.; Moore, L.B.; Galardi, C.; Wilson, J.G.; Lewis, M.C.; Roth, M.E.; et al. A Regulatory Cascade of the Nuclear Receptors FXR, SHP-1, and LRH-1 Represses Bile Acid Biosynthesis. *Mol. Cell* **2000**, *6*, 517–526. [CrossRef]
17. Sun, Y.; Demagny, H.; Schoonjans, K. Emerging Functions of the Nuclear Receptor LRH-1 in Liver Physiology and Pathology. *Biochim. Biophys. Acta (BBA)—Mol. Basis Dis.* **2021**, *1867*, 166145. [CrossRef]
18. Maliha, S.; Guo, G.L. Farnesoid X Receptor and Fibroblast Growth Factor 15/19 as Pharmacological Targets. *Liver Res.* **2021**, *5*, 142–150. [CrossRef]
19. Salhab, A.; Amer, J.; Lu, Y.; Safadi, R. Sodium $^+$/Taurocholate Cotransporting Polypeptide as Target Therapy for Liver Fibrosis. *Gut* **2022**, *71*, 1373–1385. [CrossRef]

20. Halilbasic, E.; Claudel, T.; Trauner, M. Bile Acid Transporters and Regulatory Nuclear Receptors in the Liver and Beyond. *J. Hepatol.* **2013**, *58*, 155–168. [CrossRef]
21. Cariello, M.; Piccinin, E.; Garcia-Irigoyen, O.; Sabbà, C.; Moschetta, A. Nuclear Receptor FXR, Bile Acids and Liver Damage: Introducing the Progressive Familial Intrahepatic Cholestasis with FXR Mutations. *Biochim. Biophys. Acta (BBA)—Mol. Basis Dis.* **2018**, *1864*, 1308–1318. [CrossRef] [PubMed]
22. Yang, F.; Huang, X.; Yi, T.; Yen, Y.; Moore, D.D.; Huang, W. Spontaneous Development of Liver Tumors in the Absence of the Bile Acid Receptor Farnesoid X Receptor. *Cancer Res.* **2007**, *67*, 863–867. [CrossRef] [PubMed]
23. Fiorucci, S.; Antonelli, E.; Rizzo, G.; Renga, B.; Mencarelli, A.; Riccardi, L.; Orlandi, S.; Pellicciari, R.; Morelli, A. The Nuclear Receptor SHP Mediates Inhibition of Hepatic Stellate Cells by FXR and Protects against Liver Fibrosis. *Gastroenterology* **2004**, *127*, 1497–1512. [CrossRef] [PubMed]
24. Fickert, P.; Hirschfield, G.M.; Denk, G.; Marschall, H.-U.; Altorjay, I.; Färkkilä, M.; Schramm, C.; Spengler, U.; Chapman, R.; Bergquist, A.; et al. NorUrsodeoxycholic Acid Improves Cholestasis in Primary Sclerosing Cholangitis. *J. Hepatol.* **2017**, *67*, 549–558. [CrossRef] [PubMed]
25. Fickert, P.; Fuchsbichler, A.; Moustafa, T.; Wagner, M.; Zollner, G.; Halilbasic, E.; Stöger, U.; Arrese, M.; Pizarro, M.; Solís, N.; et al. Farnesoid X Receptor Critically Determines the Fibrotic Response in Mice but Is Expressed to a Low Extent in Human Hepatic Stellate Cells and Periductal Myofibroblasts. *Am. J. Pathol.* **2009**, *175*, 2392–2405. [CrossRef]
26. Verbeke, L.; Mannaerts, I.; Schierwagen, R.; Govaere, O.; Klein, S.; Vander Elst, I.; Windmolders, P.; Farre, R.; Wenes, M.; Mazzone, M.; et al. FXR Agonist Obeticholic Acid Reduces Hepatic Inflammation and Fibrosis in a Rat Model of Toxic Cirrhosis. *Sci. Rep.* **2016**, *6*, 33453. [CrossRef]
27. Friedman, S.L. Hepatic Stellate Cells: Protean, Multifunctional, and Enigmatic Cells of the Liver. *Physiol. Rev.* **2008**, *88*, 125–172. [CrossRef]
28. Gabbia, D.; Cannella, L.; De Martin, S. The Role of Oxidative Stress in NAFLD–NASH–HCC Transition—Focus on NADPH Oxidases. *Biomedicines* **2021**, *9*, 687. [CrossRef]
29. Modica, S.; Petruzzelli, M.; Bellafante, E.; Murzilli, S.; Salvatore, L.; Celli, N.; Di Tullio, G.; Palasciano, G.; Moustafa, T.; Halilbasic, E.; et al. Selective Activation of Nuclear Bile Acid Receptor FXR in the Intestine Protects Mice Against Cholestasis. *Gastroenterology* **2012**, *142*, 355–365.e4. [CrossRef]
30. Chapman, R.W.; Lynch, K.D. Obeticholic Acid—A New Therapy in PBC and NASH. *Br. Med. Bull.* **2020**, *133*, 95–104. [CrossRef]
31. Kowdley, K.V.; Luketic, V.; Chapman, R.; Hirschfield, G.M.; Poupon, R.; Schramm, C. A randomized trial of obeticholic acid monotherapy in patients with primary biliary cholangitis. *Hepatology* **2018**, *67*, 1890–1902. [CrossRef] [PubMed]
32. Nevens, F.; Andreone, P.; Mazzella, G.; Strasser, S.I.; Bowlus, C.; Invernizzi, P.; Drenth, J.P.H.; Pockros, P.J.; Regula, J.; Beuers, U.; et al. A Placebo-Controlled Trial of Obeticholic Acid in Primary Biliary Cholangitis. *N. Engl. J. Med.* **2016**, *375*, 631–643. [CrossRef] [PubMed]
33. Trauner, M.; Nevens, F.; Shiffman, M.L.; Drenth, J.P.H.; Bowlus, C.L.; Vargas, V.; Andreone, P.; Hirschfield, G.M.; Pencek, R.; Malecha, E.S.; et al. Long-Term Efficacy and Safety of Obeticholic Acid for Patients with Primary Biliary Cholangitis: 3-Year Results of an International Open-Label Extension Study. *Lancet Gastroenterol. Hepatol.* **2019**, *4*, 445–453. [CrossRef]
34. Parés, A.; Shiffman, M.; Vargas, V.; Invernizzi, P.; Malecha, E.S.; Liberman, A.; MacConell, L.; Hirschfield, G. Reduction and Stabilization of Bilirubin with Obeticholic Acid Treatment in Patients with Primary Biliary Cholangitis. *Liver Int.* **2020**, *40*, 1121–1129. [CrossRef] [PubMed]
35. Bowlus, C.L.; Pockros, P.J.; Kremer, A.E.; Parés, A.; Forman, L.M.; Drenth, J.P.H.; Ryder, S.D.; Terracciano, L.; Jin, Y.; Liberman, A.; et al. Long-Term Obeticholic Acid Therapy Improves Histological Endpoints in Patients With Primary Biliary Cholangitis. *Clin. Gastroenterol. Hepatol.* **2020**, *18*, 1170–1178.e6. [CrossRef]
36. Hirschfield, G.M.; Floreani, A.; Tivedi, P.J.; Pencek, R.; Liberman, A.; Marmon, T.; MacConell, L. Long-term effect of obeticholic acid on transient elastography and AST to platelet ratio index in patients with PBC. *Gut* **2017**, *66* (Suppl. 2), A98–A99.
37. Younossi, Z.M.; Ratziu, V.; Loombar, R.; Rinella, M.; Anstee, Q.M.; Goodman, Z.; Bedossa, P. Obeticholic acid for the treatment of non-alcoholic steatohepatitis: Interim analysis from a multicentre, randomised, placebo-controlled phase 3 trial. *Lancet* **2019**, *394*, 2184–2196. [CrossRef]
38. Kjærgaard, K.; Frisch, K.; Sørensen, M.; Munk, O.L.; Hofmann, A.F.; Horsager, J.; Schacht, A.C.; Erickson, M.; Shapiro, D.; Keiding, S. Obeticholic Acid Improves Hepatic Bile Acid Excretion in Patients with Primary Biliary Cholangitis. *J. Hepatol.* **2021**, *74*, 58–65. [CrossRef]
39. Hirschfield, G.M.; Mason, A.; Luketic, V.; Lindor, K.; Gordon, S.C.; Mayo, M.; Kowdley, K.V.; Vincent, C.; Bodhenheimer, H.C.; Parés, A.; et al. Efficacy of Obeticholic Acid in Patients With Primary Biliary Cirrhosis and Inadequate Response to Ursodeoxycholic Acid. *Gastroenterology* **2015**, *148*, 751–761.e8. [CrossRef]
40. Obeticholic Acid. No author listed. In *LiverTox: Clinical and Research Information on Drug-Induced Liver Injury*; National Institute of Diabetes and Digestive and Kidney Diseases: Bethesda, MD, USA, 2012.
41. Roberts, S.B.; Ismail, M.; Kanagalingam, G.; Mason, A.L.; Swain, M.G.; Vincent, C.; Yoshida, E.M.; Tsien, C.; Flemming, J.A.; Janssen, H.L.A.; et al. Real-World Effectiveness of Obeticholic Acid in Patients with Primary Biliary Cholangitis. *Hepatol. Commun.* **2020**, *4*, 1332–1345. [CrossRef]

42. Gomez, E.; Garcia Buey, L.; Molina, E.; Casado, M.; Conde, I.; Berenguer, M.; Jorquera, F.; Simón, M.-A.; Olveira, A.; Hernández-Guerra, M.; et al. Effectiveness and Safety of Obeticholic Acid in a Southern European Multicentre Cohort of Patients with Primary Biliary Cholangitis and Suboptimal Response to Ursodeoxycholic Acid. *Aliment. Pharmacol. Ther.* **2021**, *53*, 519–530. [CrossRef] [PubMed]
43. D'Amato, D.; De Vincentis, A.; Malinverno, F.; Viganò, M.; Alvaro, D.; Pompili, M.; Picciotto, A.; Palitti, V.P.; Russello, M.; Storato, S.; et al. Real-World Experience with Obeticholic Acid in Patients with Primary Biliary Cholangitis. *JHEP Rep.* **2021**, *3*, 100248. [CrossRef] [PubMed]
44. Corpechot, C.; Chazouilleres, O.; Poupon, R. Early primary biliary cirrhosis: Biochemical response to treatment and prediction of long-term outcome. *J. Hepatol.* **2011**, *55*, 1361–1367. [CrossRef] [PubMed]
45. De Vincentis, A.; D'Amato, D.; Cristoferi, L.; Gerussi, A.; Malinverno, F.; Lleo, A.; Colapietro, F. Predictors of serious adverse events and non-response in cirrhotic patients with primary biliary cholangitis treated with obeticholic acid. *Liver Int.* **2022**, in press. [CrossRef] [PubMed]
46. Gulamhusein, A.F.; Roberts, S.B.; Hallidey, N.; Carbone, M.; Yimam, K.; Namphurong, T. Real World Effectiveness of Obeticholic Acid in Patients with Primary Biliary Cholangitis: The Global Experience. *Hepatology* **2020**, *S1*, 1267.
47. Gish, R.G.; Law, A.; Adekunle, F.; Wheeler, D.; Lingohr-Smith, M.; Bassanelli, C. Real-World Effectiveness of Obeticholic Acid in Patients with Primary Biliary Cholangitis. *Hepatology* **2020**, *S1*, 1268.
48. Kumagi, T.; Guindi, M.; Fischer, S.E.; Arenovich, T.; Abdalian, R.; Coltescu, C.; Heathcote, J.E.; Hirschfield, G.M. Baseline ductopenia and treatment response predict long-term histological progression in primary biliary cirrhosis. *Am. J. Gastroenterol.* **2010**, *105*, 2186–2194. [CrossRef]
49. Abbass, N.; Culver, E.L.; Thornburn, D.; Halliday, N.; Crothers, H.; Dyson, J.K.; Phaw, A.; Aspinall, R.; Khakoo, S.I.; Kallis, Y.; et al. UK-wide multicenter evaluation of second-line therapies in primary biliary cholangitis. *Clin. Gastroenterol. Hepatol.* **2022**, in press. [CrossRef]
50. Murillo Perez, C.F.; Fisher, H.; Hin, S.; Kareithi, D.; Adekunle, F.; Mayne, T.; Malecha, E.; Ness, E.; van der Meer, A.J.; Lammers, W.J.; et al. Greater Transplant-Free Survival in Patients Receiving Obeticholic Acid for Primary Biliary Cholangitis in a Clinical Trial Setting Compared to Real-World External Controls. *Gastroenterology* **2022**, S0016-5085(22)01060-5. [CrossRef]
51. Ghonem, N.S.; Ananthanarayanan, M.; Soroka, C.J.; Boyer, J.L. Peroxisome Proliferator-Activated Receptor α Activates Human Multidrug Resistance Transporter 3/ATP-Binding Cassette Protein Subfamily B4 Transcription and Increases Rat Biliary Phosphatidylcholine Secretion. *Hepatology* **2014**, *59*, 1030–1042. [CrossRef]
52. Honda, A.; Ikegami, T.; Nakamuta, M.; Miyazaki, T.; Iwamoto, J.; Hirayama, T.; Saito, Y.; Takikawa, H.; Imawari, M.; Matsuzaki, Y. Anticholestatic Effects of Bezafibrate in Patients with Primary Biliary Cirrhosis Treated with Ursodeoxycholic Acid. *Hepatology* **2013**, *57*, 1931–1941. [CrossRef] [PubMed]
53. Corpechot, C.; Chazouillères, O.; Rousseau, A.; Le Gruyer, A.; Habersetzer, F.; Mathurin, P.; Goria, O.; Potier, P.; Minello, A.; Silvain, C.; et al. A Placebo-Controlled Trial of Bezafibrate in Primary Biliary Cholangitis. *N. Engl. J. Med.* **2018**, *378*, 2171–2181. [CrossRef] [PubMed]
54. Summerfield, J.A.; Elias, E.; Sherlock, S. Effects of Clofibrate in Primary Biliary Cirrhosis Hypercholesterolemia and Gallstones. *Gastroenterology* **1975**, *69*, 998–1000. [CrossRef]
55. Soret, P.-A.; Lam, L.; Carrat, F.; Smets, L.; Berg, T.; Carbone, M.; Invernizzi, P.; Leroy, V.; Trivedi, P.; Cazzagon, N.; et al. Combination of Fibrates with Obeticholic Acid Is Able to Normalise Biochemical Liver Tests in Patients with Difficult-to-Treat Primary Biliary Cholangitis. *Aliment. Pharmacol. Ther.* **2021**, *53*, 1138–1146. [CrossRef] [PubMed]
56. Lindor, K.D.; Bowlus, C.L.; Boyer, J.; Levy, C.; Mayo, M. Primary Biliary Cholangitis: 2021 Practice Guidance Update from the American Association for the Study of Liver Diseases. *Hepatology* **2022**, *75*, 1012–1013. [CrossRef] [PubMed]

biomedicines

MDPI

Article

Diagnostic and Clinical Value of Specific Autoantibodies against Kelch-like 12 Peptide and Nuclear Envelope Proteins in Patients with Primary Biliary Cholangitis

Alicja Bauer [1,*], Andrzej Habior [2] and Damian Gawel [1,3]

1 Department of Biochemistry and Molecular Biology, Centre of Postgraduate Medical Education, 01-813 Warsaw, Poland; damian.gawel@cmkp.edu.pl
2 Clinic of Polish Gastroenterology Foundation, 02-653 Warsaw, Poland; ahab@coi.waw.pl
3 Department of Cell Biology and Immunology, Centre of Postgraduate Medical Education, 01-813 Warsaw, Poland
* Correspondence: alicja.bauer@cmkp.edu.pl

Abstract: Primary biliary cholangitis (PBC) is a chronic autoimmune liver disease characterized by the presence of antimitochondrial and antinuclear antibodies in patients' serum. Here, we analyzed the reactivity of autoantibodies against a novel autoantigen, kelch-like 12 (KLHL12) protein, in a cohort of 138 PBC and 90 non-PBC patients. Additionally, we compared the reactivity of KLHL12 with antinuclear envelope antibodies: anti-gp210, anti-p62, and anti-LBR. Commercially available kits and an 'in-house' ELISA were used in the studies. Antinuclear envelope antibodies were detected in 65% of PBC patients and the presence of these antibodies was observed more frequently in patients diagnosed with later stages (III/IV) of PBC, according to Ludwig's classification ($p < 0.05$) and were found to correlate with a higher concentration of bilirubin. Overall, anti-KLHL12 antibodies were found more frequently in PBC patients than in non-PBC controls ($p < 0.001$). Anti-KLHL12 antibodies were detected in 36% of the tested PBC cohort, including PBC patients negative for antimitochondrial antibodies. Presence of anti-KLHL12 was also associated with a higher concentration of bilirubin and correlated with fibrosis ($p < 0.05$). Anti-KLHL12 antibodies were detected in 30% of PBC individuals positive for antinuclear envelope antibodies, while anti-KLHL12 and antinuclear envelope antibodies were found in 17% of all PBC cases. Concluding, our data confirm that antibodies against the KLHL12 protein are highly specific for PBC and when used in combination with other markers, may significantly increase the diagnosis of PBC.

Keywords: PBC; autoantibodies; glycoprotein gp210; nucleoporin p62; KLHL12 peptide

Citation: Bauer, A.; Habior, A.; Gawel, D. Diagnostic and Clinical Value of Specific Autoantibodies against Kelch-like 12 Peptide and Nuclear Envelope Proteins in Patients with Primary Biliary Cholangitis. *Biomedicines* **2022**, *10*, 801. https://doi.org/10.3390/biomedicines10040801

Academic Editor: Jinghua Wang

Received: 24 January 2022
Accepted: 26 March 2022
Published: 29 March 2022

1. Introduction

Primary biliary cholangitis (PBC) is a chronic, progressive, immune-mediated cholestatic liver disease with a strong genetic basis [1–10]. The most characteristic immunological features of this entity are anti-mitochondrial antibodies [11–14]. The M2 fraction of antimitochondrial antibodies (AMA M2), directed against the 2-oxoacid-dehydrogenase complex of the inner mitochondrial membrane, is detected in up to 95% of PBC patients. In addition, different types of antinuclear antibodies (ANAs) can be found in approximately 50% of PBC patients [15–20]. There are several nuclear structures recognized as targets for ANAs in PBC [21–29]. Some ANAs specifically target nuclear envelope (NE) proteins [30–35]. ANAs directed against NE proteins, such as anti-gp210 antibodies, are not common; nevertheless, they seem to be highly specific for PBC [36,37]. Some data indicate that anti-gp210 antibodies may be used as a marker for unfavorable prognosis of PBC [38–40]. Nucleoporin p62 is another protein associated with the NE. Wesierska-Gadek et al. (2007; 2008) found anti-p62 antibodies in about 50% of PBC patients [41,42], while Miyachi et al. (2003) showed their presence in 13% of PBC cases [43].

Antibodies against the kelch-like 12 (KLHL12) peptide were recently identified as a new biomarker for PBC and notably indicate patients who are negative for conventional autoantibodies [44]. Nevertheless, the prevalence of anti-KLHL12 antibodies in different geographical areas has rarely been reported [45]. The kelch-like family of proteins, consisting of 66 KLHL genes, appears to be involved in multiple cellular functions including cell structure, cellular communication, transcriptional regulation, collagen export, and ubiquitination of proteins through interactions with the cullin-ring E3-ligases [46,47]. KLHL12, which is located inside the nucleus, is part of this evolutionarily conserved superfamily and is crucial for collagen export [46,48]. The KLHL12 antigen was detected using microarray, proteomic, and modified enzyme-linked immunosorbent assay (ELISA) analyses [49]. These new antibodies have not been widely employed in practice and only a few reports can be found [44,45,49].

In the present study, we determined specific antibodies directed against the KLHL12 peptide in sera of Polish PBC patients and compared them to autoantibodies against anti-NE proteins, including anti-gp210, anti-p62, and anti-LBR. Additionally, we compared the presence and level of all these antibodies to biochemical and histological parameters, and evaluated their significance for the diagnosis of PBC.

2. Materials and Methods

2.1. Patients

Serum samples were collected from 138 patients (131 women, 7 men; median age: 50 age range: 26–70 years), diagnosed at the Centre of Postgraduate Medical Education (Warsaw, Poland). The diagnosis of PBC was established using generally accepted criteria according to the practical guidelines of the European Association for the Study of the Liver(EASL) for PBC [50,51]. A liver biopsy was performed in all cases. Patients positive for the hepatitis B surface antigen (HBsAg), anti-hepatitis A virus IgM, hepatitis C virus, and patients with alcoholism and autoimmune hepatitis (AIH)/PBC overlap syndrome were excluded from the study. In most patients, the diagnosis was made within one year after the onset of symptoms. The main criteria for outcome measure were time of death from liver failure or time to liver transplantation. For the analysis, we selected patients who had no other comorbidities detected at the time of the study. None of the patients had previous gastrointestinal disease. However, shortly after the serum was collected, 6 patients were diagnosed with other autoimmune diseases: 3 with Sjogren's syndrome; 1 with rheumatoid arthritis; 1 with Hashimoto's disease; 1 with systemic lupus erythematosus. The tested antibodies were not detected in any of these patients.

The control group consisted of 40 patients (16 females, 24 males; median age: 47; age range: 23–67 years) with primary sclerosing cholangitis (PSC) and 20 patients with AIH (15 females, 5 men; median age: 47 years; age range: 19–67 years). Additionally, serum samples from 30 healthy adult blood donors (22 females, 8 men; median age: 33 years; age range: 20–52 years) were collected at the Warsaw Blood Bank. The study protocol was conducted in accordance with the ethical guidelines of the Declaration of Helsinki and was approved by the Ethical Committee of the Centre of Postgraduate Medical Education, Warsaw, Poland (approval number 71/PB/2019). Written informed consent was obtained from all patients.

2.2. Detection of Antibodies

2.2.1. Detection of Anti-gp210 Antibodies and AMA M2

Anti-gp210 antibodies and AMA M2 were determined using commercially available ELISA kits (QUANTA Lite® gp210; Inova Diagnostics, USA and QUANTA Lite® M2 EP-MIT3, respectively; Inova Diagnostics, San Diego, CA, USA), according to the manufacturer's instructions. Intra-assay performance of these kits was 4.6% and 2.9%, respectively, while their inter-assay performance was 5.8% and 6.1%, respectively.

2.2.2. Detection of Anti-Nucleoporin p62 Antibodies

The level of anti-nucleoporin p62 (anti-p62) was evaluated by an 'in-house' ELISA, as previously described [52]. The antibody levels were calculated with reference to standard serum. Results > 20 units/mL were considered positive. The intra-assay performance of the used 'in-house' ELISA test was on average 4.5%, while the inter-assay coefficient of variation was equal to 11%.

2.2.3. Detection of Anti-LBR Antibodies

Anti-lamin B receptor (anti-LBR) antibodies were determined using an 'in-house' ELISA. Wells of flat-bottom microtiter plates (Costar, Corning, NY, USA) were coated with the LBR recombinant protein (Abcam, Cambridge, UK) dissolved in bicarbonate buffer (pH 9.9), then saturated with 1% bovine serum albumin (BSA; Sigma-Aldrich, Steinheim, Germany) in phosphate buffered saline (PBS; pH 7.4; HyClone; Cytiva, Marlborough, MA, USA), and washed with PBS supplemented with 0.1% Tween (PBST; Sigma-Aldrich). Next, the tested sera (diluted 1:100 in PBS) were incubated in coated plates for 1 h at room temperature (RT) with horseradish peroxidase-conjugated antibodies to human IgG (dilution 1:50,000; Daco A/S; Glostrup, Denmark) in PBST. The color reaction was developed by adding 0.1 mL of tetramethylbenzidine (TMB; SERVA Electrophoresis GmbH, Heidelberg, Germany) and stopped using 0.5 M H_2SO_4. The optical density (OD) was measured at 450 nm with an automatic plate reader (Multiscan RC, Labsystem; Vantaa, Finland). The final levels of antibodies were calculated with reference to standard serum, which had been diluted to five different concentrations (10, 30, 50, 200, and 500 units/mL). Results lower than 15 units/mL were arbitrarily determined as negative. The intra-assay performance of our ELISA 'in-house' test was on average 4.8% and the inter-assay coefficient of variation was equaled to 10.5%.

2.2.4. Detection of Anti-KLHL12 Antibodies

Anti-KLHL12 antibodies were detected using an ELISA test developed at the Centre of Postgraduate Medical Education in Poland, using the recombinant KLHL12 protein (Abnova, Taipei, Taiwan). Flat-bottom microtiter plates (Costar, Corning, NY, USA) were coated with a solution of the KLHL12 recombinant protein in bicarbonate buffer (pH 9.9), then saturated with 1% BSA in PBS, and washed with PBST. The tested sera (1:100 in PBS) were incubated on coated plates for 1 h at RT with horseradish peroxidase-conjugated human IgG antibodies (Daco A/S, dilution 1:50,000 in PBST). The color reaction was developed by adding 0.1 mL of TMB (SERVA Electrophoresis GmbH) and stopped using 0.5 M H_2SO_4. The optical density (OD) was measured at 450 nm with an automatic plate reader (Multiscan RC, Labsystem, Vantaa, Finland). The levels of antibodies were calculated with reference to our standard serum diluted to: 10, 20, 50, 200, and 400 units/mL. Results lower than 30 units/mL were arbitrarily determined as negative. The intra-assay performance of the developed 'in-house' ELISA test was on average 4.3%. The calculated inter-assay coefficient of variation was equaled to 10.3%.

2.3. *Statistical Analysis*

Prevalence rates were compared between groups using the chi-squared test and Fisher's exact test. Continuous data were summarized as mean ± SD (standard deviation), and categorical data were summarized as frequencies. Continuous variables were evaluated using the Mann–Whitney test and were expressed as median ± interquartile range (IQR). A p-value below 0.05 was considered statistically significant. All statistical analyses were performed using the Statistica 8.0 software (Stat-Soft; Cracow, Poland) and MedCal for Windows, version 7.4.1.0 (MedCal Software; Mariakerke, Belgium). Statistical analysis of the ROC curve was performed using Prism software (GraphPad; La Jolla, CA, USA) and MedCal version 7.4.1.0 (MedCal Software).

3. Results

3.1. Clinical, Histological, and Laboratory Features of PBC Patients and Control Groups

The clinical, histological, and laboratory characteristics of PBC patients are presented in Table 1.

Table 1. Demographic, biochemical, immunological, and histological characteristics of PBC patients and control groups.

	Primary Biliary Cholangitis Patients (*n* = 138)	Autoimmune Hepatitis Patients (*n* = 20)	Primary Sclerosing Cholangitis Patients (*n* = 40)	Healthy Adult Blood Donors (*n* = 30)
Age, years (range)	50 (26–70)	47 (19–67)	47 (23–67)	33 (19–53)
Females/males	131/7	15/5	16/24	22/8
Bilirubin (total), mg/dL	2.4 (2.2)	2.3 (2.1)	1.4 (2.6)	0.7 (0.6)
AST, U/L	81.4 (51.2)	44.3 (71.0)	97.4 (70.1)	22.5 (21.6)
ALT, U/L	93.6 (72.5)	61.7 (52.8)	86.9 (66.0)	15.1 (26.2)
AP, U/L	506.5 (429.2)	223.3 (175.4)	345.5 (227.6)	38.7 (16.8)
γ-GT, U/L	335.5 (304.2)	231.9 (204.0)	349.2 (252.4)	18.6 (4.8)
Albumin (g/dL)	3.6 (1.2)	3.4 (2.4)	2.9 (1.1)	4.5 (2.3)
γ-globulin (g/dL)	1.8 (1.1)	1.7 (1.6)	1.5 (1.8)	1.1 (0.2)
AMA M2	113 (82%)	0 (0%)	0 (0%)	0 (0%)
Anti-gp210 antibody	65 (47%)	0 (0%)	1 (2.5%)	0 (0%)
Anti-p62 antibody	39 (28%)	1 (5%)	1 (2.5%)	0 (0%)
Anti-LBR antibody	21 (15%)	0 (0%)	0 (0%)	0 (0%)
Anti-KLHL12 antibodies	49 (36%)	1 (5%)	0 (0%)	0 (0%)
Early histological stage (I/II)	82 (59%)	6 (30%)	11 (28%)	0 (0%)
Advanced histological stage (III/IV)	52 (37%)	3 (15%)	5 (13%)	0 (0%)
Ambiguous histological stage	4 (4%)	0 (0%)	0 (0%)	0 (0%)

Data are presented as mean (± SD). Abbreviations: γ-GT, γ-glutamyl transpeptidase; ALT, alanine aminotransferase; AP, alkaline phosphatase; AST, aspartate aminotransferase; Normal value: bilirubin < 1.2 mg/dL; AST < 40 U/L; ALT < 40 U/L; AP < 115 U/mg/dL; γ-GT < 50 U/L; albumin 3.5–5.5 g/dL, γ-globulin < 3 g/dL. Conversion factors to SI units are as follows: bilirubin, 17.1; AST, ALT, AP, and γ-GT, 0.0167.

It was determined that the total bilirubin levels were higher in over 50% of the tested samples. AMA M2 was detected in 82% of patients' sera. Activity of AST and ALT was elevated in 73% and 62% of sera from PBC patients, respectively. Over 70% of patients presented increased activity of AP and γ-GT, while a decreased level of albumin was observed in 40% of PBC patients.

3.2. Occurrence and Diagnostic Value of Anti-Nuclear Envelope Antibodies

In the tested PBC patients, anti-NE antibodies were found in 76 out of 138 samples (55%). Anti-gp210 and anti-p62 antibodies were detected in 65 (47%) and in 39 (28%) out of 138 PBC patients, respectively. Among PBC patients, anti-LBR antibodies were found with a frequency of 15% (21/138), while no anti-LBR antibodies were detected in the pathological controls. None of the examined antibodies were found in any of the healthy controls. In the control group, among PSC patients, anti-gp210 and anti-p62 antibodies were found in one patient (2.5%), respectively. Among AIH patients, we also determined anti-p62 antibodies in only one sample (5%). The summary of sensitivities, specificities, and positive and negative predictive values for each detected antibody in patients with PBC is presented in Table 2.

We also checked the occurrence of the tested antibodies in the studied group of females only, as well as in the group of males. In the tested PBC female patients, anti-NE antibodies were found in 71 out of 131 samples (54%) and in the male group, anti-NE antibodies were found in 5 out of 7 samples (71%). This difference was not statistically significant. The data obtained for the female group did not differ from the data obtained for the entire PBC cohort.

Table 2. Diagnostic accuracy for anti-p62 and anti-gp210 antibodies in PBC patients.

	Anti-gp210	Anti-p62	Anti-LBR	Anti-NE
Sensitivity [%, 95% CI]	47.1 [38.6–55.8]	28.3 [20.9–36.6]	15.2 [9.7–22.3]	55.1 [46.4–63.5]
Specificity [%, 95% CI]	98.9 [93.9–99.9]	97.8 [92.2–99.7]	100.0 [96.0–100.0]	96.7 [90.6–99.3]
PPV [%, 95% CI]	98.5 [90.1–98.9]	95.1 [82.8–98.8]	100.0	96.2 [89.2–98.7]
NPV [%, 95% CI]	54.9 [51.0–58.8]	47.1 [44.4–49.8]	43.5 [41.8–45.2]	58.4 [53.8–62.9]
Positive Likelihood Ratio (LR+)	42.4 [6.0–300.1]	12.7 [3.2–51.4]	ND	16.5 [5.4–50.8]
Negative Likelihood Ratio (LR−)	0.5 [0.4–0.6]	0.7 [0.6–0.8]	0.9 [0.8–0.9]	0.5 [0.4–0.6]
Disease prevalence [%, 95% CI]	60.5 [53.4–65.9]	60.5 [53.9–65.9]	60.5 [53.9–66.9]	60.5 [53.9–66.9]
Accuracy [%, 95% CI]	67.5 [61.1–73.4]	55.7 [49.0–62.3]	48.7 [42.0–55.4]	71.5 [65.1–77.3]

ND—not defined.

Specificity of anti-NE proteins for diagnosis of PBC in the whole group of patients was 95.4%. The difference between proportions of anti-NE-positive patients and controls was 0.560 (95% C.I., 0.438–0.665, $p < 0.0001$). In our study, the positive predictive value (PPV) of anti-gp210 and/or anti-p62 was 89.2%, and the negative predictive value (NPV) was 76.4%. The accuracy of these tests and their ability to differentiate PBC patients and healthy cases was 80.3%.

The levels of anti-gp210, anti-p62, and anti-LBR antibodies in sera of PBC patients and control groups are presented in Figure 1.

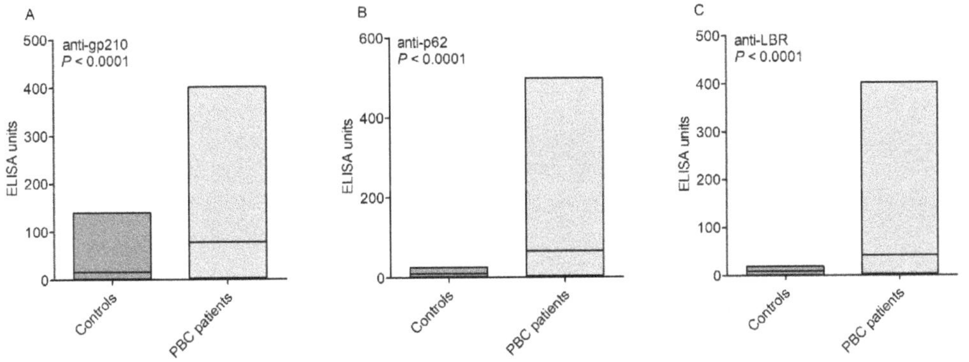

Figure 1. Levels of anti-nuclear envelope antibodies in sera of patients with PBC and the control group: (**A**) anti-gp210, (**B**) anti-p62, (**C**) anti-LBR.

There was a significant difference between PBC patients and the control group: 148 U/mL vs. 45 U/mL, $p < 0.0001$ for anti-gp120 antibodies, and 211 U/mL vs. 16 U/mL, $p < 0.0001$ for anti-p62 antibodies and 176 U/mL vs. 10 U/mL, $p < 0.0001$ for anti-LBR antibodies. Nearly 50% of patients showed a high level (above 150 U/mL) of anti-gp210, anti-p62, or anti-LBR antibodies.

Receiver operating characteristic (ROC) curve analysis for serological detection of anti-gp210 anti-p62 and anti-LBR in PBC samples is shown in Figure 2.

The determined area under the ROC curve (AUC) was greatest for anti-gp210 antibodies (0.7656). The values of AUC calculated for anti-LBR and anti-p62 autoantibodies were 0.6863 and 0.6608, respectively.

We also attempted to correlate anti-gp210, anti-p62, and anti-LBR serum antibodies with AMA M2 (Figure 3).

Anti-gp120 were detected in 52% of AMA M2-negative vs. 46% of AMA M2-positive patients. Similarly, anti-p62 were observed more frequently in AMA M2-negative (36%) than in AMA M2-positive (27%) patients. In contrast, lower levels of anti-LBR were observed in AMA M2-negative (12%) than in AMA M2-positive (22%) samples. Nevertheless, these differences were not statistically significant ($p > 0.05$).

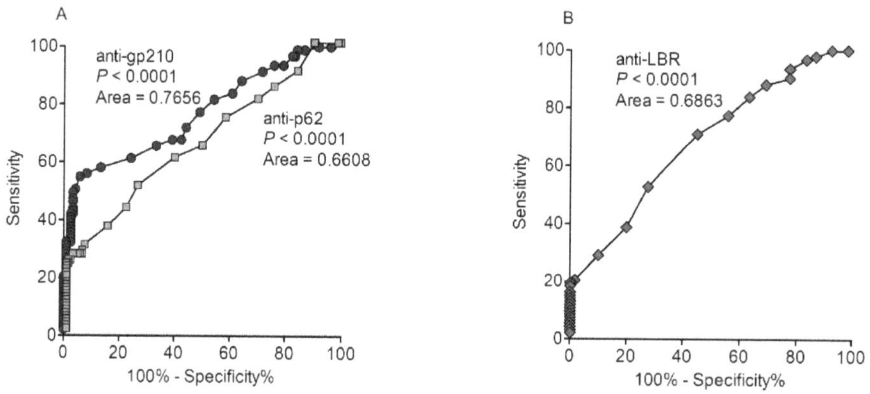

Figure 2. Receiver operating characteristic (ROC) curve analysis for serological detection of PBC anti-gp210 and anti-p62, and anti-LBR antibodies in PBC: (**A**) anti-gp210 and anti-p62, (**B**) anti-LBR.

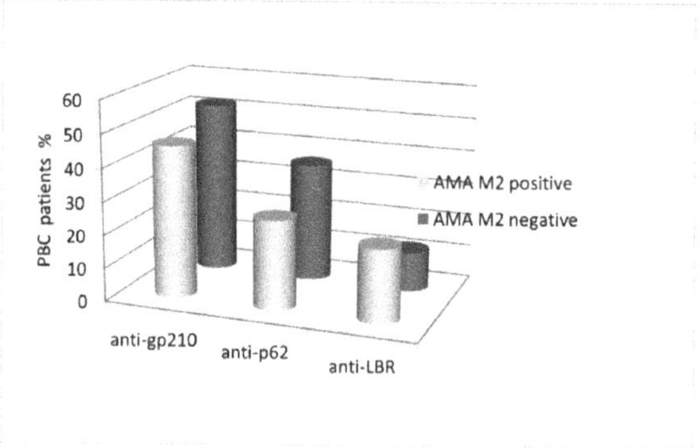

Figure 3. Prevalence of antinuclear antibodies in the studied AMA M2-positive and AMA M2-negative populations.

Among the 25 AMA M2-negative patients, two (8%) were positive for all three tested antibodies (anti-gp210, anti-p62, anti-LBR). Only four AMA M2-negative patients (16%) were positive for at least two activities. Among the 113 AMA M2-positive patients, eight (6%) presented reactivity to all three tested antibodies, while 22 patients (19%) were positive for at least two activities. In the AMA M2-negative group of PBC patients, the positive detection rate for the combined detection of anti-gp210, anti-p62, and anti-LBR antibodies was 76% (19/25) and the accuracy reached 90%.

Among the 24 AMA M2-negative female patients, 18 (75%) were positive for anti-NE antibodies.

3.3. Occurrence and Diagnostic Value of Anti-KLHL12 Antibodies

Anti-KLHL12 antibodies were detected more frequently in PBC compared to non-PBC controls ($p < 0.001$; Table 3).

In the tested PBC female patients, anti-KLHL12 antibodies were found in 47 out of 131 samples (36%), while in the male group, anti-KLHL12 antibodies were found in two out of seven samples (29%).

Specificity of anti-KLHL12 antibodies for diagnosis of PBC in the group of patients was 97%. The positive predictive value (PPV) of anti-KLHL12 antibodies in the diagnosis of PBC was 94% and the negative predictive value (NPV) was 49%. The positive and negative likelihood ratios determined from suitable sensitivities and specificities were 10.4 and 0.7, respectively. The levels of anti-KLHL12 autoantibodies in sera of PBC patients and control groups are shown in Figure 4.

Table 3. Occurrence of anti-KLHL12 antibodies in patients with PBC and control groups.

	Number of Patients	Anti-KLHL12 Antibodies
PBC	138	49 (36%)
Controls (total)	90	1 (1.1%)
PSC	40	0 (0%)
AIH	20	1 (5%)
Healthy	30	0 (0%)

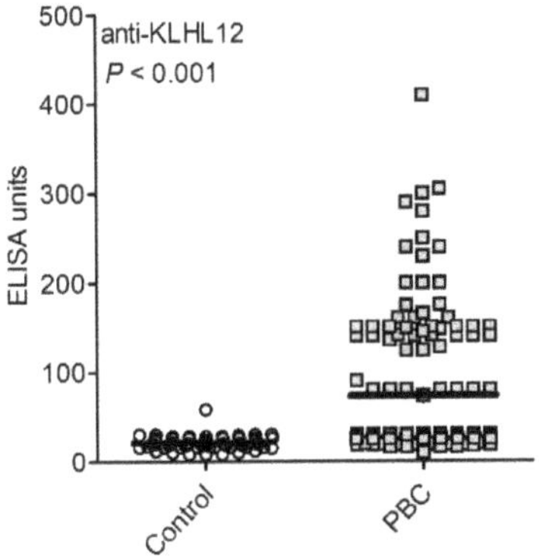

Figure 4. Anti-KLHL12 autoantibodies in sera of PBC patients.

The mean level of antibodies in the group of PBC patients was significantly higher than in the control group: 73 U/mL vs. 21 U/mL, $p < 0.001$. Over 30% of anti-KLHL12-positive PBC patients demonstrated enhanced levels of antibodies (>100 U/mL).

We generated a ROC curve. The sensitivity and specificity were calculated for the cut-off value of 30 arbitral units (Figure 5).

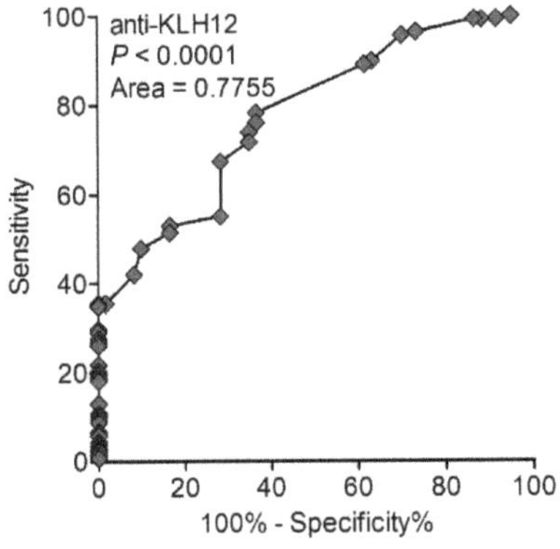

Figure 5. Receiver operating characteristic curve analysis for serological detection of anti-KLHL12 autoantibodies in PBC patients.

The analysis showed that the combined positive detection rate of anti-NE and anti-KLHL12 antibodies in PBC was 60%, while the accuracy of the tests and their ability to differentiate PBC patients and healthy cases was found to be 76%.

We also compared the presence and level of serum anti-KLHL12 antibodies with the presence of AMA M2 in PBC patients. Anti-KLHL12 antibodies were identified in 38% of AMA M2-negative vs. 30% of AMA M2-positive samples (Figure 6).

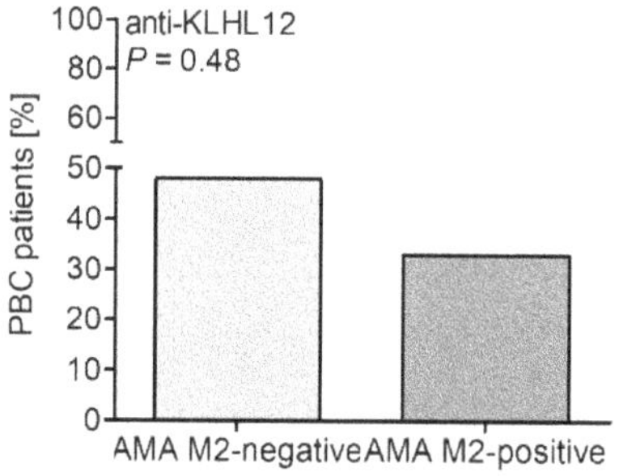

Figure 6. Prevalence of anti-KLHL12 antibodies in the AMA M2-positive and AMA M2-negative PBC cohorts.

These differences were not statistically significant, but anti-KLHL12 antibodies were more frequently detected in the AMA M2-negative group of PBC patients ($p = 0.48$).

The mean levels of the anti-KLHL12 antibodies in the AMA M2-positive and AMA M2-negative groups differed significantly (71.0 ± 57.4 vs. 48.1 ± 42.5; $p = 0.0283$). Most importantly, anti-KLHL12 antibodies were present in 38% of AMA M2-negative PBC patients. Addition of this biomarker to conventional PBC assays improves the serological sensitivity of the AMA M2-negative group of PBC subjects (from 48.3% to 68.5%).

We also studied the prevalence of anti-KLHL12 antibodies in the anti-NE-positive and anti-NE-negative PBC populations. Anti-KLHL12 antibodies were identified in 39% of the anti-NE-negative vs. 33% in the anti-NE-positive PBC samples.

We observed an autoimmune reaction against multiple nuclear components in the evaluated subgroups of PBC patients. Two (8%) out of the tested 25 AMA M2-negative patients and six (5%) out of 113 AMA M2-positive patients were positive for all four reactivities (anti-gp210; anti-p62; anti-LBR; anti-KLHL12). Interestingly, in six (4%) patients only anti-KLHL12 antibodies were found.

We evaluated the diagnosability by combining five markers: anti-gp210, anti-p62, anti-LBR, anti-KLHL12, and AMA. The test's sensitivity increased significantly from 82% to 93% for detection of AMA only ($p = 0.0093$) and a slight improvement in accuracy was also observed (from 89% to 94%).

3.4. Biochemical Features of PBC Patients According to the Status of Anti-NE and Anti-KLHL12 Antibodies

Comparison of groups of PBC patients who were positive and negative for anti-NE and/or anti-KLHL12 antibodies showed that the symptoms of the disease began at the same age in each group of patients. The results of laboratory tests performed at the time of diagnosis were comparable in patients positive and negative for both analyzed autoantibodies, with the exception of bilirubin levels. A correlation between the presence of these autoantibodies and a higher concentration of bilirubin was found. Patients with positive reactivity for anti-NE antibodies (positive for at least one of three anti-NE reactivities: anti-gp210, anti-p62, anti-LBR) and anti-KLHL12 antibodies had higher levels of total bilirubin (2.4 vs. 1.7, $p = 0.016$ and 2.6 vs. 1.5, $p = 0.037$, respectively). Data from biochemical analyses performed at the time of diagnosis in 138 PBC patients, according to the anti-NE and anti-KLHL12 antibodies status, are presented in Table 4.

Table 4. Data from biochemical analyses of 138 PBC patients, and the anti-NE and anti-KLHL12 antibodies status.

	Anti-NE Antibodies			Anti-KLHL12 Antibodies		
	Positive *n* = 25	**Negative** *n* = 68	***p*-Value**	**Positive** *n* = 37	**Negative** *n* = 56	***p*-Value**
Bilirubin (total), mg/dL	2.4 (2.2)	1.7 (1.6)	0.016	2.6 (2.6)	1.5 (1.1)	0.037
AST, U/L	108.8 (95.0)	72.5 (35.0)	0.008	86.9 (55.4)	68.8 (52.8)	ns
ALT, U/L	98.0 (95.4)	88.1 (75.1)	ns	95.3 (94.5)	89.1 (69.8)	ns
AP, U/L	586.7 (530.9)	398.9 (304.1)	0.036	557.3 (466.6)	429.8 (362.1)	ns
γ-GT, U/L	367.2 (345.8)	329.9 (327.7)	ns	343.4 (317.5)	310.8 (291.0)	ns

Data are presented as mean (± SD). Abbreviations: γ-GT, γ-glutamyl transpeptidase; ALT, alanine aminotransferase; AP, alkaline phosphatase; AST, aspartate aminotransferase; Normal value: bilirubin < 1.2 mg/dL; AST < 40 U/L; ALT < 40 U/L; AP < 115 U/mg/dL; γ-GT < 50 U/L; albumin 3.5–5.5 g/dL, γ-globulin < 3 g/dL. Conversion factors to SI units are as follows: bilirubin, 17.1; AST, ALT, AP, and γ-GT, 0.0167.

The bilirubin levels were significantly higher in the group of KLHL12-positive patients ($p < 0.05$). In patients with elevated levels of bilirubin, the mean level of antibodies was ~90 U/mL, while in patients with a normal bilirubin concentration, a level of ~50 U/mL was observed (Figure 7).

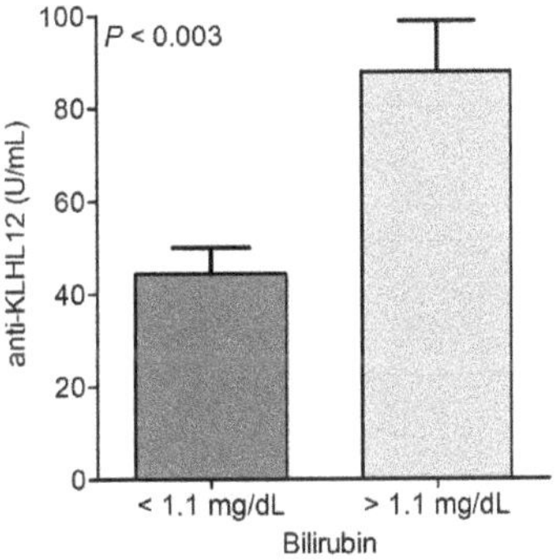

Figure 7. Level of anti-KLHL12 antibodies and bilirubin concentration in serum of PBC patients.

3.5. Autoantibodies Directed against Nuclear Envelope Proteins and KLHL12 Antibodies, and the Survival of Patients

Analysis of the survival rate performed in patients positive and negative for anti-gp210, anti-p62, and anti-LBR (Figure 8) demonstrated that these autoantibodies did not affect the length of life or time to liver transplant in PBC patients.

There was no direct association between anti-gp210, anti-p62, and anti-LBR antibodies, and the early onset or significantly shorter survival of patients. Nevertheless, in the group of patients characterized by presence of at least two types of the tested antibodies, the patient's survival time or time to liver transplant were more than 4-times shorter than in the group without anti-gp210, anti-p62, or anti-LBR antibodies (OR = 4.375; $p = 0.0432$).

Moreover, in this small group of patients characterized by presence of all three types of these antibodies, we found over 5-times more deaths or transplants than in the group without antibodies (OR = 5.200; $p = 0.036$).

Analysis of the survival of patients positive and negative for the anti-KLHL12 antibodies (Figure 9) showed that presence of these autoantibodies also does not correlate with the length of life or time to liver transplant in PBC patients ($p = 0.07$).

Although the difference was not statistically significant, the survival time of patients or the period to liver transplant was shortest for people with these antibodies, in comparison to anti-NE antibodies.

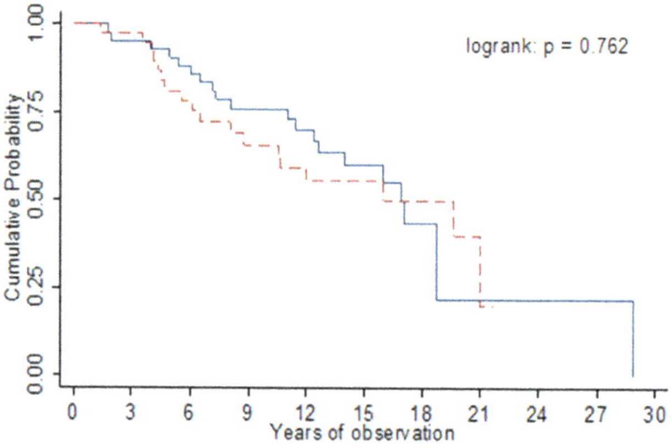

(**a**)

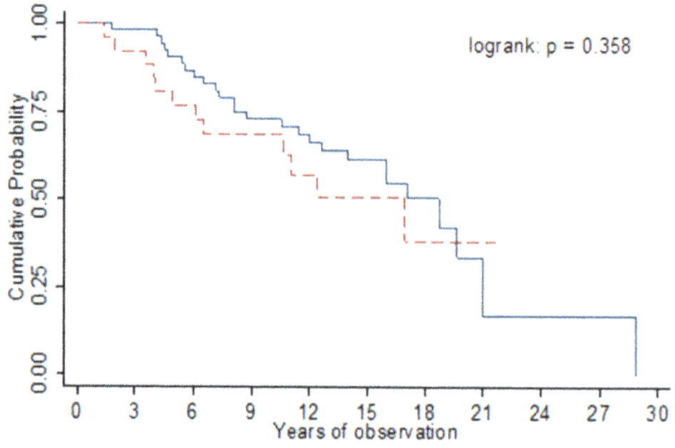

(**b**)

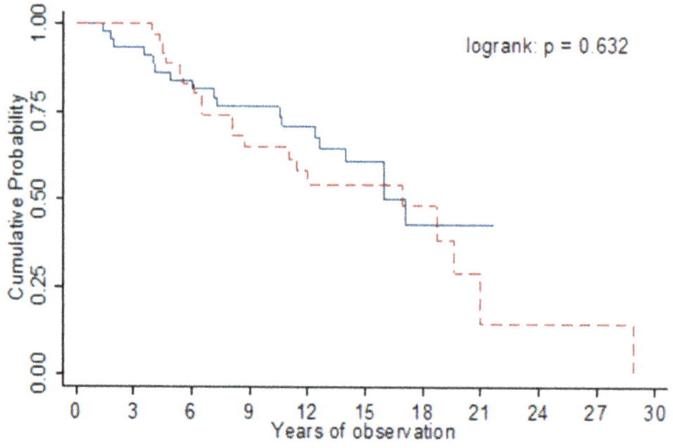

(**c**)

——— (–) - - - - - (+)

Figure 8. Kaplan–Meier curves demonstrating the survival of patients positive and negative for anti-nuclear envelope antibodies. (**a**) Anti-gp210 antibodies; (**b**) Anti-p62 antibodies; (**c**) Anti-LBR antibodies.

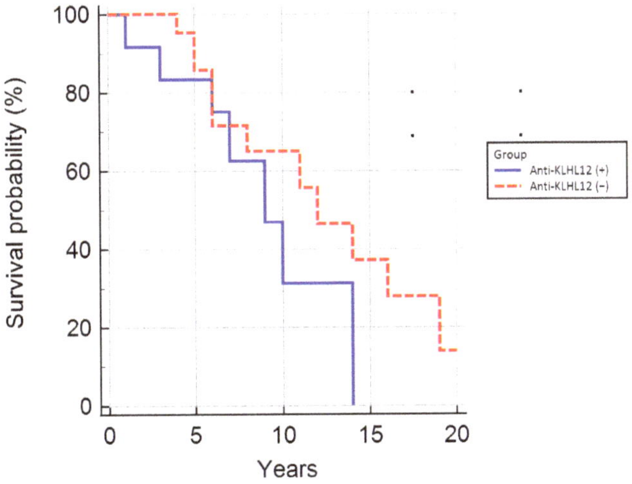

Figure 9. Kaplan–Meier curves demonstrating the survival of patients positive and negative for the anti-KLHL12 antibodies.

3.6. Analysis of the Correlation between Histological Parameters of PBC Patients, and Autoantibodies Directed against Nuclear Envelope Proteins and the KLHL12 Protein

We assessed histological material collected from PBC patients and classified it into two groups based on presence or absence of anti-NE antibodies. Among 76 anti-gp20- and/or anti-p62- and/or anti-LBR-positive PBC patients, 21% were classified into stages I/II, and 79% into stages III/IV, according to Ludwig's classification (Figure 10).

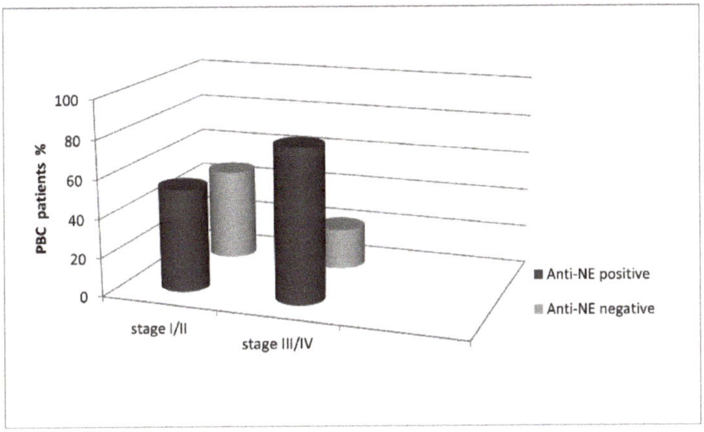

Figure 10. Prevalence of antinuclear envelope antibodies in the studied population according to stage of Ludwig's classification.

Among 82 PBC patients with early histological stages (I/II) of the disease, 43 (52%) were anti-NE-positive. In the group of PBC patients with advanced histological stages (III/IV), 41 out of 52 (79%) were anti-NE-positive ($p = 0.002$). Statistically, more patients with stages III/IV in the anti-gp210-positive than anti-gp210-negative subgroups (43% vs. 14%, $p < 0.001$) were found. The same pattern was observed for patients with anti-p62 antibodies (42% vs. 21%, $p = 0.041$ and 16% vs. 4%, $p = 0.048$) and anti-LBR antibodies (67%

vs. 31%; $p = 0.002$). Presence of the anti-KLHL12 antibodies in sera of PBC patients also correlated with the stage of liver fibrosis (Figure 11).

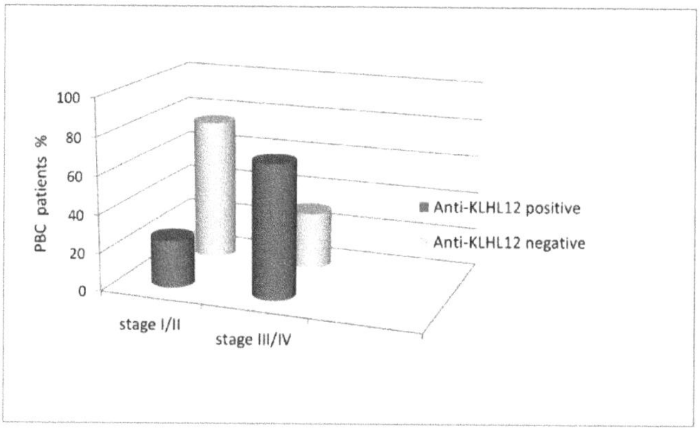

Figure 11. Presence of anti-KLHL12 antibodies and the stage of liver fibrosis in PBC patients.

Among 82 PBC patients with early histological stages (I/II) of the disease, only 20 (24%) were positive for anti-KLHL12 antibodies. We found a statistically significant difference in comparison to the group of PBC patients with advanced histological stages (III/IV), where 39 out of 52 (75%) subjects were positive for anti-KLHL12 antibodies ($p < 0.0001$).

4. Discussion

PBC is primarily characterized by presence of AMAs, with the most important antigens being PDC-E2, OGDC-E2, and BCOADC-E2 [11–13]. As non-invasive tests for identification of autoantibodies as disease markers are useful for diagnosis of patients, we analyzed the immune response against gp210, p62, and LBR antigens, and the KLHL12 protein in PBC. Anti-NE antibodies have been considered as a pathognomonic element of PBC [36], however, a significant variation in their prevalence (between 10% and 50%) has been reported. Antibodies against integral glycoproteins of the nuclear pore membrane, gp210 and p62, have been reported [16–18], and are associated with pathogenesis, progression, and severity of PBC [31–33]. Studies performed in Western Europe, North America, and East Asia have shown high levels of anti-gp210-specific antibodies in PBC patients [17–19,53,54], which has also been confirmed in the Polish population. The measured sensitivity of anti-gp210 antibodies in PBC was found to be 44% [32], which is higher than that reported from other parts of the world: Japan–26% [43], Italy–18% or 27% [30,35,55], and Spain–33% [56]. Huang et al. (2019) proposed usage of the gp210 antibody for early diagnosis of PBC [31]. In our study, antibodies directed against the p62 protein were found in 28% of the screened sera of the tested PBC patients, which was similar to the frequency reported earlier by Wesierska-Gadek et al. (2008) [41]. However, the specificity of anti-NE antibodies for PBC was greater than 97%, which seems to be remarkably high. A slightly higher prevalence of anti-gp210 and anti-p62 antibodies in AMA M2-negative PBC patients was observed. Even though this difference was not statistically significant, cases with advanced histological stages were much more common among anti-NE-positive and AMA M2-negative patients. Previous reports have highlighted the correlation between anti-gp210 and anti-p62 antibodies, and the clinical outcome of PBC. Nakamura and co-workers (2005) analyzed clinical, immunological, and histological data on 71 Japanese PBC patients in relation to the presence of the anti-gp210 antibody. They suggested that this autoantibody is a promising prognostic marker of a poor outcome of the disease [57]. Invernizzi et al. (2001) demonstrated a strong association between presence of autoantibodies against nuclear pore complexes with more active and severe cases of PBC [55]. Bogdanos et al. (2007) suggested a more progressive form of the disease in patients with ANAs [58].

Haldar et al. (2021) confirmed that presence of anti-gp210 is associated with an adverse phenotype, lack of response to treatment, and reduced transplant-free survival in the cohort of PBC patients [59]. The regional differences in the prevalence of anti-nuclear antibodies were explained by environmental and genetic factors, rather than technical differences in the determination of anti-gp210 [56]. Yang and co-workers (2004) studied presence of anti-nuclear antibodies in a large Toronto and Mayo Clinic cohort of PBC patients using immunofluorscence and found that these antibodies are associated with earlier development of liver failure [60]. They found that Wesierska-Gadek et al. (2008) reported the presence of an antibody against the nuclear pore complex in patients likely to experience an unfavorable clinical course and more rapid progression of the disease [37]. Contrary to these results, we found no direct association between presence of anti-nuclear antibodies and poor prognosis of PBC. These data stay in accordance with some of the previously published findings [43,58].

Our data also revealed that the serum bilirubin concentration at the time of diagnosis was an independent and the only risk factor for poor prognosis of PBC. Excluding bilirubin, our subjects with or without anti-gp210 or anti-p62 antibodies presented similar biochemical characteristics. Neither anti-gp210 nor anti-p62 were distinct independent risk factors for rapid progression and liver failure in PBC patients. Nevertheless, PBC patients positive for these antibodies were frequently classified into later stages (III/IV), according to Ludwig's classification. Sfakianaki et al. (2010) obtained similar results, but contrary to us, they also found a correlation between positive anti-gp210 antibodies and a short survival period of patients [61]. Therefore, it seems that presence of anti-p62 antibodies or simultaneous occurrence of anti-p62 and anti-gp210 antibodies may be of much greater significance for the prediction of a worse course of the disease. LBR autoantibodies are only rarely detected in patients with PBC (2% to 10%) [62], hence they are not of general diagnostic utility. Their prognostic significance is also unknown. Due to the low sensitivity of these antibodies in PBC, they have also not been extensively studied. We decided to analyze our relatively small group of anti-LBR positive patients in more detail. We observed that autoantibodies directed against LBR were highly specific for PBC, but were present in only 15% of our PBC patients, including AMA M2-negative subjects. In contrast, anti-LBR antibodies were not found in the pathologic and healthy controls. The detected sensitivity was higher than the values previously reported [63]. The high specificity and PPV for PBC is very interesting. Presence of anti-LBR does not correlate with patients' survival rate, but is connected with liver fibrosis.

Anti-KLHL12 antibodies have not been widely employed in practice and only a few reports can be found. The prevalence of these antibodies in different geographic areas has also not been reported and only one study demonstrated results from five different sites examined from North America and Europe [45]. Norman et al. (2015) have shown that anti-KLHL12 antibodies are present in both AMA M2-positive, and importantly, AMA M2-negative patients [40,46]. In a cohort of 366 patients with PBC, ~40% of the 277 AMA M2-positive patients were positive for anti-KLHL12 antibodies, while 53 out of 89 AMA M2-negative patients were positive for anti-KLHL12 antibodies. The specificities of antibodies were 96–97%. The Norman et al. international multi-center study included a pilot trial of 40 patients from Poland in which a commercially non-available INOVA kit was used [45]. In contrast, in our study, we analyzed sera from a larger group of Polish patients and we also developed an 'in-house' ELISA, in which a recombinant protein, KLHL12, was used to detect autoantibodies directed against KLHL12 in PBC patients and controls. We verified the seropositivity of KLHL12 in the PBC group of Polish patients and found that the frequency of these antibodies in PBC was significantly higher compared to the control groups. These anti-KLHL12 antibodies detected using the ELISA 'in-house' method presented very high specificity. In our study, the positive rate of the anti-KLHL12 antibodies was 36%, which was slightly higher than in the rest of Europe and the United States (22%, 33.3%, respectively) [45]. Norman et al. also reported that KLHL12 antibodies have higher sensitivity than anti-gp210 antibodies [44]. We have not confirmed this observation in our group of patients. A coexistence of different antibodies was observed, which suggests an autoimmune reaction against multiple nuclear components in some PBC patients. A few patients only had anti-KLHL12 antibodies. We compared the prevalence of anti-KLHL12 antibodies in the AMA M2-positive and AMA M2-negative PBC populations and no statistically significant difference was observed. The level of anti-KLHL12 antibodies was slightly enhanced in the group of AMA-positive patients.

We analyzed the immune response against the KLHL12 protein in PBC patients and linked the obtained data with biochemical and histological parameters. Interestingly, we found an association between the presence of these autoantibodies and a higher concentration of bilirubin. For the diagnosis of PBC, specificity of the disease marker is one of the most important criteria. The bilirubin levels in sera of patients positive for anti-KLHL12 antibodies were higher than those in the anti-KLH12 antibodies negative group. The level of anti-KLHL12 antibodies in sera of PBC patients was also found to correlate with the stage of liver fibrosis. Combining anti-KLHL12 antibodies with available markers (MIT3, gp210, and sp100) increased the diagnostic sensitivity for PBC. Due to the anti-NE combination and the detection of anti-KLHL12 antibodies, the diagnostic sensitivity in PBC, especially in AMA-negative PBC, can be significantly improved from 48.3% to 68.5% in ELISA. That can reduce the risk of liver biopsy. The addition of tests highly specific for anti-KLHL12 antibodies to AMA and ANA serological assays significantly improves the efficacy of clinical detection and diagnosis of PBC, especially for AMA M2-negative subjects. To become globally adopted, it is important to validate these new biomarkers in different geographical areas. It is still unclear why anti-KLHL12 antibodies are present in patients with PBC and this will require further research.

In patients with chronic intrahepatic cholestasis, determination of serum AMA and PBC-specific ANA antibodies (immunofluorescence and/or specific anti-sp100/anti-gp210 testing by Western blotting or ELISA) is recommended as the next diagnostic step [51]. AMA positivity is found in more than 90% of patients with PBC, immunofluorescence 1/40, or immunoenzymatic reactivity observed during cholestatic serum liver testing, is highly specific to the disease [64]. The EASL recommends that in patients with cholestasis and no likelihood of systemic disease, a diagnosis of PBC can be based on elevated ALP levels and presence of AMAs at a titer of 1:40 [51]. AMA reactivity is only sufficient for diagnosis of PBC when combined with abnormal serum liver tests. EASL recommends that, in the correct context, a diagnosis of AMA-negative PBC can be made in patients with cholestasis and ANA-specific immuno-fluorescence (nuclear dots or perinuclear rims) or ELISA (using sp100 or gp210 antibodies) [51,65]. In contrast to anti-gp210 antibodies, the importance of antibodies against p62 in PBC is less recognized. Although the presence of anti-p62 is fairly rare, a positive ELISA result strongly supports the diagnosis of PBC. The high specificity of anti-p62 suggests that it may be considered as a significant serological marker of PBC, even when AMA, anti-gp210, and anti-sp100 antibodies are not detectable. Our study conducted on the group of PBC patients stays in accordance with other data which confirm very high specificity of anti-p62 [33,52]. The absence of classic PBC markers, such as AMAs and anti-gp210 or anti-sp100, can lead to a delay in diagnosis and treatment. Therefore, anti-p62 detection could be of crucial importance in PBC diagnosis. The explanation as to why antibodies to KLHL12 are higher in patients with PBC remains an interesting topic, although it is still unclear. Our study, as well as Norman et al.'s results [44,45], have demonstrated that anti-KLHL12 antibodies are novel, highly specific markers of PBC and, most importantly, they have been suggested to be promising new candidates in the clinical diagnosis of PBC. The addition of tests for highly specific anti-KLHL12 antibodies to AMA and ANA serological analyses considerably improves the effectiveness of clinical detection and diagnosis of PBC [44,45,49]. The level of anti-KLHL12 antibodies in sera of PBC patients is associated with the stage of liver fibrosis, which may be important in recognition of patients at risk of advanced disease or faster disease progression. However, it must be considered that immune markers should always be interpreted together with clinical findings by an experienced practitioner to avoid misdiagnosis.

5. Conclusions

Our data confirmed that there is a correlation between the presence of anti-KLHL12 antibodies, anti-nuclear envelope antibodies, liver fibrosis, and higher bilirubin concentrations in Polish PBC patients. Antinuclear antibodies of different specificity support the autoimmunity of PBC. The ability to detect them expands the diagnostic armamentarium of PBC-specific markers, especially in cases in which AMA are not detectable, in asymptomatic patients, and for early diagnosis of PBC. High specificity of these antibodies can imply that they may take part in the pathogenesis of the disease.

It appears that KLHL12 antibodies present predictive significance for more rapid PBC progression and can be considered as a risk factor for poor prognosis. As we confirmed that these antibodies are highly specific for PBC, we propose that determination of anti-KLHL12 antibodies can be important in the diagnostic process of PBC.

Author Contributions: Conceptualization, A.B.; Methodology, A.B.; Formal analysis, A.B. and A.H.; Validation, A.B.; Investigation, A.B.; Resources, A.H.; Data curation, A.H. and A.B.; Writing—original draft preparation, A.B.; Writing—review and editing, D.G. and A.B.; Visualization, A.B. and D.G.; Project administration, A.H. and A.B.; Supervision, A.B.; Funding acquisition, A.H. and A.B.; Statistical analysis, D.G. and A.B. All authors have read and agreed to the published version of the manuscript.

Funding: The study was supported by grants: UMO-2011/01/B/NZ5/05291 from the National Centre of Science and 501-1-25-01-20 from the Centre of Postgraduate Medical Education, Warsaw, Poland.

Institutional Review Board Statement: The study protocol was conducted in accordance to the ethical guidelines of the Declaration of Helsinki and was approved by the Ethical Committee of the Centre of Postgraduate Medical Education, Warsaw (approval 12 June 2019 number 71/PB/2019).

Informed Consent Statement: Informed consent was obtained from all patients.

Data Availability Statement: All available data are presented within the article or are available on request from the corresponding author.

Acknowledgments: The authors thank Paulina Wieszczy for help in analysis of the survival.

Conflicts of Interest: The authors declare no conflict of interest.

Abbreviations

AMA: antimitochondrial antibody; AIH: autoimmune hepatitis; ALT: aspartate aminotransferase; anti-p62: anti-nucleoporin p62 antibodies ANA: antinuclear antibody, AP: alkaline phosphatase; AST: alanine aminotransferase; AUC: area under the ROC curve; EASL: European Liver Research Association; γ-GT: γ-glutamyl transpeptidase; HBsAg: hepatitis B surface antigen; IQR: interquartile range; LR−: negative likelihood ratio; NPV: negative predictive value; NE: nuclear envelope, OD: optical density; LR+: positive likelihood ratio; PPV: positive predictive value PBC: primary biliary cholangitis; PSC: primary sclerosing cholangitis; ROC: receiver operating characteristic; SD: standard deviation.

References

1. Carey, E.J.; Ali, A.H.; Lindor, K.D. Primary biliary cirrhosis. *Lancet* **2015**, *386*, 1565–1575. [CrossRef]
2. Tanaka, A.; Leung, P.S.; Young, H.A.; Gershwin, M.E. Toward solving the etiological mystery of primary biliary cholangitis. *Hepatol. Commun.* **2017**, *1*, 275–287. [CrossRef] [PubMed]
3. Chew, M.; Bowlus, C.L. Primary biliary cholangitis: Diagnosis and treatment. *Liver Res.* **2018**, *2*, 81–86. [CrossRef]
4. Beretta-Piccoli, B.T.; Mieli-Vergani, G.; Vergani, D.; Vierling, J.M.; Adams, D.; Alpini, G.; Banales, J.M.; Beuers, U.; Björnsson, E.; Bowlus, C.; et al. The challenges of primary biliary cholangitis: What is new and what needs to be done. *J. Autoimmun.* **2019**, *105*, 102328. [CrossRef] [PubMed]
5. Tsuneyama, K.; Baba, H.; Morimoto, Y.; Tsunematsu, T.; Ogawa, H. Primary Biliary Cholangitis: Its Pathological Characteristics and Immunopathological Mechanisms. *J. Med Investig.* **2017**, *64*, 7–13. [CrossRef] [PubMed]

6. Cichoż-Lach, H.; Grywalska, E.; Michalak, A.; Kowalik, A.; Mielnik, M.; Roliński, J. Deviations in Peripheral Blood Cell Populations are Associated with the Stage of Primary Biliary Cholangitis and Presence of Itching. *Arch. Immunol. Ther. Exp.* **2018**, *66*, 443–452. [CrossRef] [PubMed]
7. Hirschfield, G.M.; Chazouillères, O.; Cortez-Pinto, H.; Macedo, G.; de Lédinghen, V.; Adekunle, F.; Carbone, M. A consensus integrated care pathway for patients with primary biliary cholangitis: A guideline-based approach to clinical care of patients. *Expert Rev. Gastroenterol. Hepatol.* **2021**, *15*, 929–939. [CrossRef]
8. Younossi, Z.M.; Bernstein, D.; Shiffman, M.L.; Kwo, P.; Kim, W.R.; Kowdley, K.V.; Jacobson, I.M. Diagnosis and Management of Primary Biliary Cholangitis. *Am. J. Gastroenterol.* **2019**, *114*, 48–63. [CrossRef]
9. Paziewska, A.; Habior, A.; Rogowska, A.; Zych, W.; Goryca, K.; Karczmarski, J.; Dabrowska, M.; Ambrozkiewicz, F.; Walewska-Zielecka, B.; Krawczyk, M.; et al. A novel approach to genome-wide association analysis identifies genetic associations with primary biliary cholangitis and primary sclerosing cholangitis in Polish patients. *BMC Med. Genomics* **2017**, *10*, 2. [CrossRef]
10. Gazda, J.; Drazilova, S.; Janicko, M.; Jarcuska, P. The Epidemiology of Primary Biliary Cholangitis in European Countries: A Systematic Review and Meta-Analysis. *Can. J. Gastroenterol. Hepatol.* **2021**, *2021*, 1–11. [CrossRef]
11. Beretta-Piccoli, B.T.; Mieli-Vergani, G.; Vergani, D. The clinical usage and definition of autoantibodies in immune-mediated liver disease: A comprehensive overview. *J. Autoimmun.* **2018**, *95*, 144–158. [CrossRef] [PubMed]
12. Kouroumalis, E.; Samonakis, D.; Voumvouraki, A. Biomarkers for primary biliary cholangitis: Current perspectives. *Hepatic Med. Évid. Res.* **2018**, *10*, 43–53. [CrossRef] [PubMed]
13. Lindor, K.D.; Bowlus, C.L.; Boyer, J.; Levy, C.; Mayo, M. Primary Biliary Cholangitis: 2018 Practice Guidance from the American Association for the Study of Liver Diseases. *Hepatology* **2018**, *69*, 394–419. [CrossRef] [PubMed]
14. Cancado, E.L.R.; Harriz, M. The Importance of Autoantibody Detection in Primary Biliary Cirrhosis. *Front. Immunol.* **2015**, *6*, 309. [CrossRef] [PubMed]
15. Wang, C.; Zheng, X.; Jiang, P.; Tang, R.; Gong, Y.; Dai, Y.; Wang, L.; Xu, P.; Sun, W.; Wang, L.; et al. Genome-wide Association Studies of Specific Antinuclear Autoantibody Subphenotypes in Primary Biliary Cholangitis. *Hepatology* **2019**, *70*, 294–307. [CrossRef]
16. Cristoferi, L.; Gerussi, A.; Invernizzi, P. Anti-gp210 and other anti-nuclear pore complex autoantibodies in primary biliary cholangitis: What we know and what we should know. *Liver Int.* **2021**, *41*, 432–435. [CrossRef]
17. Rigopoulou, E.I.; Davies, E.T.; Pares, A.; Zachou, K.; Liaskos, C.; Bogdanos, D.; Rodés, J.; Dalekos, G.N.; Vergani, D. Prevalence and clinical significance of isotype specific antinuclear antibodies in primary biliary cirrhosis. *Gut* **2005**, *54*, 528–532. [CrossRef]
18. Vermeersch, P.; Bossuyt, X. Prevalence and clinical significance of rare antinuclear antibody patterns. *Autoimmun. Rev.* **2013**, *12*, 998–1003. [CrossRef]
19. Granito, A.; Yang, W.-H.; Muratori, L.; Lim, M.J.; Nakajima, A.; Ferri, S.; Pappas, G.; Quarneti, C.; Bianchi, F.B.; Bloch, D.; et al. PML Nuclear Body Component Sp140 Is a Novel Autoantigen in Primary Biliary Cirrhosis. *Am. J. Gastroenterol.* **2010**, *105*, 125–131. [CrossRef]
20. Han, E.; Jo, S.J.; Lee, H.; Choi, A.-R.; Lim, J.; Jung, E.-S.; Oh, E.-J. Clinical relevance of combined anti-mitochondrial M2 detection assays for primary biliary cirrhosis. *Clin. Chim. Acta* **2016**, *464*, 113–117. [CrossRef]
21. Hu, C.J.; Zhang, F.C.; Li, Y.Z.; Zhang, X. Primary biliary cirrhosis: What do autoantibodies tell us? *World J. Gastroenterol.* **2010**, *16*, 3616–3629. [CrossRef] [PubMed]
22. Granito, A.; Muratori, P.; Quarneti, C.; Pappas, G.; Cicola, R.; Muratori, L. Antinuclear antibodies as ancillary markers in primary biliary cirrhosis. *Expert Rev. Mol. Diagn.* **2012**, *12*, 65–74. [CrossRef] [PubMed]
23. Bogdanos, D.P.; Komorowski, L. Disease-specific autoantibodies in primary biliary cirrhosis. *Clin. Chim. Acta* **2011**, *412*, 502–512. [CrossRef] [PubMed]
24. Bauer, A.; Habior, A.; Wieszczy, P.; Gawel, D. Analysis of Autoantibodies against Promyelocytic Leukemia Nuclear Body Components and Biochemical Parameters in Sera of Patients with Primary Biliary Cholangitis. *Diagnostics* **2021**, *11*, 587. [CrossRef] [PubMed]
25. Milkiewicz, P.; Buwaneswaran, H.; Coltescu, C. Value of antibody analysis in the differential diagnosis of chronic cholestatic liver disease. *Dig. Dis.* **2009**, *7*, 1355–1360.
26. Liu, B.; Shi, X.H.; Zhang, F.C.; Zhang, W.; Gao, L.X. Anti-mitochondrial antibody-negative primary biliary cirrhosis: A subset of primary biliary cirrhosis. *Liver Int.* **2008**, *2*, 233–239. [CrossRef]
27. Agmon-Levin, N.; Shapira, Y.; Selmi, C.; Barzilai, O.; Ram, M.; Szyper-Kravitz, M.; Sella, S.; Katz, B.-S.P.; Youinou, P.; Renaudineau, Y.; et al. A comprehensive evaluation of serum autoantibodies in primary biliary cirrhosis. *J. Autoimmun.* **2010**, *34*, 55–58. [CrossRef]
28. Liu, H.; Norman, G.L.; Shums, Z.; Worman, H.J.; Krawitt, E.L.; Bizzaro, N.; Vergani, D.; Bogdanos, D.; Dalekos, G.N.; Milkiewicz, P.; et al. PBC Screen: An IgG/IgA dual isotype ELISA detecting multiple mitochondrial and nuclear autoantibodies specific for primary biliary cirrhosis. *J. Autoimmun.* **2010**, *35*, 436–442. [CrossRef]
29. Granito, A.; Muratori, L.; Tovoli, F.; Muratori, P. Autoantibodies to speckled protein family in primary biliary cholangitis. *Allergy Asthma Clin. Immunol.* **2021**, *17*, 1–4. [CrossRef]
30. Villalta, D.; Sorrentino, M.C.; Girolami, E.; Tampoia, M.; Alessio, M.G.; Brusca, I.; Daves, M.; Porcelli, B.; Barberio, G.; Bizzaro, N. Autoantibody profiling of patients with primary biliary cirrhosis using a multiplexed line-blot assay. *Clin. Chim. Acta* **2015**, *438*, 135–138. [CrossRef]

31. Huang, C.; Han, W.; Wang, C.; Liu, Y.; Chen, Y.; Duan, Z. Early Prognostic Utility of Gp210 Antibody-Positive Rate in Primary Biliary Cholangitis: A Meta-Analysis. *Dis. Markers* **2019**, *2019*, 9121207. [CrossRef] [PubMed]
32. Bauer, A.; Habior, A. Measurement of gp210 autoantibodies in sera of patients with primary biliary cirrhosis. *J. Clin. Lab. Anal.* **2007**, *21*, 227–231. [CrossRef] [PubMed]
33. Duarte-Rey, C.; Bogdanos, D.; Yang, C.-Y.; Roberts, K.; Leung, P.S.C.; Anaya, J.-M.; Worman, H.J.; Gershwin, M.E. Primary biliary cirrhosis and the nuclear pore complex. *Autoimmun. Rev.* **2012**, *11*, 898–902. [CrossRef]
34. Chantran, Y.; Ballot, E.; Johanet, C. Autoantibodies in primary biliary cirrhosis: Antinuclear envelope autoantibodies. *Clin. Res. Hepatol. Gastroenterol.* **2014**, *38*, 256–258. [CrossRef] [PubMed]
35. de Liso, F.; Matinato, C.; Ronchi, M.; Maiavacca, R. The diagnostic accuracy of biomarkers for diagnosis of primary biliary cholangitis (PBC) in anti-mitochondrial antibody (AMA)-negative PBC patients: A review of literature. *Clin. Chem. Lab. Med. (CCLM)* **2017**, *56*, 25–31. [CrossRef]
36. Hu, S.-L.; Zhao, F.-R.; Hu, Q.; Chen, W.-X. Meta-Analysis Assessment of GP210 and SP100 for the Diagnosis of Primary Biliary Cirrhosis. *PLoS ONE* **2014**, *9*, e101916. [CrossRef]
37. Zhang, Q.; Liu, Z.; Wu, S.; Duan, W.; Chen, S.; Ou, X.; You, H.; Kong, Y.; Jia, J. Meta-Analysis of Antinuclear Antibodies in the Diagnosis of Antimitochondrial Antibody-Negative Primary Biliary Cholangitis. *Gastroenterol. Res. Pr.* **2019**, *2019*, 1–12. [CrossRef]
38. Wesierska-Gadek, J.; Penner, E.; Battezzati, P.M.; Selmi, C.; Zuin, M.; Hitchman, E.; Worman, H.J.; Gershwin, M.E.; Podda, M.; Invernizzi, P. Correlation of initial autoantibody profile and clinical outcome in primary biliary cirrhosis. *Hepatology* **2006**, *43*, 1135–1144. [CrossRef]
39. Yamagiwa, S.; Kamimura, H.; Takamura, M.; Aoyagi, Y. Autoantibodies in primary biliary cirrhosis: Recent progress in research on the pathogenetic and clinical significance. *World J. Gastroenterol.* **2014**, *20*, 2606–2612. [CrossRef]
40. Nakamura, M. Clinical Significance of Autoantibodies in Primary Biliary Cirrhosis. *Semin. Liver Dis.* **2014**, *34*, 334–340. [CrossRef]
41. Wesierska-Gadek, J.; Klima, A.; Ranftler, C.; Komina, O.; Hanover, J.; Invernizzi, P.; Penner, E. Characterization of antibodies to p62 nucleoporin in primary biliary cirrhosis using human recombinant antigen. *J. Cell. Biochem.* **2008**, *104*, 27–37. [CrossRef] [PubMed]
42. Wesierska-Gadek, J.; Klima, A.; Komina, O.; Ranftler, C.; Invernizzi, P.; Penner, E. Characterization of autoantibodies against components of the nuclear pore complex, high frequency of anti-p62 nucleoporin antibodies. *Ann. N. Y. Acad. Sci.* **2007**, *1109*, 519–530. [CrossRef] [PubMed]
43. Miyachi, K.; Hankins, R.W.; Matsushima, H.; Kikuchi, F.; Inomata, T.; Horigome, T.; Shibata, M.; Onozuka, Y.; Ueno, Y.; Hashimoto, E.; et al. Profile and clinical significance of anti-nuclear envelope antibodies found in patients with primary biliary cirrhosis: A multicenter study. *J. Autoimmun.* **2003**, *20*, 247–254. [CrossRef]
44. Norman, G.L.; Yang, C.-Y.; Ostendorff, H.P.; Shums, Z.; Lim, M.J.; Wang, J.; Awad, A.; Hirschfield, G.; Milkiewicz, P.; Bloch, D.; et al. Anti-kelch-like 12 and anti-hexokinase 1: Novel autoantibodies in primary biliary cirrhosis. *Liver Int.* **2014**, *35*, 642–651. [CrossRef]
45. Norman, G.L.; Reig, A.; Viñas, O.; Mahler, M.; Wunsch, E.; Milkiewicz, P.; Swain, M.G.; Mason, A.; Stinton, L.M.; Aparicio, M.B.; et al. The Prevalence of Anti-Hexokinase-1 and Anti-Kelch-Like 12 Peptide Antibodies in Patients with Primary Biliary Cholangitis Is Similar in Europe and North America: A Large International, Multi-Center Study. *Front. Immunol.* **2019**, *10*, 662. [CrossRef]
46. Gupta, V.A.; Beggs, A.H. Kelch proteins: Emerging roles in skeletal muscle development and diseases. *Skelet. Muscle* **2014**, *4*, 11. [CrossRef]
47. Dhanoa, B.S.; Cogliati, T.; Satish, A.G.; Bruford, E.A.; Friedman, J.S. Update on the Kelch-like (KLHL) gene family. *Hum. Genom.* **2013**, *7*, 13. [CrossRef]
48. Jin, L.; Pahuja, K.B.; Wickliffe, K.E.; Gorur, A.; Baumgärtel, C.; Schekman, R.; Rape, M. Ubiquitin-dependent regulation of COPII coat size and function. *Nature* **2012**, *482*, 495–500. [CrossRef]
49. Hu, C.-J.; Song, G.; Huang, W.; Liu, G.-Z.; Deng, C.-W.; Zeng, H.-P.; Wang, L.; Zhang, F.-C.; Zhang, X.; Jeong, J.S.; et al. Identification of New Autoantigens for Primary Biliary Cirrhosis Using Human Proteome Microarrays. *Mol. Cell. Proteom.* **2012**, *11*, 669–680. [CrossRef]
50. EASL Clinical Practice Guidelines. Management of cholestatic liver diseases. *J. Hepatol.* **2009**, *51*, 237–267. [CrossRef]
51. EASL Clinical Practice Guidelines. The diagnosis and management of patients with primary biliary cholangitis. *J. Hepatol.* **2017**, *67*, 145–172.
52. Bauer, A.; Habior, A. Detection of Autoantibodies Against Nucleoporin p62 in Sera of Patients with Primary Biliary Cholangitis. *Ann. Lab. Med.* **2019**, *39*, 291–298. [CrossRef] [PubMed]
53. Nakamura, M.; Komori, A.; Ito, M.; Kondo, H.; Aiba, Y.; Migita, K.; Nagaoka, S.; Ohata, K.; Yano, K.; Abiru, S.; et al. Predictive role of anti-gp210 and anticentromere antibodies in long-term outcome of primary biliary cirrhosis. *Hepatol. Res.* **2007**, *37*, S412–S419. [CrossRef] [PubMed]
54. Kim, K.-A.; Ki, M.; Choi, H.Y.; Kim, B.H.; Jang, E.S.; Jeong, S.-H. Population-based epidemiology of primary biliary cirrhosis in South Korea. *Aliment. Pharmacol. Ther.* **2015**, *43*, 154–162. [CrossRef] [PubMed]
55. Invernizzi, P.; Podda, M.; Battezzati, P.M.; Crosignani, A.; Zuin, M.; Hitchman, E.; Maggioni, M.; Meroni, P.L.; Penner, E.; Wesierska-Gadek, J. Autoantibodies against nuclear pore complexes are associated with more active and severe liver disease in primary biliary cirrhosis. *J. Hepatol.* **2001**, *34*, 366–372. [CrossRef]

56. Bogdanos, D.; Pares, A.; Rodes, J. Vergani D Primary biliary cirrhosis specific antinuclear antibodies in patients from Spain. *Am. J. Gastroenterol.* **2003**, *99*, 763–764. [CrossRef]
57. Nakamura, M.; Shimizu-Yoshida, Y.; Takii, Y.; Komori, A.; Yokoyama, T.; Ueki, T.; Daikoku, M.; Yano, K.; Matsumoto, T.; Migita, K.; et al. Antibody titer to gp210-C terminal peptide as a clinical parameter for monitoring primary biliary cirrhosis. *J. Hepatol.* **2005**, *42*, 386–392. [CrossRef]
58. Bogdanos, D.P.; Liaskos, C.; Pares, A.; Norman, G.; Rigopoulou, E.I.; Caballeria, L.; Dalekos, G.N.; Rodes, J.; Vergani, D. Anti-gp210 antibody mirrors disease severity in primary biliary cirrhosis. *Hepatology* **2007**, *45*, 1583. [CrossRef]
59. Haldar, D.; Janmohamed, A.; Plant, T.; Davidson, M.; Norman, H.; Russell, E.; Serevina, O.; Chung, K.; Qamar, K.; Gunson, B.; et al. Antibodies to gp210 and understanding risk in patients with primary biliary cholangitis. *Liver Int.* **2020**, *41*, 535–544. [CrossRef]
60. Yang, W.-H.; Yu, J.H.; Nakajima, A.; Neuberg, D.; Lindor, K.; Bloch, D.B. Do antinuclear antibodies in primary biliary cirrhosis patients identify increased risk for liver failure? *Clin. Gastroenterol. Hepatol.* **2004**, *2*, 1116–1122. [CrossRef]
61. Sfakianaki, O.; Koulentaki, M.; Tzardi, M.; Tsangaridou, E.; Theodoropoulos, P.A.; Castanas, E.; Kouroumalis, E.A. Peri-nuclear antibodies correlate with survival in Greek primary biliary cirrhosis patients. *World J. Gastroenterol.* **2010**, *16*, 4938–4943. [CrossRef] [PubMed]
62. Nakamura, M.; Kondo, H.; Tanaka, A.; Komori, A.; Ito, M.; Yamamoto, K.; Ohira, H.; Zeniya, M.; Hashimoto, E.; Honda, M.; et al. Autoantibody status and histological variables influence biochemical response to treatment and long-term outcomes in Japanese patients with primary biliary cirrhosis. *Hepatol. Res.* **2014**, *45*, 846–855. [CrossRef] [PubMed]
63. Tsangaridou, E.; Polioudaki, H.; Sfakianaki, R.; Samiotaki, M.; Tzardi, M.; Koulentaki, M.; Panayotou, G.; Kouroumalis, E.; Castanas, E.; Theodoropoulos, P.A. Differential detection of nuclear envelope autoantibodies in primary biliary cirrhosis using routine and alternative methods. *BMC Gastroenterol.* **2010**, *10*, 28. [CrossRef] [PubMed]
64. Vergani, D.; Alvarez, F.; Bianchi, F.B.; Cancado, E.L.; Mackay, I.R.; Manns, M.P.; Nishioka, M.; Penner, E. Liver autoimmune serology, a consensus statement from the committee for of the International Autoimmune Hepatitis Group. *J. Hepatol.* **2004**, *41*, 677–683. [PubMed]
65. Dahlqvist, G.; Gaouar, F.; Carrat, F.; Meurisse, S.; Chazouillères, O.; Poupon, R.; Johanet, C.; Corpechot, C.; The French Network of Immunology Laboratories. Large-scale characterization study of patients with antimitochondrial antibodies but nonestablished primary biliary cholangitis. *Hepatology* **2016**, *65*, 152–163. [CrossRef]

biomedicines

MDPI

Article

Hepatitis B Virus Variants with Multiple Insertions and/or Deletions in the X Open Reading Frame 3′ End: Common Members of Viral Quasispecies in Chronic Hepatitis B Patients

Selene García-García [1,2,3,†], Andrea Caballero-Garralda [1,4,†], David Tabernero [1,2,*], Maria Francesca Cortese [1,2,*], Josep Gregori [2,5], Francisco Rodriguez-Algarra [6], Josep Quer [2,3,5], Mar Riveiro-Barciela [2,7], Maria Homs [8,9], Ariadna Rando-Segura [1,10], Beatriz Pacin-Ruiz [1,2,3], Marta Vila [1], Roser Ferrer-Costa [1], Tomas Pumarola [10], Maria Buti [2,7] and Francisco Rodriguez-Frias [1,2,3,*]

1 Liver Pathology Unit, Departments of Biochemistry and Microbiology, Vall d'Hebron University Hospital, 08035 Barcelona, Spain; selene.garcia@vhir.org (S.G.-G.); acaballero@laboratorioechevarne.com (A.C.-G.); a.rando@vhebron.net (A.R.-S.); beatriz.pacin@vhir.org (B.P.-R.); marta.vila.salvador@vhir.org (M.V.); roferrer@vhebron.net (R.F.-C.)

2 Centro de Investigación Biomédica en Red de Enfermedades Hepáticas y Digestivas (CIBERehd), Instituto de Salud Carlos III, 28029 Madrid, Spain; josep.gregori@gmail.com (J.G.); josep.quer@vhir.org (J.Q.); mmriveir@vhebron.net (M.R.-B.); mbuti@vhebron.net (M.B.)

3 Biochemistry and Molecular Biology Department, Universitat Autònoma de Barcelona (UAB), 08193 Bellaterra, Spain

4 Echevarne Laboratory, Department of Biochemistry, 08037 Barcelona, Spain

5 Liver Diseases-Viral Hepatitis, Liver Unit, Vall d'Hebron Institute of Research (VHIR), Vall d'Hebron University Hospital, 08035 Barcelona, Spain

6 Blizard Institute, Barts and the London School of Medicine and Dentistry, Queen Mary University of London, London E1 2AT, UK; f.rodriguez-algarra@qmul.ac.uk

7 Liver Unit, Department of Internal Medicine, Vall d'Hebron University Hospital, 08035 Barcelona, Spain

8 Anoia Primary Care Service, Territorial Management of Central Catalonia, Catalan Institute of Health, 08700 Igualada, Spain; mhoms.cc.ics@gencat.cat

9 Health Promotion in Rural Areas Research Group, Territorial Management of Central Catalonia, Catalan Institute of Health, 08272 Sant Fruitós de Bages, Spain

10 Department of Microbiology, Vall d'Hebron University Hospital, 08035 Barcelona, Spain; tpumarola@vhebron.net

* Correspondence: david.tabernero@ciberehd.org (D.T.); maria.cortese@vhir.org (M.F.C.); frarodri@vhebron.net (F.R.-F.)

† These authors contributed equally to this work.

Citation: García-García, S.; Caballero-Garralda, A.; Tabernero, D.; Cortese, M.F.; Gregori, J.; Rodriguez-Algarra, F.; Quer, J.; Riveiro-Barciela, M.; Homs, M.; Rando-Segura, A.; et al. Hepatitis B Virus Variants with Multiple Insertions and/or Deletions in the X Open Reading Frame 3′ End: Common Members of Viral Quasispecies in Chronic Hepatitis B Patients. *Biomedicines* **2022**, *10*, 1194. https://doi.org/10.3390/biomedicines10051194

Academic Editor: Jinghua Wang

Received: 31 March 2022
Accepted: 19 May 2022
Published: 21 May 2022

Abstract: Deletions in the 3′ end region of the hepatitis B virus (HBV) X open reading frame (*HBX*) may affect the core promoter (Cp) and have been frequently associated with hepatocellular carcinoma (HCC). The aim of this study was to investigate the presence of variants with deletions and/or insertions (Indels) in this region in the quasispecies of 50 chronic hepatitis B (CHB) patients without HCC. We identified 103 different Indels in 47 (94%) patients, in a median of 3.4% of their reads (IQR, 1.3–8.4%), and 25% (IQR, 13.1–40.7%) of unique sequences identified in each quasispecies (haplotypes). Of those Indels, 101 (98.1%) caused 44 different altered stop codons, the most commonly observed were at positions 128, 129, 135, and 362 (putative position). Moreover, 39 (37.9%) Indels altered the TATA-like box (TA) sequences of Cp; the most commonly observed caused TA2 + TA3 fusion, creating a new putative canonical TATA box. Four (8%) patients developed negative clinical outcomes after a median follow-up of 9.4 (8.7–12) years. In conclusion, we observed variants with Indels in the *HBX* 3′ end in the vast majority of our CHB patients, some of them encoding alternative versions of HBx with potential functional roles, and/or alterations in the regulation of transcription.

Keywords: hepatitis B virus; hepatitis B X open reading frame; *HBX* 3′ end region; insertions; deletions; quasispecies; next-generation sequencing

1. Introduction

Hepatitis B remains a major global health problem. This infectious disease is estimated to have caused 820,000 deaths in 2019, mostly from cirrhosis and hepatocellular carcinoma (HCC), while 296 million people were chronically infected with hepatitis B virus (HBV) [1]. Neither of the current antiviral therapies (nucleoside/nucleotide analogs [NAs] and pegylated interferon alpha [IFN]) is able to achieve a complete cure of the infection. This is mainly due to the persistence of the HBV genome in the nuclei of infected hepatocytes [2], both as an episomal chromosome-like structure called covalently closed circular DNA (cccDNA) and integrated into the host's genome. Both cccDNA and integrated forms of the viral genome are the sources of all HBV transcripts [3,4]. The HBV genome is about 3.2 Kb in length and, due to this small size, in the same nucleotide (nt) sequence, it contains four highly overlapped open reading frames (ORFs), the regulatory elements to control their transcription, and structural elements essential for viral replication [5]. The packing of information is notable in the X ORF (*HBX*, nt 1374–1838), especially in its 3′ end region (nt 1523–1838), a sequence that also contains the Core promoter (Cp), which controls the transcription of pregenomic RNA (pgRNA), an intermediate in viral replication that is also translated to HBcAg and the viral polymerase, and pre-core RNA (pcRNA), which is translated to HBeAg. This promoter includes sequence and structural motifs such as the four TATA-like boxes (TA) 1 to 4, the enhancer II (ENHII), and the direct repeat 1 (DR1), all essential for viral replication [6,7].

The *HBX* gene encodes the HBV X protein (HBx), a 17-kilodalton (KDa) protein composed of 154 amino acids (aa) [8]. This protein is characterized by an astonishing pleiotropic function thanks to its direct interactions with multiple cellular proteins. Specifically, HBx is capable of promoting HBV replication by epigenetic stimulation of cccDNA transcription [3]. Moreover, it is able to facilitate the interaction of stimulating cellular transcriptional factors to this episome, in order to regulate the transcription of host genes, disrupt protein degradation, modulate signaling pathways, manipulate cell death, and deregulate the cell cycle [9]. The HBx C-terminal end plays a key role in controlling these functions owing to its transactivating activity [10]. This region of HBx is encoded by the *HBX* 3′ end region, where deletions (Del) have been more frequently detected in the tumor than in the adjacent non-tumor tissues from HCC patients by population sequencing [11]. These Del, along with insertions (Ins) in this region of *HBX* may yield significantly altered HBx due to *HBX* frameshifts. HBx with truncations in the C-terminal end (hereinafter referred to as HBxCtermTrunc) has been associated with a critical role in HCC carcinogenesis [12]. In addition, these Indels may affect not only HBx but also the properties of the multiple important regulatory and structural motifs (Cp, ENHII, DR1, etc.), overlapped with it. Viral populations (variants) with insertions and/or deletions (Indels) contribute to the high genetic variability of HBV, which leads to a highly heterogeneous viral infection distributed as a quasispecies: a mixture or swarm of variants genetically closely related but not identical [13]. Interestingly, previous studies using clone sequencing identified variants with Indels in the *HBX* 3′ end region, both in patients with severe liver disease [14,15] and in chronic hepatitis B (CHB) patients without HCC [16,17]. This suggests that these variants are usually present in HBV quasispecies, in both severe and mild forms of liver disease, despite the possible alterations of the HBx caused by Indels in the *HBX* 3′ region, or the effects on the promoter activity of Cp. Many of these variants may even play some functional role.

The aim of this study was to investigate the presence of variants with Indels in the *HBX* 3′ end region in CHB patients without HCC using next-generation sequencing (NGS). This high-throughput technology can reveal these kinds of variants even if they are present as minor variants in the quasispecies, undetectable using Sanger or clone sequencing. We identified variants with Indels in the *HBX* 3′ end region in most of our CHB patients, and potential alterations to HBx and Cp and functional consequences of the most relevant of those Indels have been discussed.

2. Materials and Methods

2.1. Patients and Samples

In this retrospective study, CHB patients who attended the outpatient clinic of Vall d'Hebron University Hospital (Barcelona, Spain) were selected according to the following inclusion criteria: age over 18 years; available serum sample with HBV-DNA levels of 1000 IU/mL or higher (to ensure sufficient HBV-DNA levels to study their quasispecies) obtained after more than 6 months with detectable HBsAg, in a period without antiviral treatment and no evidence of HCC; negative test for hepatitis C virus (HCV), human immunodeficiency virus (HIV), and hepatitis D virus (HDV) infections; written informed consent for participation provided.

2.2. Serological and Virological Determinations

Serological markers of HBV and HCV infections [HBsAg, HBeAg, and antibodies against HCV (anti-HCV)] were tested using commercial electrochemiluminescence immunoassays on a COBAS 8000 instrument (Roche Diagnostics, Rotkreuz, Switzerland). Anti-HDV antibodies were tested using the HDV Ab kit (Dia.Pro Diagnostics Bioprobes, Sesto San Giovanni, Italy), and anti-HIV antibodies with the Liaison XL murex HIV Ab/Ag kit (DiaSorin, Saluggia, Italy). HBV-DNA was measured in the Cobas 6800 System (Roche Diagnostics, Mannheim, Germany), with a detection limit of 10 IU/mL. HBV genotyping was performed using a line-probe assay (INNO-LiPA HBV Genotyping Assay; Fujirebio Europe N.V., Ghent, Belgium).

2.3. Amplification of HBV Genome Region Analyzed and Next-Generation Sequencing

In this study, a fragment of the HBV genome located between nt 1596 and 1912 was amplified using an in-house nested PCR and sequenced on forward and reverse strands by means of NGS, using ultra-deep pyrosequencing (UDPS) technology [Genome Sequencer FLX and Junior systems (454 Life Sciences-Roche, Branford, CT, USA)], as previously described [18]. Briefly, HBV-DNA was extracted from 200 μL of serum using QIAamp DNA Mini Kit (QIAGEN, Hilden, Germany) as per the manufacturer's instructions. Nested PCRs were performed using the PfuUltra II Fusion HS DNA polymerase (Agilent technologies, Santa Clara, CA, USA), using the following primers: outer PCR, forward 5′-*GTTGTAAAACGACGGCCAGT*TGTGCACTTCGCYTCACC-3′ and reverse 5′-*CACAGGAAACAGCTATGACC*AGWAGCTCCAAATTCTTTATAAGG-3′. These primers contain an M13 universal adaptor sequence at the 5′ end (in italics) and the template-specific sequence. The nested PCR primers contained 5′ 25-nt sequences A and B, which are adaptors for the elements of the 454 Life Sciences-Roche UDPS system, followed by a 10-nt sequence used as a unique identifier for each sample (multiplex identifier), and the same M13 universal adaptor sequences included in the outer PCR primers at the 3′ ends. Finally, 468 base pairs (bp) amplicons were obtained, which were pooled and processed according to the 454 Life Sciences-Roche UDPS protocol.

The NGS raw data presented in this study are openly available in the NCBI database Sequence Read Archive (SRA), at BioProject accession number PRJNA625435. The BioSample accession numbers are included in Table S1.

2.4. Next-Generation Sequencing Data Treatment

The HBV genomic fragment analyzed was sequenced on both strands, forward and reverse. The sequences obtained by NGS (referred to as reads) were processed using a data treatment workflow, established in previous studies with HBV [19] and HCV controls [20] to minimize the scoring of PCR artifacts and sequencing errors: the reads obtained were demultiplexed by identifying the multiplex identifier and the template specific primer sequences. Primers were then trimmed and both strands were treated separately. First, the reverse reads were reverse complemented, and all (forward and reverse) reads that (1) did not cover the full amplicon, (2) had more than one indetermination, and (3) had an identity relative to the reference sequence below 70% were discarded. The resulting sequences were collapsed to haplotypes (HPL), i.e., unique sequences covering the full amplicon with their corresponding frequencies, thus each HPL corresponds to a quasispecies variant.

Multiple alignments of the forward and reverse HPL of each sample, with abundances not below 0.1%, were then performed with a reference sequence of the corresponding genotype (Table S2), using the MUSCLE software package (version 3.8.31) [21]. Only those HPL common to both strands were retained, and those unique to a single strand were removed. The resulting HPLs were called consensus HPLs and their final frequencies were taken as the sum of the read counts in each strand. The multiple alignments of the consensus HPLs with the corresponding reference sequence were used to report Indels.

All computations were performed with the R environment and language [22], using in-house scripts with the help of the Biostrings [23] and ape packages [24].

2.5. Cloning to Confirm NGS Results

The presence of variants with Indels identified in this study was confirmed by cloning and sequencing of some selected samples. The same PCR products obtained from these samples and analyzed by NGS were also cloned using Zero Blunt TOPO PCR cloning Kit (Life Technologies, Carlsbad, CA, USA), following the manufacturer's instructions. Briefly, the 468-bp amplicons obtained using nested PCR were cloned into pCR™4Blunt-TOPO® vector and the resulting constructs were used to chemically transform *Escherichia coli* competent cells using the heat shock method. The transformed bacteria were incubated on a Luria–Bertani (LB) broth agar plate overnight at 37 °C and 18–29 clones/samples were selected for sequencing.

In those selected clones, the pCR™4Blunt-TOPO® vectors containing a 468-bp amplicon sequence were isolated with the QIAprep Miniprep kit (QIAGEN, Hilden, Germany), following the manufacturer's instructions. Finally, the amplicon sequences were directly sequenced using the BigDye Terminator v3.1 Cycle Sequencing Kit (Thermo Fisher Scientific, Waltham, MA, USA), with the primers M13-Fw and TOPO Rv provided in the Zero Blunt TOPO PCR cloning Kit, on an ABI PRISM 3130xl Genetic Analyzer (Thermo Fisher Scientific, Waltham, MA, USA).

2.6. RNA Structural Modelling

The structure of significant sequence motifs included in the analyzed region, with or without Indels identified, was analyzed at the theoretical level. To this end, the local RNA structures obtained from the sequence of selected HPL were modeled using the RNAfold Webserver (http://rna.tbi.univie.ac.at/cgi-bin/RNAWebSuite/RNAfold.cgi (accessed on 28 March 2022)), from the Vienna RNA Websuite [25]. The Vienna RNA WebServers are based on the latest Vienna RNA Package (Version 2.4.18). All parameters of the web application were set to default. Secondary RNA structure was predicted using generalized centroid estimators.

2.7. Statistical Analysis

All statistical analyses were performed in R [26]. Proportions of cases showing a specific Indel have been compared between HBeAg-positive and negative patients using Fisher's exact test. The percentages of reads and HPL with Indels were shown as median and interquartile range (IQR). Statistical comparisons between median percentages of reads and HPL with Indels in HBeAg-positive and HBeAg-negative patients were performed using the Kruskal–Wallis test. Correlation of these median percentages with HBV-DNA levels were assessed by Spearman's correlation coefficient. P values of less than 0.05 were considered significant.

3. Results

3.1. Patients and Samples

A group of 50 CHB patients was selected, most of whom were HBeAg-negative and did not show a significant fibrosis degree (≤F3). Demographical, clinical, virological, serological, and biochemical markers from the patients included in this study are summarized in Table 1.

Table 1. Characteristics of patients on obtaining the sample analyzed.

	Patients (*N* = 50)
Age (median years, IQR)	43 (35–55)
Gender (*N* Male, %)	42 (84)
HBV-DNA (median logIU/mL, IQR)	5.9 (5.3–7.9)
HBV genotype	
A (*N*, %)	39 (78)
D (*N*, %)	8 (16)
F (*N*, %)	3 (6)
HBeAg-negative (*N*, %)	33 (66)
ALT (median IU/L, IQR)	80 (57–115)
Liver fibrosis [1]	
≤F3 (%)	45 (90)
>F3 (%)	5 (10)
Treatment history	
Previous NA (*N*, %)	17 (34)
Previous IFN (*N*, %)	2 (4)

[1] Ishak fibrosis stage (F), assessed by liver biopsy. Abbreviations: N indicates number; IQR, interquartile range; HBV, hepatitis B virus; IU, international units; HBeAg, hepatitis B e antigen; ALT, alanine aminotransferase; NA, nucleoside/nucleotide analogs; IFN, interferon.

3.2. *Overview of Next-Generation Data Analyses*

The fragment of the HBV genome between nt 1596 and 1912 encodes from aa 75 to 154 of HBx, along with the last 8 aa of the RNAse H in the polymerase ORF and the pre-core and the first 5 aa of the core region in the pre-core/core ORF (Figure 1). In this study, we focused on the effects of Indels on *HBX* and the overlapped Cp; their effects on these short polymerase and core ORFs stretches were considered beyond the scope of this study and were not explored.

NGS and bioinformatics processing of the amplicon libraries of this fragment of HBV genome, obtained from the 50 included samples yielded a total of 960,921 reads, a median of 16,735/sample (IQR, 9277–24,668). Of those 960,921 reads, 70,278 (7.3%) showed Indels, including single Ins, Del, or combinations of them, affecting the HBx coding sequence. Interestingly, those reads were found in 47/50 (94%) patients, mainly in small percentages (median of 3.4% per sample [IQR, 1.3–8.4%]). HBeAg-positive patients showed higher percentages of Indel reads than HBeAg-negative patients (median of 6.1% versus [vs.] 1.5%, respectively; $p = 0.03$). The percentage of reads with Indels did not show any statistically significant correlation with HBV-DNA levels, whether considering all patients together or separating them according to HBeAg status.

Those reads were grouped in a total of 1039 HPL (median of 17/sample [IQR, 11–28]), of which 288 (27.7%) showed Indels and represented a median of 25% (IQR, 13.1–40.7%) of HPL found in each sample. Among the Indels identified in those 288 HPL, 103 different single Ins or Del, or combinations of them affected the HBx coding region (named as ID: 1–103, Table S3). While median percentages of Indel HPL were higher in HBeAg-positive patients than in HBeAg-negative (33.3% vs. 25%, respectively), the differences were not statistically significant. The correlation between Indel HPL and HBV-DNA levels was also not statistically significant.

Of those Indels, 12 (11.7%) were observed in at least 10% of patients (Table 2). Of these Indels, ID: 11 and 30 were only present in HBeAg-negative patients; however, the percentages of cases showing these Indels showed no statistically significant differences between HBeAg-positive and HBeAg-negative patients. ID: 85, on the other hand, showed a lower median percentage of reads in HBeAg-positive patients than in HBeAg-negative patients (0.4% vs. 1.1%, respectively; $p = 0.01$), although no statistical difference in terms of proportion of positive cases had been observed. No other statistically significant differences between HBeAg-positive and HBeAg-negative patients were observed in this group of Indels. No significant correlation was observed with HBV-DNA levels.

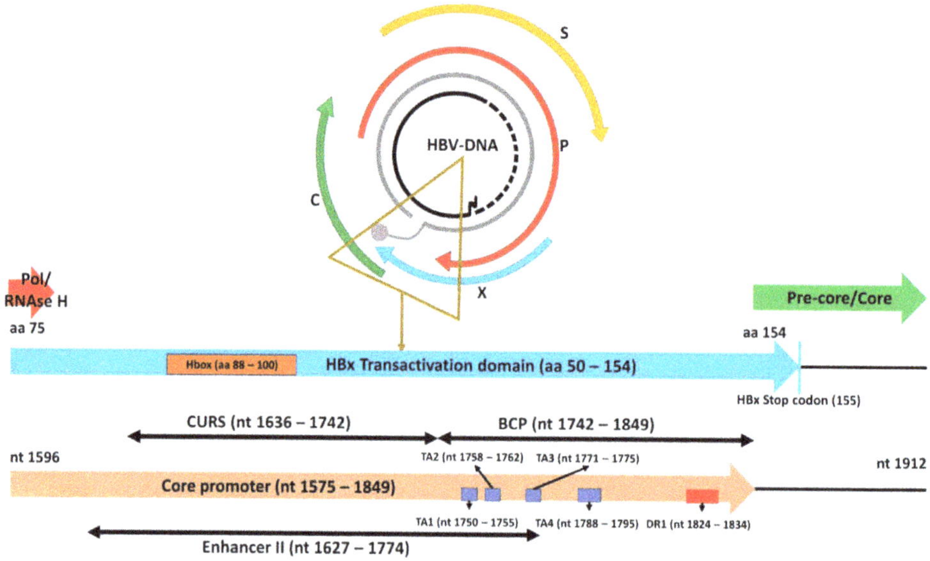

Figure 1. Fragment of hepatitis B virus (HBV) genome analyzed in this study. It encompasses parts of the Polymerase, X (*HBX*), and pre-core/core open reading frames (ORF). The fragment of *HBX* analyzed encodes most of hepatitis B X protein (HBx) transactivating C-terminal domain, including its essential α-helical motif (Hbox) [27]. In addition, the nucleotide (nt) sequence of that fragment (nts 1596 to 1912) contains most of the core promoter sequence, including the core upstream regulatory sequence (CURS) and the basic core promoter (BCP) with the TATA-like boxes 1–4 (TA1–TA4); nt positions are shown as described in [6]. It also includes the Enhancer II and the direct repeat 1 (DR1) sequences; nt positions are shown as described in [7].

Table 2. Description and frequencies of reads and haplotypes of the insertions, deletions or combinations of both, identified in more than 10% of the 50 patients studied.

ID	Deletions	Insertions	N Patients (%)	Median % Reads/Patient (IQR)	Median % HPL/Patient (IQR)
11	1646	-	6 (12)	0.5 (0.4–0.6)	6.5 (2.8–10.4)
30	1692	1697TT	6 (12)	0.5 (0.4–0.6)	7.5 (6.1–14.6)
37	-	1739G	9 (18)	0.3 (0.3–0.5)	8.3 (7.1–14.3)
38	-	1746G/T	7 (14)	0.4 (0.3–0.4)	10 (6.7–12.7)
40	1749	-	7 (14)	0.4 (0.3–0.5)	6.7 (5.2–11.3)
51	1763–1770	-	10 (20)	1.7 (0.9–2.1)	5.5 (3.0–8.2)
59	-	1781C	5 (10)	0.6 (0.6–0.7)	8.3 (4.8–8.3)
74	-	1820C	7 (14)	0.4 (0.4–0.9)	4.3 (1.9–4.8)
84	-	1825T	19 (38)	1.5 (0.7–2.1)	4.8 (2.8–6.9)
85	1825	-	10 (20)	0.4 (0.4–0.8)	4.1 (2.8–5.1)
88	-	1826C/T	9 (18)	0.6 (0.4–0.9)	4.8 (2.6–8.3)
103	-	1838A	5 (10)	1.2 (0.9–2.7)	2.3 (2.2–5.9)

Abbreviations: ID indicates code to identify single insertion or deletion, or combinations of them (see Table S3); N, number; IQR, interquartile range; HPL, haplotypes.

3.3. Alternative HBX Stop Codons

Almost all the different Indels identified (101/103, 98.1%) altered the position of the wild-type (WT) *HBX* stop codon 155 (Table S3). These 101 Indels were detected in all

47 patients showing Indel reads, causing 44 different altered stop codons, 15 (34.1%) of which were identified in more than 10% of patients (Table 3). Of these codons 23 (52.3%) were located before the WT position, leading to a HBxCtermTrunc, while 21 (47.7%) were located beyond the WT position, leading to an elongated HBx (HBxLong).

Table 3. Description and frequencies of reads and haplotypes of the altered stop codons identified in more than 10% of the 50 patients studied.

HBX Stop Codon	IDs	N Patients (%)	Median % Reads/Patient (IQR)	Median % HPL/Patient (IQR)
95	2, 3, 7, 8	5 (10)	0.4 (0.3–0.5)	5.9 (5.3–8.3)
109	28, 29, 30, NA	9 (18)	0.5 (0.4–0.6)	6.7 (4.3–16.7)
125	18, NA	8 (16)	1.9 (0.6–3.8)	3.8 (2.2–5.8)
128	37, 38, 41	15 (30)	0.4 (0.3–0.6)	8.3 (5.6–18.3)
129	6, 11, 23, 25, 34, 35, 36, 39, 40	21 (42)	0.5 (0.4–0.6)	7.1 (4.8–11.1)
132	45, 46, 49, 57	5 (10)	0.5 (0.5–0.8)	2.6 (2.6–4.3)
135	14, 15, 22, 47, 48, 51, 53, 55, 80, 81, 87, 90, 100	14 (28)	2.0 (0.5–4.9)	6.1 (3.0–11.8)
138	59	5 (10)	0.6 (0.6–0.7)	8.3 (4.8–8.3)
149	63, 72	5 (10)	0.7 (0.4–1.0)	4.5 (4.2–4.8)
156	12, 13, 27, 58, 76, 82, 89	7 (14)	2.6 (0.7–7.3)	7.1 (5.5–7.7)
179	85	10 (20)	0.4 (0.4–0.8)	4.1 (2.8–5.1)
180 *	75, 86, 98	5 (10)	0.9 (0.6–1.2)	5.1 (3.6–5.9)
207 *	101, NA	6 (12)	0.5 (0.4–0.6)	3 (2.4–4.4)
360 *	70, 92	5 (10)	0.6 (0.6–1.1)	2.6 (2.3–4.3)
362 *	74, 78, 84, 88	24 (48)	1.6 (0.8–2.1)	5.8 (3.1–10.7)

Abbreviations: *HBX* indicates hepatitis B X open reading frame; IDs, code to identify single insertion or deletion, or combinations of them, described in Table S3; N, number; IQR, interquartile range; HPL, haplotypes; NA, haplotype/s without insertions and/or deletions. * Putative stop codons of the HPL without stop codon in *HBX*, obtained by extension of those HPL with reference sequences V01460 (for genotype D HPL) and X02763 (for genotype A HPL) and continue translation.

The most frequent premature stop codons among patients were those in positions 128, 129, and 135, associated with several different Indels (Table 3). Interestingly, while the premature stop codon 128 was associated with single nt Ins in positions 1739, 1746, and 1751 (ID: 37, 38, and 41, respectively), stop codon 129 was associated with 9 different single nt Dels between positions 1630–1749 (Table S3). Therefore, both stop codons were associated with single nt Ins or Del in a region just before TA region, or inside TA1 (Figure 1). On the other hand, stop codon 135 was associated with 13 different Indels affecting the TA region, as discussed below (Section 3.4. Indels Affecting the TATA-Like Box Region).

In relation to the stop codons beyond the WT position, it must be borne in mind that the fragment of HBV genome analyzed made it possible to continue translation in the same ORF as *HBX* until codon 179, which allowed us to identify 9 stop codons between positions 155 and 179 (in codons 156, 157, 158, 173, 174, 175 176, 177 and 179). However, some HPLs with Indels did not show any stop codon. In those cases, a reference HBV genome sequence of the same genotype was added after nt 1912, and translation was continued in the same ORF until the appearance of a stop codon. The accession numbers of reference sequences used were V01460 (for genotype D HPL) and X02763 (for genotype A HPL); no genotype F HPL showed stop codons beyond 179. Thanks to this, 12 additional putative stop codons have been identified (in codons 180, 181, 182, 183, 207, 355, 356, 357, 360, 361, 362 and 363). The putative stop codon located at position 362 was the most frequently altered stop codon identified and was observed in almost half of the patients (Table 3). Interestingly, the elongation of *HBX* to codon 362 shifted this reading frame to the core ORF, thus resulting in a putative fusion protein, which would include from aa 1 to 149 or 150 of HBx plus aa 3 or 4 to 214 of the pre-core protein. This stop codon was associated with single nt Ins located within or adjacent to a five T region (1821–1825), partially overlapped with the DR1 motive. Of note, one of these Ins was the ID: 84 (Ins 1825T), the most prevalent in patients of the 103 different Indels identified (Table 2), found in 13049/960921 (1.4%) and 23/1039 (2.2%) of total reads and HPL obtained, respectively. However, the Ins ID: 84 (and also ID: 74) are not strictly associated with the stop codon before position 362; a few HPL with both Ins showed a stop codon in position 175 (Table S3). In fact, HPL with a putative stop codon between positions 355 to 363, potentially encoding an HBx + pre-core fusion protein, were identified in 25/50 (50%) patients, in a median of 1.6% (1.2–3%) of their reads and 7.7% (4.3–14.3%) of their HPL. These putative stop codons were associated with Dels between positions 1805 and 1843 (ID: 64, 67, 69, 70, 73, 83, 92, 94, and 97), and Ins within or very close to the five T region between positions 1821–1825 (ID: 20, 74, 77, 78, 84 and 88) (Table S3).

Interestingly, the Ins events in this polyT homopolymeric region would have similar consequences to the programmed −1 ribosomal frameshifting (PRF) mRNA signals. These signals are used by many viruses, such as Rous sarcoma virus and HIV-1, to induce a proportion of translating ribosomes to slip back by 1 nt into an overlapping ORF and to continue the translation, thus producing coordinated expression of two or more proteins from a single mRNA [28–30]. Of note, the region involving this polyT homopolymeric region in HBV showed RNA folding highly similar to that predicted for the HIV-1 PRF signal, which includes a heptanucleotide slippery sequence (UUUUUUA) followed by a spacer region and a downstream RNA stem-loop structure [29] (Figure 2). Additionally, of note in the same five T region is the single nt Del 1825 (ID: 85), present in 20% of patients (Table 2) and associated with a stop codon at position 179 (Table 3).

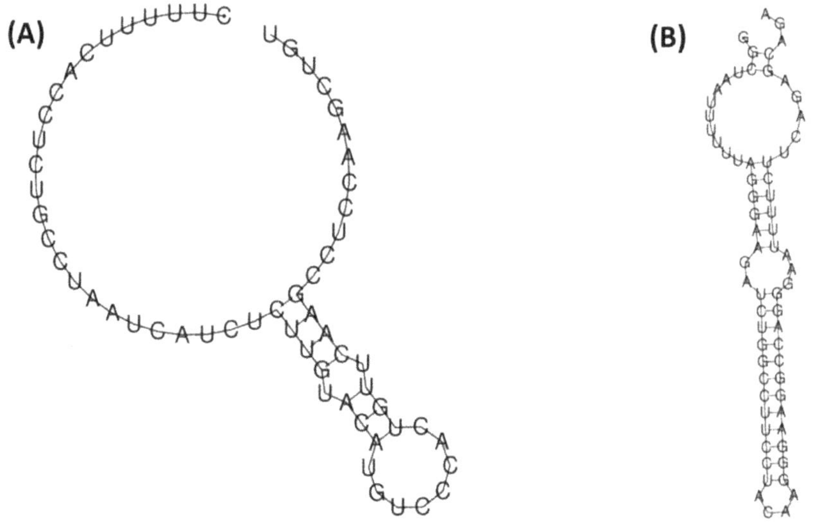

Figure 2. Comparison between the predicted local RNA folding of the region between nucleotides 1820 and 1880 of the hepatitis B virus (HBV) genome, including the polyT homopolymeric region between positions 1821–1825 (**A**); the region between nucleotides 1625 to 1691 of the human immunodeficiency virus-1 (HIV), including the Programmed −1 ribosomal frameshifting mRNA signal (**B**). The HBV sequence has been modeled from the genotype A reference sequence used to report Indels, included in Table S2. The HIV sequence has been modeled from the Genbank pattern with accession number NC_001802.1.

3.4. Indels Affecting the TATA-Like Box Region

A group of 39/103 (37.9%) identified Indels were located in the TA region (Figure 1). Altogether, these Indels were found in 28,628/960,921 (3%) of total reads obtained, which were grouped in 111/1039 (10.7%) HPL, and were present in 25/50 (50%) patients. Notably, these Indels were included in the region between nt 1751 and 1787; none of them affected the TA4 sequence (nt 1788–1795). The effects of these 39 Indels on the TA region are summarized in Table 4.

Table 4. Alterations in the core promoter TATA-like boxes caused by insertions and deletions identified between nucleotides 1751 and 1787 in the 50 patients studied.

TA Alteration	Cause of Alteration and Indels Involved	N Patients (%)	Median % Reads/Patient (IQR)	Median % HPL/Patient (IQR)
Insertion in TA1 (nt 1750–1755)	**Ins:** ID: 41 (Ins 1751G)	3 (6)	0.3–0.4 *	3.4–5.9 *
Partial or total TA1 or TA2 (nt 1758–1762) elimination	7 to 10 nt Del between nt 1754 and 1767: **Dels:** ID: 42, 45, 47, 48, 49, 50	5 (10)	0.5 (0.4–2.0)	3.6 (2.2–4.5)
Partial or total TA2 + TA3 (nt 1758–1775) elimination	**Ins + Del**: ID: 16 Dels between nt 1756 and 1787: **Dels**: ID: 43, 44, 46 **Ins + Dels:** ID: 9, 12, 13, 14, 15, 17, 18, 19, 20, 22, 26, 27	3 (6)	0.9–71.2 *	2.3–61.8 *
TA2 + TA3 Fusion	8 nt Del between nt 1763 and 1770: **Del:** ID: 51 **Ins + Dels:** ID: 24, 80, 81, 87, 90, 100	10 (20)	1.8 (0.9–4.3)	5.5 (3.0–17.5)
Partial or total TA3 (nt 1771–1775) elimination	8 to 10 nt Del between nt 1763 and 1776 **Dels:** ID: 52, 53, 55, 56, 57	7 (14)	0.4 (0.4–2.1)	2.6 (2.4–5.6)
No TA affected	**Ins:** ID: 58 (Ins 1768GTT/ATT), 59 (Ins 1781C), 60 (Ins 1785C) **Del**: ID: 54 (Del 1766)	10 (20)	0.6 (0.4–0.9)	6.5 (4.3–8.3)

Abbreviations: TA indicates TATA-like boxes; N, number; IQR, interquartile range; HPL, haplotypes; nt, nucleotides; Ins, insertions; Del, deletions; IDs, code to identify single Ins or Del, or combinations of them, described in Table S4. * No median was calculated due to low number of patients, instead the maximum and minimum percentage of reads and haplotypes per patient are shown.

All Indels affecting the TA region also altered the WT *HBX* stop codon, showing 17 different stop codons, 12 (70.6%) of which led to HBxLong (Table S4). Of note among them is the stop codon in position 135, which was caused by 13/39 (33.3%) of those Indels. Of those 13 Indels, 10 (76.9%) contained 8 nt deletions (Del8nt) between positions 1757 and 1773, which eliminated TA2, caused the fusion of TA2 + TA3, or partially eliminated TA3. The stop codon in position 135 was also associated with 3 Indel combinations including Del 1758–1777, which eliminated TA2 + TA3 (Table S4). Altogether, these 13 Indels causing stop codon 135 were identified in 14 patients, 56% of 25 patients with Indels in the TA region, and 28% of the 50 patients included. These patients showed a relatively high median percentage of reads with this stop codon compared to the other stop codons associated with Indels (Table 3), even reaching 20.8% of reads obtained in a single case.

Of the 39 Indels affecting the TA region, we identified 14 (35.9% ID: 9, 12–20, 22, 24, 26, and 27) complex Indel combinations, present in 4 patients, 16% of 25 patients with Indels in the TA region, and 8% of 50 patients included. These combinations included Del which, in most cases, caused a total or partial elimination of TA2 + TA3, linked to additional big Ins (24–28 nt) in a region of the core upstream regulatory sequence (CURS) (Table S4). The CURS contains several sequence motifs that positively regulate the activity of the basal core promoter (BCP), which includes the TA (Figure 1). Notably, most of these variants contained a duplication in the motif known as α box (nts 1646–1668) [6], overlapping the *HBX* region encoding an α-helical motif (Hbox, between aa 88–100), which binds to the DNA damage-binding protein 1 (DDB1) [27], an essential interaction for HBV replication [31]. It is worth mentioning that, in a single patient, 72.9% of reads and 65.5% of HPL showed these complex Indel combinations. In particular, more than a half (51.9%) of reads obtained corresponded to Indel combination ID: 12, constituted by the 24 nt Ins 1647TCTTACATAAGAGGACTCTTGGAC, and Del 1627 + 1758 − 1777 which eliminates TA2 + TA3. Ins 1647 is a duplication of the contiguous sequence which causes the duplication of regulatory motifs in Cp such as the α box and binding sites for CCAAT/enhancer-binding protein α (C/EBPα) [6,32]. This duplication also results in a strong modification of the HBx Hbox (88SCPRSYIRGLLDS100 instead of 88ILPKVLHKRTLGLP100) [27].

The most common alteration of a TA sequence observed among patients showing Indels in that region was the fusion of TA2 and TA3 sequences due to a Del8nt between nt 1763 and 1770 (ID: 51) (Table 4). This Del8nt was among the most prevalent in the 50 patients included, with a relatively high median percentage of reads compared to the other Indels identified in more than 10% of patients (Table 2). Interestingly, the fusion of TA2 + TA3 due to Del 1763–1770 created the sequence TTAAATATTA. This sequence was coincident with that of a canonical/true TATA box [33], as the TA4, which we named TA23. Similar to the TA4 sequence, when viral genome double-stranded DNA is separated into single strands, (e.g., during cccDNA transcription), TA23 was found to be completely unpaired (Figure 3). In addition, the Del 1763–1770 was also present in Indel combinations identified in single patients. In Indels ID: 80, 81, 87, 90, and 100, this Del8nt was linked to an additional Ins around or inside DR1, and in ID: 24 to a big Ins at CURS. This last Indel caused the appearance of a premature stop codon in position 144, while the remaining Indels showing the Del 1763–1770 were associated with the prevalent altered *HBX* stop codon at position 135. However, it should be noted that this Del8nt was not strictly associated with the stop codon at position 135, as shown in a single HPL with the Del ID: 51, which showed the *HBX* stop codon at position 122 instead of 135 (Table S4).

3.5. Confirmation of Indel Variants by Cloning

Four patients with important percentages of variants with Indels by NGS were selected for cloning/sequencing analysis. The results of this additional analysis are shown in Table 5. In patient 2, cloning/sequencing confirmed the presence of the major complex Indel combination ID: 12 in a similar percentage to that found using NGS. In addition, cloning analysis also showed the presence of minor Indels such as the Ins ID: 74, and complex Indel combinations not identified by NGS. The presence of Ins 1825T (ID: 84) and Del 1825T (ID: 85), both highly prevalent in the included patients, was confirmed in patients 17 and 39, and in patient 20, respectively. Of note, the percentages of reads and clones that did not show any Indels were similar (indicated with a—in the Deletions and Insertions columns in Table 5).

Table 5. Description of the insertions, deletions, or combinations of both, identified by cloning/sequencing analysis in the 4 patients selected.

Patient (N Clones Analyzed)	Deletions	Insertions	N Clones (%)	ID	N Reads (%)
2 (24)	1627 + 1758 − 1777	1647 TCTTA-CATAAGAG-GACTCTTGGAC	12 (50)	12	9554 (51.9)
	-	1820 C	1 (4.2)	74	75 (0.4)
	1627 + 1726 + 1758 − 1777	1647 TCTTA-CATAAGAG-GACTCTTGGAC	2 (8)	-	-

Table 5. *Cont.*

Patient (N Clones Analyzed)	Deletions	Insertions	N Clones (%)	ID	N Reads (%)
	1627 + 1758 − 1777	1647 TCTTA-CATAAGAG-GACTCTTGGAC + 1822 ATTCAA + 1825 T	1 (4.2)	-	-
	1627	1600T + 1647 TCT-TACATAAGAG-GACTCTTGGAC	1 (4.2)	-	-
	-	-	7 (29.2)	-	4692 (25.5)
17 (29)	-	1825 T	2 (6.9)	84	3140 (14.2)
	-	1909 TG	1 (3.4)	*	*
	-	-	26 (89.7)	-	18736 (84.8)
20 (18)	1825	-	1 (5.6)	85	3011 (15.5)
	-	1826 TTC	6 (33.3)	89	2171 (11.2)
	-	-	11 (61)	-	14064 (72.5)
39 (19)	-	1605 T	1 (5.3)	-	-
	-	1825 T	7 (36.8)	84	3242 (22.9)
	-	1895 T	1 (5.3)	*	*
	-	-	10 (52.6)	-	9701 (68.5)

Abbreviations: N Clones indicates number of clones showing a specific insertion, deletion or combination of both; ID, code to designate single insertion or deletion, or combinations of them identified by next-generation sequencing (see Table S3); N Reads, number of next-generation sequencing reads showing a specific single insertion or deletion, or a combination of both. * Insertions that have not been assessed in next-generation sequencing reads since they are located out of hepatitis B X gene open reading frame.

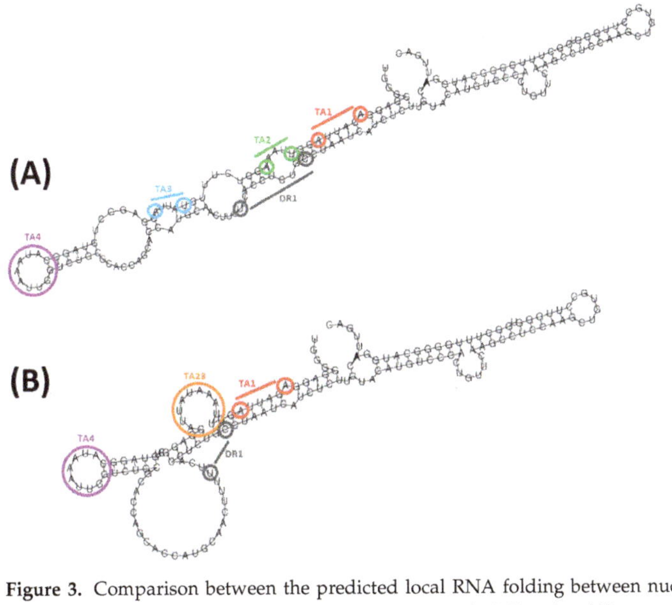

Figure 3. Comparison between the predicted local RNA folding between nucleotides 1741 and 1912 encompassing the TA region of the core promoter, of a WT variant (**A**) versus a variant including the deletion 1763–1770 (ID: 51) (**B**). Both variants have been modeled from the genotype A reference sequence used to report Indels, included in Table S2. In red, TA1 sequence (AGAUUA); in green, TA2 sequence (UUAAA); in blue, TA3 sequence (UAUUA); in purple, TA4 sequence (CAUAAAUU); in grey, DR1 sequence (UUCACCUCUGC); in orange, TA23 sequence (UUAAAUAUUA).

3.6. Clinical Outcome of Patients Studied

Development of negative clinical outcomes associated with CHB was assessed in each of the 50 patients included for a median of 9.4 (IQR 8.7–12) years after obtaining selected samples. During this time, all patients received antiviral treatment, and only the five patients with advanced fibrosis (Ishak score > F3) on enrolment in the study developed negative clinical outcomes. One of these progressed to cirrhosis after superinfection with HCV 6.3 years after the sample analyzed was obtained and was excluded from further analysis. Two of the remaining four cases progressed to cirrhosis 3.9 and 3 years after the sample analyzed was obtained, respectively. The other two cases progressed to HCC 9.5 and 10.2 years after the sample analyzed was obtained, respectively; none of them showed cirrhosis at the time of HCC diagnosis.

All four patients showed variants encoding HBxCtermTrunc. Interestingly, a patient who progressed to cirrhosis and another who progressed to HCC, showed the Ins ID: 37 (Ins 1739G) and 38 (Ins 1746G/T), causing the highly prevalent stop codon at position 128 (Table 3). Notably, both patients showed higher percentages of reads and HPL harboring this stop codon than the median of all 50 patients, especially the patient who developed HCC: 0.9% vs. 1.5% vs. 0.4% of reads; and 20% vs. 33.3% vs. 8.3% of HPL in the cirrhotic, the HCC and median of all patients, respectively. The other patient who progressed to HCC showed the single nt Del ID: 36 (Del 1727), leading to the also prevalent *HBX* stop codon at position 129 (Table 3). Again, this patient showed higher percentages of reads and HPL harboring this stop codon than the median of all 50 patients: 1% vs. 0.5% of reads and 12.5% vs. 7.1%, respectively. The second patient who progressed to cirrhosis did not show any HPL with Indels, but one of them encoded a HBxCtermTrunc ending at codon 148.

4. Discussion

Indels in the *HBX* 3′ end region may lead to severe alterations in the HBx C-terminal end. Variants with Dels in that region and HBxCtermTrunc have been typically linked to HCC carcinogenesis [11,12]. However, the NGS analysis of the HBV quasispecies identified variants with 103 different Indels through the *HBX* 3′ end region in almost all (94%) of the 50 patients without HCC included in our study, most of them with no significant liver fibrosis. Previous studies by clone sequencing [16,17] and NGS [34] including CHB patients without HCC support these results. Peng et al. [16], reported 42 different variants with Indels in the Cp quasispecies, virtually all of them affecting *HBX*, in all 12 untreated HBeAg-positive CHB patients included. Hao et al. [17] characterized the Indels along the full-length HBV genome of 30 HBeAg-positive untreated CHB patients, of which 33/125 (26.4%) Dels and 14/45 (31.1%) Ins were within the *HBX* 3′ end region encoding aa 75–154 which we analyzed in this study. Li et al. [34] used NGS to analyze genome-wide mutation profiles, including deletion patterns, in 17 patients with advanced liver disease and 30 chronic HBV carriers. Interestingly, despite the younger age and absence of severe liver disease in the chronic carrier group, 11/21 (52%) Del validated in that group were in *HBX* 3′ end, while none of the patients with the advanced liver disease showed Dels in this region. Notably, the cut-off to eliminate technical artifacts adopted in that study was 1% in quasispecies, while in our study, it was 0.1% (as long as the sequence was present in both forward and reverse strands), thanks to the adaptation of our previously-described bioinformatics algorithm [19,20]. Additionally, the average sequencing coverage was 2047× and 687× in advanced liver disease and chronic carrier patients, respectively, while in our study, we obtained a median of 16735 reads [IQR, 9277–24,668]. The lower cut-off to eliminate technical artifacts along with higher sequencing coverages may explain why we detected a higher variability of Indels in the *HBX* 3′ end, even taking into account only single Dels (46 of 103 Indels identified in our study vs. 21 Dels identified in the study by Li et al.). Moreover, cloning/sequencing analysis of samples from four patients with important percentages of variants with Indels by NGS confirmed the presence of some Indels identified by NGS in their quasispecies. Importantly, this analysis confirmed the existence of Ins and Del around and inside the five T homopolymer between positions 1821 and 1825 identified by NGS (ID: 74, 84, 85, and 89), a region where the UDPS technology may introduce deletion and insertion sequencing errors [35]. Cloning/sequencing even confirmed the complex combination of Ins and Dels ID: 12. Altogether, suggests that Indel variants are usually present in HBV quasispecies, even in CHB patients without HCC.

HBx (only 154 aa long) is characterized by an astonishing pleiotropic function, which mainly relies on its interactions with cellular proteins that take part in HBV replication, transactivation, signaling pathway, protein degradation, cell death, and cell cycle [9]. In this regard, HBx C-terminal end contains sequence motifs essential for its transactivating activity [10], (i.e., protein–protein interactions), which may be affected by Indels identified in this study. In fact, almost all Indels identified altered the WT *HBX* stop codon, giving rise to variants encoding 44 different HBxCtermTrunc or HBxLong, making it reasonable to speculate that at least some of those Indels may develop different functions to WT HBx. For instance, we identified Indel variants potentially encoding different HBx + core fusion proteins, which would include almost the entire HBx and pre-core/core aa sequences, ending at 7 putative *HBX* stop codons between codons 355 to 363. These stop codons were associated with 15 different single or combined Indels between nt positions 1805 and 1843, detected in half of the patients included in this study. The fusion protein encoded by variants with these Indels may be relevant for the HBV replicative cycle: HBx is essential for initiating and maintaining transcription from cccDNA templates in de novo infected cells [36], but it is not clear how the nascent cccDNA can acquire this protein if the HBx mRNA is not able to be transcribed from this episome. This apparent contradiction may be explained by the existence of HBx forms with fused core aa sequences, which suggests that the resulting protein may be a "traveler HBx" form which, hypothetically, would reach infected cells to supply them with HBx. In support of this hypothesis, HBx has been detected in the serum of hepatitis B patients using ELISA [37], and HBx reactive determinants have been described in liver-derived HBcAg particles from human HBV and other hepadnaviruses [38]. However, it is important to note that the relevance to HBV infection and pathogenesis of this theoretical "traveler HBx" form is yet to be confirmed experimentally.

Additionally, in support of this hypothesis, Kim et al. [39] described the in vitro expression of a 40 KDa protein resulting from the fusion of *HBX* + core ORFs, which showed transactivating activity. Interestingly, the expression of this protein revealed the Ins 1821T, within the five T region where it has been described as highly prevalent Indels among our patients, Ins 1825T (ID: 84, observed in 38% of our patients), and Del 1825T (ID: 85, observed in 20% of our patients). It is likely that this T homopolymeric region facilitates polymerase slipping as a possible event responsible for Indels in this position, which would explain the high prevalence of Indels in position 1825, which were also reported in CHB patients quasispecies by clone sequencing [16,17]. The Ins 1825T is very often associated with the putative codon 362, which was indeed very common among our patients (observed in 48%) and represented a relatively high percentage of their reads compared to other stop codons. Indels in this five T homopolymeric region shift ORF from *HBX* to the core and continue translation until the stop codon of this last ORF, the stop codon 362, which may be an alternative mechanism similar to the frameshifts produced by PRF signals. Interestingly, the polyT homopolymeric sequence is highly conserved among other hepadnaviruses, and its predicted RNA folding is similar to that of HIV-1 PRF. For this reason, we considered that this polyT region might also be a potential HBV PRF signal, which may act as a mechanism to produce HBx + core fusion proteins, in addition to Ins in that region.

Another group of Indels that may play a functional role in the HBV replication cycle are those located in the TA region. We identified 39 Indels located between nt 1751 and 1787, many of which affected TA2 and TA3 sequences of the BCP, which are required for the optimal transcription of pcRNA [6]. Although these data showed high variability in the TA region, TA4 was completely preserved, suggesting a more essential role for this TA than the remaining ones. Previous studies performed by population (Sanger) sequencing [40,41] described frequent Del affecting TA1 to TA3 sequences showing two patterns: around 8 to 10, and around 19–21 Del, very similar to patterns observed in this study, as shown in Table 4, thus further supporting our results. Most of the Indels identified in the TA region led to HBxCtermTrunc and, interestingly, approximately a third of them were associated with a premature *HBX* stop codon at position 135, which has been identified in 28% of the 50 patients included. This premature stop codon was principally (but not exclusively) associated with the Del8nt between positions 1757 and 1773, among which Del8nt 1763–1770 (ID: 51) stands out, identified in 20% of patients studied. Interestingly, ID: 51 caused the fusion of TA2 and TA3 sequences, creating a sequence motif that coincided with that of a true (canonical) TATA box [33], which we named TA23. The structural prediction of this putative new TA revealed a complete unpairing, similar to the other true or canonical TA box in the BCP, TA4, and it maintains the same distance as TA3 to the pcRNA start sites, while it is located around 40 nt upstream of the pgRNA starting point [6]. Although this distance is slightly larger than the optimal TATA box position for achieving high tissue specificity (31 and 30 nt upstream of the RNA transcription starting site), the liver tissue-specific expression of pgRNA from TA23 would still be feasible [42]. This potential role as a true TA would explain the 1.8-fold increase in Cp activity relative to WT observed by Peng et al. [16] with TA1 deleted + Del8nt 1763–1770. Moreover, despite its association with HBxCtermTrunc, none of the patients who showed this Del8nt in our study experienced negative clinical outcomes. In previous studies, the Del 1763–1770 was identified in the HBV quasispecies of patients who progressed to cirrhosis or end-stage liver disease and patients who did not [15]. Thus, ID:51 did not appear to be associated with severe liver disease per se.

In the TA region, our attention was also drawn to the 14 complex Indel combinations containing Dels between nt 1756 and 1787 (affecting TA2 and TA3 sequences) and large Ins (24–28 nt) at CURS. Several of those variants showed a duplication in the sequence containing the α box motif (nts 1646–1668) and binding sites for C/EBPα (BCP positive regulatory motifs located in the CURS) [6,32]. This duplication also caused a drastic change in the HBx Hbox sequence, which may affect its predicted α helix structure [27], which would, in turn, hamper or eliminate the essential HBx-DDB1 interaction. DDB1 is a linker protein for the assembly of a large number of proteins to Cullin 4 (CUL4)-based E3 ubiquitin ligase [43]. The interaction of HBx with DDB1-CUL4-ROC1 (CRL4) E3 ligase is critical for ubiquitination and degradation of structural maintenance chromosome complex proteins 5 and 6 (Smc5/6), which antagonize HBV replication [31]. It would thus be logical to think that HPL with these Indels would be negatively selected. In fact, we found them in only four (8%) of the fifty patients studied; however, in one of them (patient 2), HPL with those complex Indel combinations represented the master sequence (more than 50% of reads obtained showed Ins: 1647 TCTTACATAAGAGGACTCTTGGAC Del: 1627 + 1758 − 1777, ID: 12) and their presence in the quasispecies of that patient was confirmed by cloning and sequencing. In addition, variants with duplications in the α box were reported earlier using cloning and sequencing studies [14,16]. This suggests a mechanism of these variants to initiate and maintain a productive HBV infection, an alternative to overcoming the Smc5/6 inhibitory effects. A possible explanation may be that expression of HBV cccDNA may be favored by the duplication of the C/EBPα binding site. This de novo C/EBP target may increase transcriptional activity, compensating for the decrease in HBV replication by alterations of the HBx coding sequence, which potentially impair HBx-DDB1 interaction.

The vast majority of the 103 Indels identified in this study altered the *HBX* stop codon, yielding a total of 44 different stop codons, 23 (52.3%) of which caused HBxCtermTrunc, and 9 (39.1%) of them were identified in more than 10% of patients. The truncated HBx forms have been reported to lose their transcriptional activity and their inhibitory effects on cell proliferation and transformation, as well as to enhance metastasis compared to full-length HBx, thus playing a critical role in HCC carcinogenesis [12,44,45]. However, in our patient cohort, only five patients experienced negative clinical outcomes after a median follow-up of 9.4 (IQR, 8.7–12) years, and this outcome may be associated solely with CHB infection in only four cases. Notably, three of them showed HPL with Ins ID: 36,

37, and 38, associated with *HBX* stop codons at positions 128 and 129. Interestingly, these three patients showed higher percentages of reads and HPL with these stop codons than the median reads and HPL/patient. It thus seems possible that the proportions of Indel variants encoding HBxCtermTrunc at positions 128 and 129 in the HBV quasispecies, rather than their mere presence, may contribute to their pathological effects. However, it was not possible to further explore this hypothesis in our study, as too few of the patients included experienced negative outcomes to allow for reliable statistical comparisons with those who experienced benign outcomes. In addition, we were not able to assess percentages of variants with Indels in the quasispecies of those four patients in serum samples obtained closer in time to a diagnosis of cirrhosis or HCC, as these additional serum samples were not available to us.

So far, we have discussed some possible functional roles of some of the 103 Indels identified in 94% of 50 patients analyzed. In this cohort of patients, we found that variants showing Indels were usually present as minor ones (median, 3.4% [IQR, 1.3–8.4%] of reads in each sample), and their median percentages were significantly higher in HBeAg-positive patients than in HBeAg-negative patients. However, when assessing individual Indels, due to disparities in the number of HBeAg-positive vs. HBeAg-negative patients (17 vs. 33), we found no significant differences between those groups. In fact, it must be remembered that this study is essentially descriptive, and further studies with larger and more balanced groups of patients, as well as in vitro phenotypic analyses, are required to confirm the functional roles of the Indels identified. For instance, the association of Dels between nt 1805 and 1843, and Ins within or very close to the five poly-T region between nt 1821–1825, with putative stop codons between positions 355 to 363 should be confirmed with longer NGS reads, encompassing at least the entire 3′ *HBX* and pre-core/core ORFs. In this regard, it would be ideal to provide confirmation using a third-generation NGS platform, applying error-correction procedures [35]. It would also be interesting to determine whether variants with combinations of Dels in the TA region and big Ins at CURS, such as ID: 12, with a highly altered HBx sequence, are able to sustain HBV replication, and perform additional studies assessing the effects over HBV replication and Cp activity of the new TA23 sequence motif due to the prevalent Del8nt 1763–1770 (ID: 51). Nevertheless, it seems reasonable to hypothesize that Indel events may be used as a strategy for increasing the coding capacity of the *HBX* 3′ end. Multiple examples exist of smart mechanisms for synthesizing new proteins from single genomic sequences in RNA viruses, which allow them to maximize genomic information content with a limited genome size. For instance, in bovine viral diarrhea virus, a 27-nt Ins in the NS2 protein-coding region has been associated with the cytopathogenic form of this virus [46], and a 15-nt Del in NS gene of H5N1 subtype avian influenza virus was associated with increased virulence of this subtype in chickens and mice [47]. However, Indel events are not necessarily associated with increases in virulence, as in the case of the SARS-CoV-2 spike gene, where minor quasispecies variants with an accumulation of Dels upstream and very close to the S1/S2 cleavage site have been associated with mild COVID-19 [48]. Thus, viruses can use Indels as mechanisms to encode alternative proteins, with important functional roles in the natural history of their infections. In line with this, our results suggest that at least some of the Indels that we identified in the quasispecies of the *HBX* 3′ end, may be linked to functional roles in the HBV replicative cycle. This suggests a general *HBX* multicoding mechanism, which would enable the characteristic HBx pleiotropic function.

5. Conclusions

In summary, the common presence in HBV quasispecies of HPL, equivalent to variants, with Indels in the 3′ end of *HBX* in CHB patients with nonsevere liver disease, suggests that these variants are "normal members". Such Indels usually result in modification of the *HBX* stop codon, giving rise to truncated or long putative HBx versions with possible functional roles in the HBV replicative cycle. We also hypothesize that some of those HBx versions associated with Indels may be linked to severe progression in the case of high proportions. In addition, these Indels may also have consequences for transcription regulation of this virus due to sequence overlapping with regulatory elements such as Cp, ENH II, etc. Therefore, the phenotypical effects of these variants with Indels deserve further study. Altogether, this suggests that the production of 3′ *HBX* Indels is the origin of an HBx multicoding mechanism to increase the coding capacity for the small HBV genome and may be important for the extremely complex multifunctional activity of the HBx protein.

Supplementary Materials: The following supporting information can be downloaded at: https://www.mdpi.com/article/10.3390/biomedicines10051194/s1. Table S1. Biosample accession numbers of next-generation sequencing raw data. Table S2. Reference sequences of hepatitis B virus genotypes A, D/E and F used for alignining forward and reverse haplotypes of each sample, with abundances not below 0.1%. Table S3. Description of 103 different single insertions (Ins) or deletions (Del), or combinations of them that affected the HBx coding region, identified in the 50 patients studied. Table S4. Description of 39 different single insertions (Ins) or deletions (Del), or combinations of them that affected the region encompassing the four TATA-like boxes (TA) of the core promoter, between nucleotides 1751 and 1787.

Author Contributions: Conceptualization, F.R.-F., M.B. and T.P.; methodology, S.G.-G., A.C.-G., M.H., B.P.-R. and M.V.; software, J.G. and F.R.-A.; validation, D.T., M.F.C., J.Q. and M.R.-B.; formal analysis, D.T., M.F.C. and R.F.-C.; investigation, S.G.-G., A.C.-G., B.P.-R., M.V. and A.R.-S.; resources, F.R.-F. and M.B.; data curation, J.G. and F.R.-A.; writing—original draft preparation, S.G.-G., A.C.-G., D.T. and M.H.; writing—review and editing, M.F.C., J.Q., M.R.-B., A.R.-S. and F.R.-F.; visualization, D.T., M.F.C., J.G., R.F.-C. and T.P.; supervision, D.T. and F.R.-F.; project administration, D.T. and M.F.C.; funding acquisition, F.R.-F. All authors have read and agreed to the published version of the manuscript.

Funding: This research was funded by Instituto de Salud Carlos III and co-financed by the European Regional Development Fund (ERDF), grant number PI18/01436; PI19/00301; and by the Centro para el Desarrollo Tecnológico Industrial (CDTI) from the Spanish Ministry of Economy and Business, grant number IDI-20200297. The APC was funded by the grant PI18/01436.

Institutional Review Board Statement: The study was conducted according to the guidelines of the Declaration of Helsinki, and approved by the Ethics Committee of the Vall d'Hebron Research Institute (protocol code PR(AG)146/2020, approved on 4 March 2020).

Informed Consent Statement: Informed consent was obtained from all subjects involved in the study.

Data Availability Statement: The next-generation sequencing raw data presented in this study are openly available in NCBI's Sequence Read Archive (SRA), at BioProject reference number PRJNA625435. BioSample reference numbers are provided in Table S1.

Conflicts of Interest: The authors declare no conflict of interest. The funders had no role in the design of the study; in the collection, analyses, or interpretation of data; in the writing of the manuscript, or in the decision to publish the results.

References

1. World Health Organization. Hepatitis B. Available online: https://www.who.int/news-room/fact-sheets/detail/hepatitis-b (accessed on 3 March 2022).
2. Martinez, M.G.; Testoni, B.; Zoulim, F. Biological Basis for Functional Cure of Chronic Hepatitis B. *J. Viral Hepat.* **2019**, *26*, 786–794. [CrossRef]
3. Nassal, M. HBV CccDNA: Viral Persistence Reservoir and Key Obstacle for a Cure of Chronic Hepatitis B. *Gut* **2015**, *64*, 1972–1984. [CrossRef]
4. Tu, T.; Budzinska, M.A.; Shackel, N.A.; Urban, S. HBV DNA Integration: Molecular Mechanisms and Clinical Implications. *Viruses* **2017**, *9*, 75. [CrossRef]
5. Panjaworayan, N.; Roessner, S.K.; Firth, A.E.; Brown, C.M. HBVRegDB: Annotation, Comparison, Detection and Visualization of Regulatory Elements in Hepatitis B Virus Sequences. *Virol. J.* **2007**, *4*, 136. [CrossRef]
6. Quarleri, J. Core Promoter: A Critical Region Where the Hepatitis B Virus Makes Decisions. *World J. Gastroenterol.* **2014**, *20*, 425–435. [CrossRef]
7. Kramvis, A.; Kew, M.C. The Core Promoter of Hepatitis B Virus. *J. Viral Hepat.* **1999**, *6*, 415–427. [CrossRef]
8. Levrero, M.; Zucman-Rossi, J. Mechanisms of HBV-Induced Hepatocellular Carcinoma. *J. Hepatol.* **2016**, *64*, S84–S101. [CrossRef]

9. Xie, N.; Chen, X.; Zhang, T.; Liu, B.; Huang, C. Using Proteomics to Identify the HBx Interactome in Hepatitis B Virus: How Can This Inform the Clinic? *Expert Rev. Proteom.* **2014**, *11*, 59–74. [CrossRef]
10. Kumar, V.; Jayasuryan, N.; Kumar, R. A Truncated Mutant (Residues 58–140) of the Hepatitis B Virus X Protein Retains Transactivation Function. *Proc. Natl. Acad. Sci. USA* **1996**, *93*, 5647–5652. [CrossRef]
11. Zhang, A.Y.; Lai, C.L.; Poon, R.T.P.; Huang, F.Y.; Seto, W.K.; Fung, J.; Wong, D.K.H.; Yuen, M.F. Hepatitis B Virus Full-Length Genomic Mutations and Quasispecies in Hepatocellular Carcinoma. *J. Gastroenterol. Hepatol.* **2016**, *31*, 1638–1645. [CrossRef]
12. Ning-Fang, M.; Lau, S.H.; Hu, L.; Xie, D.; Wu, J.; Yang, J.; Wang, Y.; Wu, M.C.; Fung, J.; Bai, X.; et al. COOH-Terminal Truncated HBV X Protein Plays Key Role in Hepatocarcinogenesis. *Clin. Cancer Res.* **2008**, *14*, 5061–5068. [CrossRef]
13. Rodriguez-Frias, F.; Buti, M.; Tabernero, D.; Homs, M. Quasispecies Structure, Cornerstone of Hepatitis B Virus Infection: Mass Sequencing Approach. *World J. Gastroenterol.* **2013**, *19*, 6995–7023. [CrossRef]
14. Günther, S.; Piwon, N.; Iwanska, A.; Schilling, R.; Meisel, H.; Will, H. Type, Prevalence, and Significance of Core Promoter/Enhancer II Mutations in Hepatitis B Viruses from Immunosuppressed Patients with Severe Liver Disease. *J. Virol.* **1996**, *70*, 8318–8331. [CrossRef] [PubMed]
15. Preikschat, P.; Günther, S.; Reinhold, S.; Will, H.; Budde, K.; Neumayer, H.H.; Krüger, D.H.; Meisel, H. Complex HBV Populations with Mutations in Core Promoter, C Gene, and Pre-S Region Are Associated with Development of Cirrhosis in Long-Term Renal Transplant Recipients. *Hepatology* **2002**, *35*, 466–477. [CrossRef]
16. Peng, Y.; Liu, B.; Hou, J.; Sun, J.; Hao, R.; Xiang, K.; Yan, L.; Zhang, J.; Zhuang, H.; Li, T. Naturally Occurring Deletions/Insertions in HBV Core Promoter Tend to Decrease in Hepatitis B e Antigen-Positive Chronic Hepatitis B Patients during Antiviral Therapy. *Antivir. Ther.* **2015**, *20*, 623–632. [CrossRef]
17. Hao, R.; Xiang, K.; Peng, Y.; Hou, J.; Sun, J.; Li, Y.; Su, M.; Yan, L.; Zhuang, H.; Li, T. Naturally Occurring Deletion/Insertion Mutations within HBV Whole Genome Sequences in HBeAg-Positive Chronic Hepatitis B Patients Are Correlated with Baseline Serum HBsAg and HBeAg Levels and Might Predict a Shorter Interval to HBeAg Loss and Seroconversi. *Infect. Genet. Evol.* **2015**, *33*, 261–268. [CrossRef]
18. Caballero, A.; Gregori, J.; Homs, M.; Tabernero, D.; Gonzalez, C.; Quer, J.; Blasi, M.; Casillas, R.; Nieto, L.; Riveiro-Barciela, M.; et al. Complex Genotype Mixtures Analyzed by Deep Sequencing in Two Different Regions of Hepatitis B Virus. *PLoS ONE* **2015**, *10*, e0144816. [CrossRef]
19. Ramírez, C.; Gregori, J.; Buti, M.; Tabernero, D.; Camós, S.; Casillas, R.; Quer, J.; Esteban, R.; Homs, M.; Rodríguez-Frías, F.; et al. A Comparative Study of Ultra-Deep Pyrosequencing and Cloning to Quantitatively Analyze the Viral Quasispecies Using Hepatitis B Virus Infection as a Model. *Antivir. Res.* **2013**, *98*, 273–283. [CrossRef]
20. Gregori, J.; Esteban, J.I.; Cubero, M.; Garcia-Cehic, D.; Perales, C.; Casillas, R.; Alvarez-Tejado, M.; Rodríguez-Frías, F.; Guardia, J.; Domingo, E.; et al. Ultra-Deep Pyrosequencing (UDPS) Data Treatment to Study Amplicon HCV Minor Variants. *PLoS ONE* **2013**, *8*, e83361. [CrossRef]
21. Edgar, R.C.; Drive, R.M.; Valley, M. MUSCLE: Multiple Sequence Alignment with High Accuracy and High Throughput. *Nucleic Acids Res.* **2004**, *32*, 1792–1797. [CrossRef]
22. R Core Team. *R: A Language and Environment for Statistical Computing*; R Foundation for Statistical Computing. Vienna, Austria, 2013. Available online: https://www.yumpu.com/en/document/view/6853895/r-a-language-and-environment-for-statistical-computing (accessed on 18 May 2022).
23. Pages, H.; Aboyoun, P.; Gentleman, R.; DebRoy, S. *Biostrings: String Objects Representing Biological Sequences, and Matching Algorithms*; R Package Version. 2.31.14; Fred Hutchinson Cancer Research Center: Seattle, WA, USA, 2011.
24. Paradis, E.; Claude, J.; Strimmer, K. APE: Analyses of Phylogenetics and Evolution in R Language. *Bioinformatics* **2004**, *20*, 289–290. [CrossRef] [PubMed]
25. Gruber, A.R.; Lorenz, R.; Bernhart, S.H.; Neuböck, R.; Hofacker, I.L. The Vienna RNA Websuite. *Nucleic Acids Res.* **2008**, *36*, 70–74. [CrossRef] [PubMed]
26. R Core Team. *A Language and Environment for Statistical Computing*; R Foundation for Statistical Computing. Vienna, Austria, 2021. Available online: https://cran.asia/web/packages/dplR/vignettes/chron-dplR.pdf (accessed on 18 May 2022).
27. Li, T.; Robert, E.I.; van Breugel, P.C.; Strubin, M.; Zheng, N. A Promiscuous Alpha-Helical Motif Anchors Viral Hijackers and Substrate Receptors to the CUL4-DDB1 Ubiquitin Ligase Machinery. *Nat. Struct. Mol. Biol.* **2010**, *17*, 105–111. [CrossRef] [PubMed]
28. Firth, A.E.; Brierley, I. Non-Canonical Translation in RNA Viruses. *J. Gen. Virol.* **2012**, *93*, 1385–1409. [CrossRef] [PubMed]
29. Mouzakis, K.D.; Lang, A.L.; Vander Meulen, K.A.; Easterday, P.D.; Butcher, S.E. HIV-1 Frameshift Efficiency Is Primarily Determined by the Stability of Base Pairs Positioned at the MRNA Entrance Channel of the Ribosome. *Nucleic Acids Res.* **2013**, *41*, 1901–1913. [CrossRef] [PubMed]
30. Belew, A.T.; Meskauskas, A.; Musalgaonkar, S.; Adnavi, V.M.; Sulima, S.O.; Kasprzak, W.K.; Shapiro, B.A.; Dinman, J. Ribosomal Frameshifting in the CCR5 MRNA Is Regulated by MiRNAs and the NMD Pathway. *Nature* **2014**, *512*, 265–269. [CrossRef] [PubMed]
31. Murphy, C.M.; Xu, Y.; Li, F.; Nio, K.; Reszka-Blanco, N.; Li, X.; Wu, Y.; Yu, Y.; Xiong, Y.; Su, L. Hepatitis B Virus X Protein Promotes Degradation of SMC5/6 to Enhance HBV Replication. *Cell Rep.* **2016**, *16*, 2846–2854. [CrossRef]
32. Choi, B.H.; Park, G.T.; Rho, H.M. Interaction of Hepatitis B Viral X Protein and CCAAT/ Enhancer-Binding Protein Alpha Synergistically Activates the Hepatitis B Viral Enhancer II/Pregenomic Promoter. *J. Biol. Chem.* **1999**, *274*, 2858–2865. [CrossRef]

33. Lee, T.Y.; Chang, W.C.; Hsu, J.B.K.; Chang, T.H.; Shien, D.M. GPMiner: An Integrated System for Mining Combinatorial Cis-Regulatory Elements in Mammalian Gene Group. *Ser. Adv. Bioinform. Comput. Biol.* **2012**, *13*, S3. [CrossRef]
34. Li, F.; Zhang, D.; Li, Y.; Jiang, D.; Luo, S.; Du, N.; Chen, W.; Deng, L.; Zeng, C. Whole Genome Characterization of Hepatitis B Virus Quasispecies with Massively Parallel Pyrosequencing. *Clin. Microbiol. Infect.* **2015**, *21*, 280–287. [CrossRef]
35. Garcia-Garcia, S.; Cortese, M.F.; Rodríguez-Algarra, F.; Tabernero, D.; Rando-Segura, A.; Quer, J.; Buti, M.; Rodríguez-Frías, F. Next-Generation Sequencing for the Diagnosis of Hepatitis B: Current Status and Future Prospects. *Expert Rev. Mol. Diagn.* **2021**, *21*, 381–396. [CrossRef] [PubMed]
36. Lucifora, J.; Arzberger, S.; Durantel, D.; Belloni, L.; Strubin, M.; Levrero, M.; Zoulim, F.; Hantz, O.; Protzer, U. Hepatitis B Virus X Protein Is Essential to Initiate and Maintain Virus Replication after Infection. *J. Hepatol.* **2011**, *55*, 996–1003. [CrossRef] [PubMed]
37. Pál, J.; Nyárády, Z.; Marczinovits, I.; Pár, A.; Ali, Y.S.; Berencsi, G.; Kvell, K.; Németh, P. Comprehensive Regression Analysis of Hepatitis B Virus X Antigen Level and Anti-HBx Antibody Titer in the Sera of Patients with HBV Infection. *Pathol. Oncol. Res.* **2006**, *12*, 34–40. [CrossRef] [PubMed]
38. Feitelson, M.A. Products of the "X" Gene in Hepatitis B and Related Viruses. *Hepatology* **1986**, *6*, 191–198. [CrossRef]
39. Kim, S.K.; Jang, S.K.; Rho, H.M. Effect of Frameshift Mutation in the Pre-C Region of Hepatitis B Virus on the X and C Genes. *J. Gen. Virol.* **1994**, *75*, 917–923. [CrossRef]
40. Deng, H.; Dong, J.; Cheng, J.; Huangfu, K.J.; Shi, S.S.; Hong, Y.; Ren, X.M.; Li, L. Quasispecies Groups in the Core Promoter Region of Hepatitis B Virus. *Hepatobiliary Pancreat. Dis. Int.* **2002**, *1*, 392–396.
41. Zhang, D.; Dong, P.; Zhang, K.; Deng, L.; Bach, C.; Chen, W.; Li, F.; Protzer, U.; Ding, H.; Zeng, C. Whole Genome HBV Deletion Profiles and the Accumulation of PreS Deletion Mutant during Antiviral Treatment. *BMC Microbiol.* **2012**, *12*, 307. [CrossRef]
42. Ponjavic, J.; Lenhard, B.; Kai, C.; Kawai, J.; Carninci, P.; Hayashizaki, Y.; Sandelin, A. Transcriptional and Structural Impact of TATA-Initiation Site Spacing in Mammalian Core Promoters. *Genome Biol.* **2006**, *7*, R78. [CrossRef]
43. Angers, S.; Li, T.; Yi, X.; MacCoss, M.J.; Moon, R.T.; Zheng, N. Molecular Architecture and Assembly of the DDB1-CUL4A Ubiquitin Ligase Machinery. *Nature* **2006**, *443*, 590–593. [CrossRef]
44. Li, W.; Li, M.; Liao, D.; Lu, X.; Gu, X.; Zhang, Q. Carboxyl-Terminal Truncated HBx Contributes to Invasion and Metastasis via Deregulating Metastasis Suppressors in Hepatocellular Carcinoma. *Oncotarget* **2016**, *7*, 55110–55127. [CrossRef]
45. Tu, H.; Bonura, C.; Giannini, C.; Mouly, H.; Soussan, P.; Kew, M.; Paterlini-Bréchot, P.; Bréchot, C.; Kremsdorf, D. Biological Impact of Natural COOH-Terminal Deletions of Hepatitis B Virus X Protein in Hepatocellular Carcinoma Tissues. *Cancer Res.* **2001**, *61*, 7803–7810. [PubMed]
46. Tautz, N.; Meyers, G.; Stark, R.; Dubovi, E.J.; Thiel, H.J. Cytopathogenicity of a Pestivirus Correlates with a 27-Nucleotide Insertion. *J. Virol.* **1996**, *70*, 7851–7858. [CrossRef] [PubMed]
47. Long, J.X.; Peng, D.X.; Liu, Y.L.; Wu, Y.T.; Liu, X.F. Virulence of H5N1 Avian Influenza Virus Enhanced by a 15-Nucleotide Deletion in the Viral Nonstructural Gene. *Virus Genes* **2008**, *36*, 471–478. [CrossRef] [PubMed]
48. Andres, C.; Garcia-Cehic, D.; Gregori, J.; Piñana, M.; Rodriguez-Frias, F.; Guerrero-Murillo, M.; Esperalba, J.; Rando, A.; Goterris, L.; Codina, M.G.; et al. Naturally Occurring SARS-CoV-2 Gene Deletions Close to the Spike S1/S2 Cleavage Site in the Viral Quasispecies of COVID19 Patients. *Emerg. Microbes Infect.* **2020**, *9*, 1900–1911. [CrossRef] [PubMed]

biomedicines

MDPI

Article

Baseline Circulating miR-125b Levels Predict a High FIB-4 Index Score in Chronic Hepatitis B Patients after Nucleos(t)ide Analog Treatment

Jyun-Yi Wu [1,†], Yi-Shan Tsai [1,†], Chia-Chen Li [1], Ming-Lun Yeh [1,2], Ching-I Huang [1,2], Chung-Feng Huang [1,2,3], Jia-Ning Hsu [1], Meng-Hsuan Hsieh [1,2,3,4], Yo-Chia Chen [5], Ta-Wei Liu [1], Yi-Hung Lin [1], Po-Cheng Liang [1], Zu-Yau Lin [1,2], Wan-Long Chuang [1,2], Ming-Lung Yu [1,2,6] and Chia-Yen Dai [1,2,3,4,7,8,*]

1 Hepatobiliary Division, Department of Internal Medicine and Hepatitis Center, Kaohsiung Medical University Hospital, Kaohsiung Medical University, Kaohsiung 807, Taiwan
2 Faculty of Internal Medicine and Graduate Institute of Clinical Medicine, College of Medicine, Kaohsiung Medical University, Kaohsiung 807, Taiwan
3 Department of Occupational Medicine, Kaohsiung Medical University Hospital, Kaohsiung Medical University, Kaohsiung 807, Taiwan
4 Health Management Center, Kaohsiung Medical University Hospital, Kaohsiung Medical University, Kaohsiung 807, Taiwan
5 Department of Biological Science and Technology, National Pingtung University of Science and Technology, Pingtung 912, Taiwan
6 School of Medicine, College of Medicine and Center of Excellence for Metabolic Associated Fatty Liver Disease, National Sun Yat-Sen University, Kaohsiung 804, Taiwan
7 College of Professional Studies, National Pingtung University of Science and Technology, Pingtung 912, Taiwan
8 Drug Development and Value Creation Research Center, Kaohsiung Medical University, Kaohsiung 807, Taiwan
* Correspondence: daichiayen@gmail.com
† These authors contributed equally to this work.

Citation: Wu, J.-Y.; Tsai, Y.-S.; Li, C.-C.; Yeh, M.-L.; Huang, C.-I.; Huang, C.-F.; Hsu, J.-N.; Hsieh, M.-H.; Chen, Y.-C.; Liu, T.-W.; et al. Baseline Circulating miR-125b Levels Predict a High FIB-4 Index Score in Chronic Hepatitis B Patients after Nucleos(t)ide Analog Treatment. *Biomedicines* **2022**, *10*, 2824. https://doi.org/10.3390/biomedicines10112824

Academic Editor: Giovanni Squadrito

Received: 29 September 2022
Accepted: 3 November 2022
Published: 5 November 2022

Abstract: The regulatory role of microRNAs (miRNAs) in HBV-associated HCC pathogenesis has been reported previously. This study aimed to investigate the association between serum miR-125b and liver fibrosis progression in chronic hepatitis B (CHB) patients after nucleos(t)ide analog (NA) treatment. Baseline serum miR-125b levels and other relevant laboratory data were measured for 124 patients who underwent 12-month NA therapy. Post-12-month NA therapy, serum miR-125, platelet, AST, and ALT levels were measured again for post-treatment FIB-4 index calculation. Univariate and multivariate logistic regression analyses were performed to identify independent risk factors for a higher post-treatment FIB-4 index. Results showed that baseline miR-125b levels were inversely correlated with the post-treatment FIB-4 index ($\rho = -0.2130$, $p = 0.0082$). In logistic regression analyses, age (OR = 1.17, $p < 0.0001$), baseline platelet level (OR = 0.98, $p = 0.0032$), and ALT level (OR = 1.00, $p = 0.0241$) were independent predictors of FIB-index > 2.9 post-12-month treatment. The baseline miR-125b level was not significantly associated with a higher post-treatment FIB-4 index ($p = 0.8992$). In 59 patients receiving entecavir (ETV) monotherapy, the alternation of serum miR-125b in 12 months and age were substantially associated with a higher post-treatment FIB-4 index (>2.9), suggesting that miR-125b is a reliable biomarker for detecting early liver fibrosis under specific anti-HBV NA treatments (e.g., ETV).

Keywords: chronic hepatitis B; nucleos(t)ide analogs; miR-125b; hepatitis B virus; biomarker; fibrosis score

1. Introduction

The prevalence of chronic hepatitis B infection is 4.1%, corresponding to 316 million infected people [1]. It remains an incurable viral disease that can only be controlled by certain medications prescribed in different combinations [2]. There is a significant correlation between hepatitis B viral infection, liver cirrhosis, and hepatocellular carcinoma (HCC). Moreover, hepatitis B virus (HBV) infection and liver fibrosis predispose patients to develop hepatocellular carcinoma (HCC) [3,4]. HCC accounts for 85–90% of all primary liver cancers and is the third most common cause of cancer-related deaths; the five-year survival rate for HCC is 6.9%. The high mortality and poor survival associated with HCC have prompted research on the progression of HBV infection and liver cirrhosis. Liver cirrhosis is characterized by liver tissue fibrosis, which results in the formation of abnormal nodules [5]. As a common consequence of chronic hepatitis B (CHB), it promotes the development of HCC through several possible mechanisms. Molecular mechanisms have been discussed, including identifying HCC driver genes, the p53-RB pathway, and the WNT pathway [6]. Moreover, the long period of hepatic inflammation, as one of the immune responses during chronic HBV infection, increases the hepatocyte turnover rate and gene mutation, which facilitates progression to liver fibrosis, liver cirrhosis, and HCC [3]. Therefore, controlling HBV infection and the early prediction of subsequent possible liver fibrosis are crucial strategies to prevent high-mortality HCC.

Circulating miR-125b levels can inhibit HBV expression in vitro [7] and have long been investigated as an innovative treatment and noninvasive biomarker for CHB, liver fibrosis, and HCC [8,9]. Several studies have illustrated a correlation between miR-125b expression and CHB and its role as a tumor suppressor in several cancers [10–12]. Few studies have focused on the role of miR-125b in hepatic inflammation [13]. Zhou et al. demonstrated its ability as a reliable biomarker to predict the virologic response to nucleos(t)ide analog (NA) treatment, which has become the standard of care for patients with CHB [14]. For HCC, studies have described the regulatory role of miRNAs in HBV-associated HCC pathogenesis [8,15]. The ability of miR-125b to act as a novel biomarker for HBV-positive HCC has been demonstrated [16]. Nonetheless, relatively fewer studies have focused on the relationship between miR-125b and liver fibrosis, especially after anti-HBV nucleos(t)ide analog (NA) treatment.

Previous studies have shown that miR-125b can promote hepatic stellate cell activation and liver fibrosis by activating RhoA signaling, and antagonizing miR-125b can significantly alleviate liver fibrosis in CCl4-treated mice [17]. However, there is no corresponding clinical research on the correlation between circulating miR-125b levels and the development of liver fibrosis, especially with anti-HBV NA therapy. The only study that discussed the miR-125b level post-NA therapy mainly focused on HBV/HCV-coinfected patients, rather than HBV infection alone, and there was no evaluation of the correlation between the post-treatment miR-125b level and liver fibrosis [18]. Hence, to further clarify the clinical correlation between circulating miR-125b and the formation of liver fibrosis in post-NA therapy CHB patients, we designed this study to investigate whether baseline and post-treatment serum miR-125b levels can be a reliable predictor of new-onset liver fibrosis after 12-month CHB NA treatment.

2. Material and Methods

2.1. Study Design

We conducted a retrospective cohort study based on circulating miR125-b levels and serum markers among patients diagnosed with liver fibrosis from stage F0 to F4 after a 12-month NA treatment and patients without a new diagnosis of liver fibrosis after a 12-month NA treatment. The diagnosis and staging of liver fibrosis were made based on the METAVIR score [19], which was applied based on the liver biopsy results, FIB-4 index calculation [20,21], and a FibroScan® (Echosens, Paris, France). We also found an association between serum miR-125b levels and the clinical characteristics of CHB patients, identifying its predictive ability for liver fibrogenesis after NA treatment.

2.2. Patients

Patients were recruited from 2004 to 2020 from the medical center of Kaohsiung Medical University Hospital. A total of 127 HBeAg-negative patients underwent NA therapy for HBV infection, according to the Asian-Pacific Association for the Study of the Liver recommendations [22]. The exclusion criteria included patients with other hepatobiliary diseases (e.g., hepatitis C virus (HCV) infection), autoimmune hepatitis, other etiologies of cirrhosis (e.g., primary biliary cirrhosis), primary sclerosing cholangitis, Wilson disease, and α1-antitrypsin deficiency. Three patients were lost to follow-up. Ultimately, 124 patients were included in the analysis. Among the 124 patients, 59 of them received entecavir (ETV) monotherapy, 53 patients received lamivudine (LAM) therapy, and the remaining 12 patients received adefovir, telbivudine (LDT), or tenofovir (TDF) monotherapy or combined therapy. Signed informed consent was obtained from these patients for all interviews, anthropomorphic measurements, blood sampling, and medical record review. This study was approved by the ethics committee of Kaohsiung Medical University Hospital (KMUHIRB-E(II)-20190405).

2.3. Laboratory Data

Serum markers, such as aspartate aminotransferase (AST) (Roche Cobas GOT/AST IFCC, Via Casa Sicignano, Sant'Antonio Abate, Italy), alanine transaminase (ALT) (Roche Cobas GPT/ALT IFCC, Via Casa Sicignano, Sant'Antonio Abate, Italy), international normalized ratio (INR), blood urea nitrogen, creatinine, bilirubin, platelets, and albumin, were measured by standard biochemistry tests. HBsAg, HBeAg, and anti-HBe were examined using an enzyme immunoassay (EIA; Abbott Laboratories, North Chicago, IL, USA), and a quantitative HBV DNA analysis was performed using the Roche Cobas Apliprep/Cobas Taqman HBV Test (Roche Molecular System, Roche, Branchburg, NJ, USA).

2.4. Extraction of MicroRNAs

The miRNAs were extracted from 200 μL of serum using TRIzol LS (Thermo Scientific, Waltham, MA, USA). The detection of miRNAs was performed by RT-qPCR using TaqMan® MicroRNA assays and measured using a 7900® Sequence Detection System (Applied Biosystems, Lincoln Centre Drive, Foster City, CA, USA). The expression levels of miRNAs in each sample were normalized to the corresponding spike-in cel-39 level [23].

2.5. Questionnaire Interview for Patient Profiles

All participants were personally interviewed using structured questionnaires to collect information on demographic characteristics, including alcohol consumption and personal histories of diseases such as previous diagnoses of diabetes, hypertension, heart disease, liver disease, and cardiovascular disease.

2.6. Statistical Analysis

We analyzed basic demographic data, including case number, sex, age, body mass index, and the presence of hypertension, diabetes, and metabolic syndrome. Student's *t*-test, the Mann–Whitney U test, chi-squared test, and Fisher's exact test were used for statistical tests. All tests were two-sided, and a probability value (p value) < 0.05 was considered statistically significant. A 95% confidence interval (CI) for these covariates was calculated. Linear regression analysis was adopted to assess the correlation between variables, as determined by Spearman's rank correlation coefficient (ρ). Multivariate logistic regression analysis was used to evaluate the odds ratio (OR).

3. Results

3.1. Characteristics of Patients and Changes in the Parameters

Table 1 summarizes the characteristics of the entire cohort, as well as of the two subgroups divided by the baseline FIB-4 index of 2.9, which has been reported to be the cut-off for advanced fibrosis in patients with CHB [24]. Compared with patients who had a FIB-4 index less than 2.9, those who had a FIB-4 index more than 2.9 were older (53.72 ± 9.76 vs. 43.59 ± 11.26 years, $p < 0.0001$), more likely to have hypertension (28.6% vs. 16.2%, $p = 0.0226$), had higher AST levels (377.9 ± 405.6 vs. 111.7 ± 137.9 U/I, $p < 0.0001$), higher ALT levels (509.1 ± 541.8 vs. 215.2 ± 272.5 U/I, $p < 0.0001$), a lower WBC count (4961.3 ± 1552.9 vs. 6072.5 ± 1753.2 × $10^3/mm^3$, $p = 0.0004$), a lower platelet count (125.7 ± 41.2 vs. 204.9 ± 70.3 × $10^3/mm^3$, $p < 0.0001$), a higher bilirubin level (2.69 ± 3.37 vs. 1.37 ± 1.48 mg/dL, $p = 0.0045$), and a lower albumin level (3.72 ± 0.54 vs. 4.26 ± 0.36 gm/dL, $p < 0.0001$). After a follow-up period of 12 months after initial treatment, the alterations in the FIB-4 index and miRNA125b levels are shown in Figure 1. Compared to the baseline FIB-4 index, the FIB-4 index attained after the 12-month treatment demonstrated a significant reduction ($p < 0.0001$). Such a significant difference was not observed regarding mi125b between the baseline and post-treatment levels. The baseline miRNA-125b level and post-treatment FIB-4 indices were significantly and inversely correlated (ρ = −0.2130, $p = 0.0082$) (Figure 2A). However, the alteration in miRNA-125b level during the 12 months was not correlated with the post-treatment FIB-4 index (ρ = −0.1041, $p = 0.2719$) (Figure 2B). Between subgroups divided by a post-treatment FIB-4 index of 2.9, neither baseline miRNA-125b ($p = 0.2322$) nor alteration of miRNA-125b ($p = 0.2498$) showed significant differences (Figure 3).

Table 1. Patient's characteristics.

Variable	Overall	FIB-4 Score ≤ 2.9	FIB-4 Score > 2.9 (*n* = 54)	*p* Value
	(*n* = 124)	(*n* = 70)		
Mean age (years)	47.95 (11.75)	43.49 (11.26)	53.72 (9.76)	<0.0001 *
Gender				0.3810
Male	95	52	43	
Female	29	18	11	
BMI (kg/m^2)	23.99 (3.59)	24.10 (3.37)	23.88 (3.87)	0.7620
BH (cm)	166.59 (8.02)	168.23 (7.60)	164.52 (8.13)	0.0060 *
BW (kg)	66.75 (12.20)	68.25 (11.22)	64.92 (13.18)	0.0746
HBV DNA > 2000 IU/mL (%)	76.61	70.00	85.19	0.0476 *
HBeAg(+)	30.89 (38/123)	31.88 (22/69)	29.63 (17/54)	0.7883
Lab data (mean, SD)				
WBCs ($\times 10^3/mm^3$)	5585.79 (1751.43)	6072.50 (1753.19)	4961.32 (1552.85)	0.0004 *
Platelet ($\times 10^3/mm^3$)	170.43 (71.12)	204.93 (70.29)	125.70 (41.18)	<0.0001 *
AST (U/L)	227.64 (314.82)	111.69 (137.87)	377.94 (405.57)	<0.0001 *
ALT (U/L)	343.16 (435.35)	215.17 (272.48)	509.07 (541.77)	0.0001 *
Creatinine (mg/dL)	0.89 (0.48)	0.86 (0.24)	0.92 (0.66)	0.5363
Bilirubin (mg/dL)	2.00 (2.57)	1.37 (1.48)	2.69 (3.37)	0.0045 *
Albumin (gm/dL)	4.02 (0.53)	4.26 (0.36)	3.72 (0.54)	<0.0001 *
HB (g/dL)	13.95 (1.56)	14.20 (1.60)	13.64 (1.46)	0.0512
Log $2^{-\text{delta miRNA 125b}}$	−1.21 (0.85)	−1.20 (0.84)	−1.22 (0.88)	0.8992
Ct values of cel-39 (internal control; mean ± SD)	27.35 (1.65)	27.34 (1.74)	27.36 (1.55)	0.9673
Comorbidities	(*n* = 98)	(*n* = 56)	(*n* = 42)	
Diabetes mellitus (%)	10.20	8.93	11.90	0.6300
Hypertension (%)	17.34	8.93	28.57	0.0110 *
	(*n* = 122)	(*n* = 68)	(*n* = 54)	
Alcohol use (%)	16.40	16.18	16.67	0.9421

BMI, body mass index; BH, body height; BW, body weight; WBC, white blood cell count; PLT, platelet count; AST, aspartate aminotransferase; ALT, alanine aminotransferase; Cr, creatinine; HB, hemoglobin level; delta miRNA 125b represents $Ct_{miR-125b}$-Ct_{cel-39}. All values are expressed as the mean (standard deviation (SD)). The p value was calculated for the continuous variables using Student's t-test or the Mann–Whitney test, and the $\chi 2$ test was used for the categorical variables, with $\alpha = 0.05$. * = $p < 0.05$.

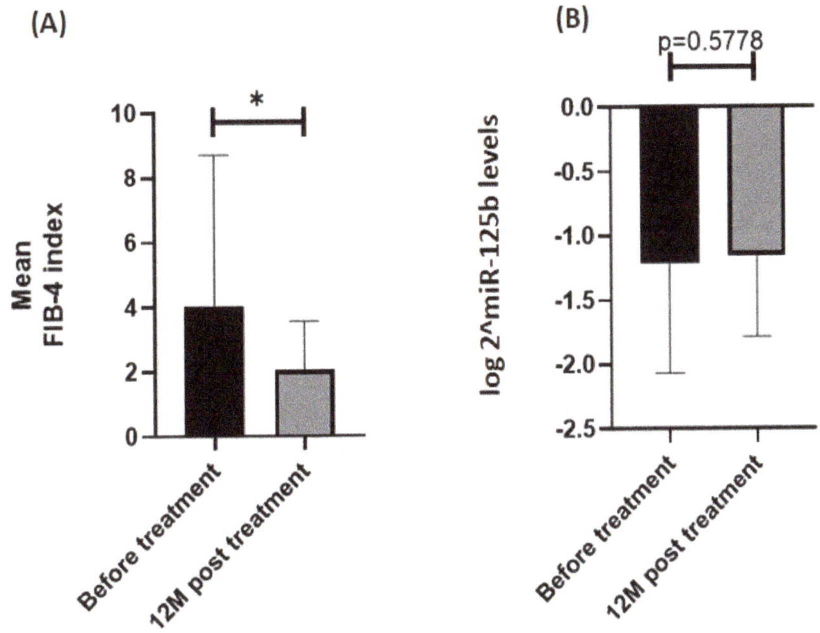

Figure 1. Comparing the differences in the (**A**) mean FIB−4 index and (**B**) log 2^miR−125b levels at the baseline and post−treatment. Error bars show mean ± standard deviation. *p* value from the Mann–Whitney test is shown. * = $p < 0.05$.

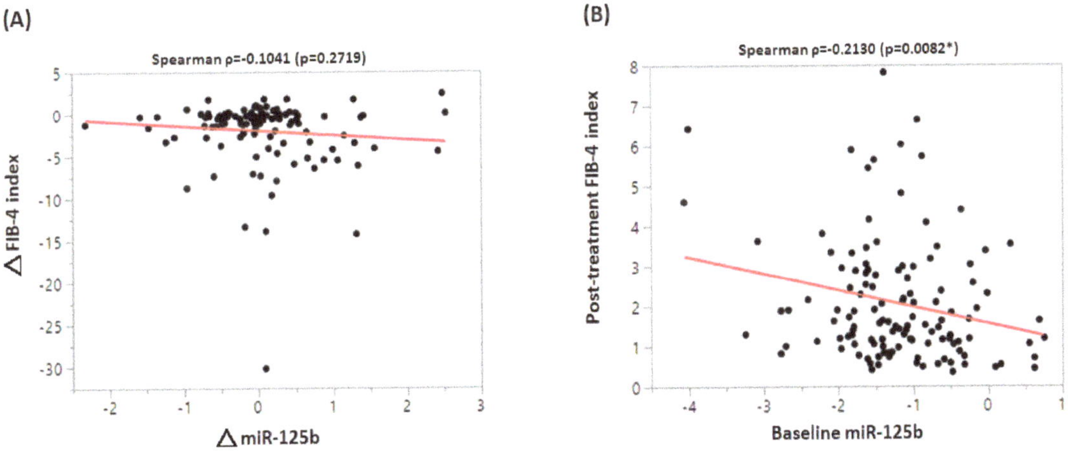

Figure 2. Linear regression analysis was used to assess the correlation between (**A**) the change in miRNA−125b and the change in the FIB−4 index, and (**B**) the baseline miRNA−125b (serum miRNA−125b, i.e., log 2^baseline miR−125b) and post-treatment FIB−4 index. △FIB−4 index, 12-month FIB−4 index; △miRNA−125b, log $2^{-\text{delta post-miR-125b}}$ − log $2^{-\text{delta pre-miR-125b}}$. * = $p < 0.05$.

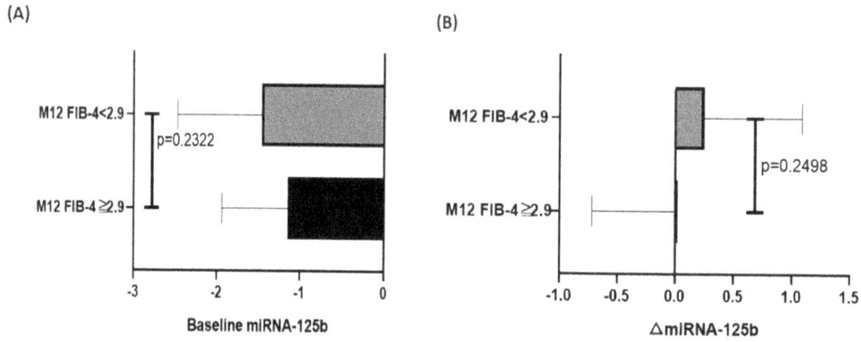

Figure 3. Comparing two subgroups divided by a post-treatment FIB−4 index of 2.9, showing the differences in the (**A**) baseline miRNA−125b (log 2^baseline miR−125b) and (**B**) △miRNA−125b (log $2^{-\text{delta post-miR-125b}}$ − log $2^{-\text{delta pre-miR-125b}}$). Error bars show mean ± standard deviation. *p* value from the Mann–Whitney test is shown.

3.2. Baseline and Clinical Parameters Associated with FIB-4 Index after NA Treatment

Table 2 illustrates the results of the univariate logistic regression FIB-4 index analysis. Neither baseline miRNA-125b nor alteration of miRNA-125b during the 12-month treatment period was associated with the risk of the post-treatment FIB-4 index being higher than 2.9. With regard to initial laboratory findings, a higher WBC count (p = 0.0156), lower platelet count (< 0.0001), and higher ALT level (p = 0.0496) were significantly associated with the risk of a FIB-4 index > 2.9 after 12-month anti-HBV medication treatment. Older age (p < 0.0001) was also associated with an increased risk of a FIB-4 index of more than 2.9. Such a significant association was not found for the other variables. Multivariate logistic regression analyses showed that older age (p < 0.0001), lower platelet count (p = 0.0032), and higher ALT level (p = 0.0241), but not lower WBC count, remained significant predictors of a FIB-4 index > 2.9.

Table 2. Predictor of 12M FIB-4 index analysis.

	Univariate Analyses		Multivariate Analyses	
Variable	**OR (95%CI)**	***p* Value**	**OR (95%CI)**	***p* Value**
Age	1.17 (1.09–1.25)	<0.0001 *	1.17 (1.09–1.26)	<0.0001 *
Gender (male/female)	0.89 (0.33–2.37)	0.8188		
HBV DNA > 2000 IU/mL	2.11 (0.67–6.69)	0.2034		
HBeAg(+)	0.41 (0.14–1.17)	0.0963		
Lab data				
WBCs	1.00 (1.00–1.00)	0.0156 *	1.00 (1.00–1.00)	0.1562
Platelet	0.98 (0.97–0.99)	<0.0001 *	0.98 (0.96–0.99)	0.0032 *
AST	1.00 (1.00–1.00)	0.7116		
ALT	1.00 (1.00–1.00)	0.0496 *	1.00 (1.00–1.00)	0.0241 *
Creatinine	0.87 (0.31–2.45)	0.7900		
Bilirubin	1.08 (0.93–1.25)	0.3138		
Albumin (gm/dL)	0.51 (0.23–1.15)	0.1058		
HB (g/dL)	0.77 (0.58–1.01)	0.0601		
Log $2^{-\text{delta pre-miR-125b}}$	0.65 (0.40–1.08)	0.0938		
Δ Log $2^{-\text{delta miRNA 125b}}$	0.65 (0.37–1.13)	0.1270		
Comorbidities				
Diabetes mellitus	1.37 (0.32–5.76)	0.6699		
Hypertension	1.91 (0.62–5.88)	0.2596		
Alcohol use	0.86 (0.80–0.26)	0.8019		

BMI, body mass index; BH, body height; BW, body weight; WBC, white blood cell count; PLT, platelet count; AST, aspartate aminotransferase; ALT, alanine aminotransferase; Cr, creatinine; HB, hemoglobin level; delta miRNA 125b represents Ct $_{\text{miR-125b}}$-Ct $_{\text{cel-39}}$; Δlog $2^{-\text{delta miR-125b}}$ = Log $2^{-\text{delta post-miR-125b}}$ − Log $2^{-\text{delta pre-miR-125b}}$. * = $p < 0.05$.

3.3. miR-125b Predicts Liver Fibrosis Stratified by ETV and LAM Response

Of the 124 analyzed patients, 59 were treated with entecavir and 53 were treated with lamivudine. Tables 3 and 4 depict the univariate and multivariate logistic regression models in these subgroups. In 59 patients treated with entecavir for 12 months, older age ($p = 0.0078$) and alteration of miRNA-125b levels during treatment ($p = 0.0157$) were substantially associated with a FIB-4 index of more than 2.9 in both univariate and multivariate analyses. A lower baseline platelet level ($p = 0.0109$) was also a risk factor for a high FIB-4 index in the univariate analysis. The baseline miRNA-125b levels were not associated with a high FIB-4 index. In 53 patients treated with lamivudine, older age and lower baseline platelet levels were independently associated with a higher FIB-4 index (≥2.9) in both the univariate and multivariate analyses. Neither baseline miRNA-125b nor alteration of miRNA-125b during treatment was associated with any degree of a high post-treatment FIB-4 index in univariate analyses.

Table 3. Baseline vs. 12M FIB-4 index analysis in ETV ($n = 59$).

	Univariate Analyses		Multivariate Analyses	
Variable	**OR (95%CI)**	***p* Value**	**OR (95%CI)**	***p* Value**
Age	1.14 (1.05–1.25)	0.0033 *	1.17 (1.04–1.32)	0.0078 *
Gender (male/female)	1.27 (0.30–5.42)	0.7442		
HBV DNA > 2000 IU/mL	1.76 (0.33–9.32)	0.5036		
HBeAg(+)	0.19 (0.02–1.65)	0.1332		
Lab data				
WBCs	1.00 (1.00–1.00)	0.2872		
Platelet	0.98 (0.97–0.99)	0.0109 *	0.99 (0.98–1.00)	0.1522
AST	1.00 (1.00–1.00)	0.6767		
ALT	1.00 (1.00–1.00)	0.2354		
Creatinine	0.89 (0.32–2.44)	0.8213		
Bilirubin	1.06 (0.90–0.12)	0.4909		
Albumin (gm/dL)	0.42 (0.13–1.31)	0.1362		
HB (g/dL)	0.66 (0.42–1.03)	0.0718		
Log $2^{-\text{delta pre-miR-125b}}$	0.52 (0.25–1.06)	0.0727		
Δ Log $2^{-\text{delta miRNA 125b}}$	0.34 (0.13–0.88)	0.0268 *	0.22 (0.06–0.75)	0.0157 *
Comorbidities				
Diabetes mellitus	1.38 (0.30–6.36)	0.6756		
Hypertension	2.00 (0.48–8.30)	0.3400		
Alcohol use	1.27 (0.33–4.95)	0.7314		

BMI, body mass index; BH, body height; BW, body weight; WBC, white blood cell count; PLT, platelet count; AST, aspartate aminotransferase; ALT, alanine aminotransferase; Cr, creatinine; HB, hemoglobin level; delta miRNA 125b represents $Ct_{miR-125b}$-Ct_{cel-39}; Δ Log $2^{-\text{delta post-miR-125b}}$ − Log $2^{-\text{delta pre-miR-125b}}$. * = $p < 0.05$.

Table 4. Baseline vs. 12M FIB-4 index analysis in LAM ($n = 53$).

	Univariate Analyses		Multivariate Analyses	
Variable	**OR (95%CI)**	***p* Value**	**OR (95%CI)**	***p* Value**
Age	1.18 (1.06–1.32)	0.0030 *	1.22 (1.06–1.41)	0.0068 *
Gender (male/female)	0.22 (0.04–1.05)	0.0579		
HBV DNA > 2000 IU/mL	1.22 (0.22–6.84)	0.8222		
HBeAg(+)	0.82 (0.17–3.86)	0.8030		
Lab data				
WBCs	1.00 (1.00–1.00)	0.0503		
Platelet	0.97 (0.95–0.99)	0.0094 *	0.95 (0.90–1.00)	0.0314 *
AST	1.00 (1.00–1.00)	0.9120		
ALT	1.00 (1.00–1.00)	0.1204		

Table 4. *Cont.*

	Univariate Analyses		Multivariate Analyses	
Variable	**OR (95%CI)**	***p* Value**	**OR (95%CI)**	***p* Value**
Creatinine	0.59 (0.03–13.72)	0.7413		
Bilirubin	1.17 (0.82–0.12)	0.3856		
Albumin (gm/dL)	0.48 (0.12–1.93)	0.3026		
HB (g/dL)	0.74 (0.46–1.19)	0.2139		
Log $2^{-\text{delta pre-miR-125b}}$	0.82 (0.34–1.97)	0.6508		
Δ Log $2^{-\text{delta miRNA 125b}}$	1.10 (0.45–2.71)	0.8338		
Comorbidities				
Diabetes mellitus	1.10 (0.30–6.36)	0.9945		
Hypertension	0.90 (0.08–9.97)	0.9316		
Alcohol use	1.50 (0.33–4.95)	0.9980		

BMI, body mass index; BH, body height; BW, body weight; WBC, white blood cell count; PLT, platelet count; AST, aspartate aminotransferase; ALT, alanine aminotransferase; Cr, creatinine; HB, hemoglobin level; delta miRNA 125b represents Ct $_{\text{miR}-125\text{b}}$-Ct $_{\text{cel}-39}$; Δ Log $2^{-\text{delta post}-\text{miR}-125\text{b}}$ − Log $2^{-\text{delta pre}-\text{miR}-125\text{b}}$. * = $p < 0.05$.

4. Discussion

The micro-RNA cluster, miR-125b, is a potential noninvasive biomarker for chronic hepatitis, liver fibrosis, and HCC. In this 1-year retrospective cohort study, we investigated the association between circulating miR-125b levels and liver fibrosis progression in HBV-infected patients treated with oral antiviral medications. We found no significant difference between the miR-125b levels at the baseline and those at the end of the 12th month after initial treatment. Neither the baseline miR-125b level nor miR-125b variation during the 12-month treatment period was associated with a higher FIB-4 index (>2.9). However, baseline miR-125b levels remained significantly and inversely correlated with the FIB-4 index after 12 months of treatment in the overall cohort. The miR-125b variation in 59 patients treated with lamivudine for 12 months was independently associated with a high FIB-4 index (>2.9) risk through univariate and multivariate logistic regression analyses. These real-world findings implicate an association between the alteration of miR-125b levels during certain anti-HBV treatments and possible changes in liver fibrosis.

Different potential noninvasive biomarkers have been investigated for HCC, but they poorly detect early HCC and liver fibrosis. Currently, alpha-fetoprotein is the only reliable marker for diagnosing HCC. Yet, its low specificity, especially in chronic liver disease, limits its application in real-world settings [25]. Given the high correlation between liver cirrhosis and HBV-related HCC, early prediction of liver fibrosis occurrence in HBV patients is an efficient strategy to prevent HBV-related HCC.

Previous studies have shown that the expression levels of miR-125b are serum miRNAs that represent potential biomarkers for hepatocellular carcinoma in patients with chronic hepatitis B virus infection [16,26–29]. In contrast, the association between miR-125b and early fibrosis has not yet been fully investigated. There is also no evidence demonstrating a correlation between direct-acting HBV treatment and alteration of miR-125b. Giray et al. carried out a study to investigate 24 miRNAs as a potential biomarker for the diagnosis of early liver fibrosis. The study was performed in three patient groups: CHB (n = 24), HBV-positive cirrhosis (n = 22), and HBV-positive HCC (n = 20), along with one control group (n = 28). In all these three patient groups, the expression level of miR-125b-5p was reported to be significantly upregulated (1.904–2.854-fold changes) compared to the control group by the Mann–Whitney *U* test.

Nevertheless, when all groups were compared with the control group using a one-way ANOVA test, the expression levels of miR-125b only showed an upregulated tendency without a statistically significant difference (p = 0.07192) [16]. Intriguingly, in our study, although the FIB-4 index showed a substantial decrease after 12 months of HBV treatment, the alteration in miR-125b was not significant. Between the two subgroups, divided by a post-treatment FIB-4 index of 2.9, neither the baseline miR-125b level nor the alternation showed significant differences. Our findings indicate that NA therapy for CHB might prevent the progression of liver fibrosis by counteracting upregulated miR-125b levels.

In line with our hypothesis, Yeh et al. carried out a prospective single-center study to investigate the outcomes of HBV infection in 79 HBV/HCV-coinfected patients after 1 year of DAA therapy [18]. This study reported reduced serum levels of miR-125b in HBV/hepatitis C virus (HCV)-coinfected patients after direct antiviral agents (DAAs) were administered for HCV infection and a continuous decline in miR-125b levels after stopping DAAs in patients with HBV reactivation, compared with no change in miR-125b levels in patients without HBV reactivation. This partially explains the miR125b alternation in our study as not only related to the progression of liver fibrosis but also to viral replication and involving more complex virus–host interactions, which require further investigation.

Zhou et al. conducted a retrospective cohort study to investigate the predictive value of baseline miR-125b levels for NA therapy in patients with CHB. A total of 66 HBeAg-positive CHB patients who had received LDT-optimized therapy ($n = 39$) or TDF monotherapy ($n = 27$) for 144 weeks were analyzed. Their results indicated that the baseline serum miR-125b level is an independent predictor of a complete response (defined as HBV DNA < 500 IU/mL and HBeAg seroconversion). This finding suggests that baseline miRNA-125b is a satisfying biomarker for HBeAg seroconversion following 144-week NA treatment [14].

In the present study, although baseline miR-125b was not an independent predictor for a FIB-4 index higher than 2.9 after 12 months of NA treatment in the overall HBV-positive cohort, there was a significant inverse correlation between the baseline serum miR-125b and post-treatment FIB-4 index. After we further analyzed 59 patients treated with LAM monotherapy for 12 months, the multivariate logistic regression model confirmed the substantial association between serum miR-125b alteration (OR = 0.22, $p = 0.0157$) and the risk of a higher FIB-4 index. In the same analysis, the baseline miR-125b level showed borderline significance ($p = 0.0727$) in univariate analyses. The major difference between our study and that of Zhou et al. is the duration of NA treatment. With a one-year therapy shorter than the duration of Zhou et al.'s study, the association between serum miR-125b alteration and fibrosis has been elucidated. Further studies are needed to validate the findings concerning long-term NA therapy.

After further interpretation of the comparison between 59 patients receiving ETV and 53 patients receiving LAM, we found that older age was a common independent predictor of a higher post-treatment FIB-4 index in both treatment groups and all cohorts. In all 124 patients, lower baseline platelet levels and higher baseline ALT levels were also significantly associated with the risk of a higher post-treatment FIB-4 index in both univariate and multivariate analyses.

However, the baseline serum ALT level was no longer a significant predictor in either the ETV or LAM group. The baseline platelet level remained an independent risk factor in the LAM group for a higher FIB-4 index after 12 months of treatment. Instead of platelet levels, the alteration of miR-125b during 12-month treatment can substantially and independently predict a higher post-treatment FIB-4 index, as discussed above. These findings suggest that the risk factors for liver fibrosis progression may differ between different NA treatment groups. Circulating miR-125b, a noninvasive and an easily accessible molecule, can be a reliable biomarker for predicting early liver fibrosis in HBV-positive patients, particularly those receiving specific NA treatment, such as ETV. Further large-scale studies with longer follow-up periods are needed to validate this finding.

This study had some limitations. First, it was a retrospective study conducted in a single center, although there has been no previous retrospective or prospective multicenter study with the same study design. Second, we did not generally define liver cirrhosis with a liver biopsy, given the standardized strategies that aim to prevent unnecessary healthcare-associated risks. Instead, we analyzed the FIB-4 index, validated in various patient settings with patient age and laboratory profiles [22,30–33]. Third, our analysis did not include some liver-disease-relevant data, such as INR, due to incomplete collection. However, data analyzed in a real clinical setting remain crucial in CHB and liver fibrosis.

In conclusion, the baseline serum miR-125b level was significantly and inversely correlated with the post-treatment FIB-4 index. Furthermore, the alteration in miR-125b levels during specific NA therapy, such as ETV, may be associated with the FIB-4 index after 12-month treatment. These findings are fundamental in recognizing miR-125b as a biomarker for the early progression of liver fibrosis during HBV treatment, especially the widely adopted ETV. Additionally, given that the long-term goal of surveillance for liver cirrhosis and HCC is to prevent the occurrence of early liver fibrosis, instead of monitoring miR-125b alone, our findings merit further studies to validate the role of different NA treatments in affecting serum miR-125b levels and their relationship to liver fibrosis.

Author Contributions: Investigation: Y.-S.T., Y.-C.C. and J.-N.H.; formal analysis: J.-Y.W., Y.-S.T. and C.-C.L.; patient sample collection: C.-I.H., M.-L.Y. (Ming-Lun Yeh), C.-F.H., M.-H.H., T.-W.L., Y.-H.L., P.-C.L., Z.-Y.L., C.-Y.D., M.-L.Y. (Ming-Lung Yu) and W.-L.C.; writing—original draft preparation: J.-Y.W., Y.-S.T. and C.-Y.D.; writing—review and editing: Y.-C.C., C.-Y.D. and M.-L.Y. All authors have read and agreed to the published version of the manuscript.

Funding: This work was supported by grants from the National Science Council of Taiwan (grant numbers MOST 109-2314-B-037-045-MY3 and 111-2314-B-037-102), the National Pingtung University of Science and Technology, and Kaohsiung Medical University (NPUST kmU-111-P009).

Institutional Review Board Statement: The study was conducted in accordance with the Declaration of Helsinki, and approved by the Institutional Review Board of Kaohsiung Medical University Hospital (KMUHIRB-E(II)-20190405).

Informed Consent Statement: Informed consent was obtained from all subjects involved in the study.

Conflicts of Interest: The guarantor of the article is Chia-Yen Dai, M.D., Ph.D. The authors declare that they have no conflicts of interest. Ethics approval and consent to participate were obtained. This study was reviewed and approved by the IRB ethics committee (KMUHIRB-E(II)-201904054).

References

1. GBD 2019 Hepatitis B Collaborators. Global, regional, and national burden of hepatitis B, 1990-2019: A systematic analysis for the Global Burden of Disease Study 2019. *Lancet Gastroenterol. Hepatol.* **2022**, *7*, 796–829. [CrossRef]
2. Fanning, G.C.; Zoulim, F.; Hou, J.; Bertoletti, A. Therapeutic strategies for hepatitis B virus infection: Towards a cure. *Nat. Rev. Drug Discov.* **2019**, *18*, 827–844. [CrossRef] [PubMed]
3. Kanda, T.; Goto, T.; Hirotsu, Y.; Moriyama, M.; Omata, M. Molecular Mechanisms Driving Progression of Liver Cirrhosis towards Hepatocellular Carcinoma in Chronic Hepatitis B and C Infections: A Review. *Int. J. Mol. Sci.* **2019**, *20*, 1358. [CrossRef] [PubMed]
4. Chen, C.J.; Yang, H.I.; Su, J.; Jen, C.L.; You, S.L.; Lu, S.N.; Huang, G.T.; Iloeje, U.H.; Group, R.-H.S. Risk of hepatocellular carcinoma across a biological gradient of serum hepatitis B virus DNA level. *JAMA* **2006**, *295*, 65–73. [CrossRef] [PubMed]
5. Gines, P.; Krag, A.; Abraldes, J.G.; Sola, E.; Fabrellas, N.; Kamath, P.S. Liver cirrhosis. *Lancet* **2021**, *398*, 1359–1376. [CrossRef]
6. Llovet, J.M.; Kelley, R.K.; Villanueva, A.; Singal, A.G.; Pikarsky, E.; Roayaie, S.; Lencioni, R.; Koike, K.; Zucman-Rossi, J.; Finn, R.S. Hepatocellular carcinoma. *Nat. Rev. Dis. Prim.* **2021**, *7*, 6. [CrossRef]
7. Zhang, Z.; Chen, J.; He, Y.; Zhan, X.; Zhao, R.; Huang, Y.; Xu, H.; Zhu, Z.; Liu, Q. miR-125b inhibits hepatitis B virus expression in vitro through targeting of the SCNN1A gene. *Arch. Virol.* **2014**, *159*, 3335–3343. [CrossRef]
8. Sartorius, K.; Makarova, J.; Sartorius, B.; An, P.; Winkler, C.; Chuturgoon, A.; Kramvis, A. The Regulatory Role of MicroRNA in Hepatitis-B Virus-Associated Hepatocellular Carcinoma (HBV-HCC) Pathogenesis. *Cells* **2019**, *8*, 1504. [CrossRef]
9. Xu, J.; An, P.; Winkler, C.A.; Yu, Y. Dysregulated microRNAs in Hepatitis B Virus-Related Hepatocellular Carcinoma: Potential as Biomarkers and Therapeutic Targets. *Front. Oncol.* **2020**, *10*, 1271. [CrossRef]
10. Jia, H.Y.; Wang, Y.X.; Yan, W.T.; Li, H.Y.; Tian, Y.Z.; Wang, S.M.; Zhao, H.L. MicroRNA-125b functions as a tumor suppressor in hepatocellular carcinoma cells. *Int. J. Mol. Sci.* **2012**, *13*, 8762–8774. [CrossRef]
11. Zhao, L.; Wang, W. miR-125b suppresses the proliferation of hepatocellular carcinoma cells by targeting Sirtuin7. *Int. J. Clin. Exp. Med.* **2015**, *8*, 18469–18475. [PubMed]
12. Wang, Y.; Wei, Y.; Fan, X.; Zhang, P.; Wang, P.; Cheng, S.; Zhang, J. MicroRNA-125b as a tumor suppressor by targeting MMP11 in breast cancer. *Thorac. Cancer* **2020**, *11*, 1613–1620. [CrossRef] [PubMed]
13. Chaudhuri, A.A.; So, A.Y.; Sinha, N.; Gibson, W.S.; Taganov, K.D.; O'Connell, R.M.; Baltimore, D. MicroRNA-125b potentiates macrophage activation. *J. Immunol.* **2011**, *187*, 5062–5068. [CrossRef] [PubMed]
14. Zhou, P.; Dong, M.; Wang, J.; Li, F.; Zhang, J.; Gu, J. Baseline serum miR-125b levels predict virologic response to nucleos(t)ide analogue treatment in patients with HBeAg-positive chronic hepatitis B. *Exp. Ther. Med.* **2018**, *16*, 3805–3812. [CrossRef]
15. Li, F.; Zhou, P.; Deng, W.; Wang, J.; Mao, R.; Zhang, Y.; Li, J.; Yu, J.; Yang, F.; Huang, Y.; et al. Serum microRNA-125b correlates with hepatitis B viral replication and liver necroinflammation. *Clin. Microbiol. Infect.* **2016**, *22*, 384.e1–384.e10. [CrossRef]

16. Giray, B.G.; Emekdas, G.; Tezcan, S.; Ulger, M.; Serin, M.S.; Sezgin, O.; Altintas, E.; Tiftik, E.N. Profiles of serum microRNAs; miR-125b-5p and miR223-3p serve as novel biomarkers for HBV-positive hepatocellular carcinoma. *Mol. Biol. Rep.* **2014**, *41*, 4513–4519. [CrossRef] [PubMed]
17. You, K.; Li, S.Y.; Gong, J.; Fang, J.H.; Zhang, C.; Zhang, M.; Yuan, Y.; Yang, J.; Zhuang, S.M. MicroRNA-125b Promotes Hepatic Stellate Cell Activation and Liver Fibrosis by Activating RhoA Signaling. *Mol. Ther. Nucleic Acids* **2018**, *12*, 57–66. [CrossRef]
18. Yeh, M.L.; Huang, C.F.; Huang, C.I.; Holmes, J.A.; Hsieh, M.H.; Tsai, Y.S.; Liang, P.C.; Tsai, P.C.; Hsieh, M.Y.; Lin, Z.Y.; et al. Hepatitis B-related outcomes following direct-acting antiviral therapy in Taiwanese patients with chronic HBV/HCV co-infection. *J. Hepatol.* **2020**, *73*, 62–71. [CrossRef]
19. Jieanu, C.F.; Ungureanu, B.S.; Sandulescu, D.L.; Gheonea, I.A.; Tudorascu, D.R.; Ciurea, M.E.; Purcarea, V.L. Quantification of liver fibrosis in chronic hepatitis B virus infection. *J. Med. Life* **2015**, *8*, 285–290.
20. Vallet-Pichard, A.; Mallet, V.; Nalpas, B.; Verkarre, V.; Nalpas, A.; Dhalluin-Venier, V.; Fontaine, H.; Pol, S. FIB-4: An inexpensive and accurate marker of fibrosis in HCV infection. comparison with liver biopsy and fibrotest. *Hepatology* **2007**, *46*, 32–36. [CrossRef]
21. Sterling, R.K.; Lissen, E.; Clumeck, N.; Sola, R.; Correa, M.C.; Montaner, J.; Mark, S.S.; Torriani, F.J.; Dieterich, D.T.; Thomas, D.L.; et al. Development of a simple noninvasive index to predict significant fibrosis in patients with HIV/HCV coinfection. *Hepatology* **2006**, *43*, 1317–1325. [CrossRef] [PubMed]
22. Shiha, G.; Ibrahim, A.; Helmy, A.; Sarin, S.K.; Omata, M.; Kumar, A.; Bernstien, D.; Maruyama, H.; Saraswat, V.; Chawla, Y.; et al. Asian-Pacific Association for the Study of the Liver (APASL) consensus guidelines on invasive and non-invasive assessment of hepatic fibrosis: A 2016 update. *Hepatol. Int.* **2017**, *11*, 1–30. [CrossRef] [PubMed]
23. Tsai, Y.S.; Yeh, M.L.; Tsai, P.C.; Huang, C.I.; Huang, C.F.; Hsieh, M.H.; Liu, T.W.; Lin, Y.H.; Liang, P.C.; Lin, Z.Y.; et al. Clusters of Circulating let-7 Family Tumor Suppressors Are Associated with Clinical Characteristics of Chronic Hepatitis C. *Int. J. Mol. Sci.* **2020**, *21*, 4945. [CrossRef] [PubMed]
24. Parikh, P.; Ryan, J.D.; Tsochatzis, E.A. Fibrosis assessment in patients with chronic hepatitis B virus (HBV) infection. *Ann. Transl. Med.* **2017**, *5*, 40. [CrossRef] [PubMed]
25. Liu, Y.; He, J.; Li, C.; Benitez, R.; Fu, S.; Marrero, J.; Lubman, D.M. Identification and confirmation of biomarkers using an integrated platform for quantitative analysis of glycoproteins and their glycosylations. *J. Proteome Res.* **2010**, *9*, 798–805. [CrossRef]
26. Li, L.M.; Hu, Z.B.; Zhou, Z.X.; Chen, X.; Liu, F.Y.; Zhang, J.F.; Shen, H.B.; Zhang, C.Y.; Zen, K. Serum microRNA profiles serve as novel biomarkers for HBV infection and diagnosis of HBV-positive hepatocarcinoma. *Cancer Res.* **2010**, *70*, 9798–9807. [CrossRef]
27. Auvinen, E. Diagnostic and Prognostic Value of MicroRNA in Viral Diseases. *Mol. Diagn. Ther.* **2017**, *21*, 45–57. [CrossRef]
28. Chen, S.; Chen, H.; Gao, S.; Qiu, S.; Zhou, H.; Yu, M.; Tu, J. Differential expression of plasma microRNA-125b in hepatitis B virus-related liver diseases and diagnostic potential for hepatitis B virus-induced hepatocellular carcinoma. *Hepatol. Res.* **2017**, *47*, 312–320. [CrossRef]
29. Jin, Y.; Wong, Y.S.; Goh, B.K.P.; Chan, C.Y.; Cheow, P.C.; Chow, P.K.H.; Lim, T.K.H.; Goh, G.B.B.; Krishnamoorthy, T.L.; Kumar, R.; et al. Circulating microRNAs as Potential Diagnostic and Prognostic Biomarkers in Hepatocellular Carcinoma. *Sci. Rep.* **2019**, *9*, 10464. [CrossRef]
30. Kawata, N.; Takahashi, H.; Iwane, S.; Inoue, K.; Kojima, M.; Kohno, M.; Tanaka, K.; Mori, H.; Isoda, H.; Oeda, S.; et al. FIB-4 index-based surveillance for advanced liver fibrosis in diabetes patients. *Diabetol. Int.* **2021**, *12*, 118–125. [CrossRef]
31. Li, Y.; Regan, J.; Fajnzylber, J.; Coxen, K.; Corry, H.; Wong, C.; Rosenthal, A.; Atyeo, C.; Fischinger, S.; Gillespie, E.; et al. Liver Fibrosis Index FIB-4 Is Associated With Mortality in COVID-19. *Hepatol. Commun.* **2021**, *5*, 434–445. [CrossRef] [PubMed]
32. Lee, J.; Vali, Y.; Boursier, J.; Spijker, R.; Anstee, Q.M.; Bossuyt, P.M.; Zafarmand, M.H. Prognostic accuracy of FIB-4, NAFLD fibrosis score and APRI for NAFLD-related events: A systematic review. *Liver Int.* **2021**, *41*, 261–270. [CrossRef] [PubMed]
33. Mallet, V.; Parlati, L.; Vallet-Pichard, A.; Terris, B.; Tsochatzis, E.; Sogni, P.; Pol, S. FIB-4 index to rule-out advanced liver fibrosis in NAFLD patients. *Presse Med.* **2019**, *48*, 1484–1488. [CrossRef] [PubMed]

biomedicines

Article

Long-Term Persistence of Mitochondrial DNA Instability among HCV-Cured People Who Inject Drugs

Mélusine Durand [1], Nicolas Nagot [1], Quynh Bach Thi Nhu [2], Amélie Vizeneux [1], Linh Le Thi Thuy [2], Huong Thi Duong [2], Binh Nguyen Thanh [2], Delphine Rapoud [1], Roselyne Vallo [1], Catherine Quillet [1], Hong Thi Tran [2], Laurent Michel [3], Thanh Nham Thi Tuyet [4], Oanh Khuat Thi Hai [4], Vinh Vu Hai [5], Jonathan Feelemyer [6], Philippe Vande Perre [1], Don Des Jarlais [6], Khue Pham Minh [2], Didier Laureillard [1,7] and Jean-Pierre Molès [1,*]

1 Pathogenesis and Control of Chronic and Emerging Infections, University of Montpellier, INSERM, 34000 Montpellier, France
2 Faculty of Public Health, Hai Phong University of Medicine and Pharmacy, Hai Phong 180000, Vietnam
3 Pierre Nicole Center, French Red Cross, 75005 Paris, France
4 Supporting Community Development Initiatives, Hanoi 111000, Vietnam
5 Infectious Diseases Department, Viet Tiep Hospital, Hai Phong 180000, Vietnam
6 College of Global Public Health, New York University, New York, NY 10012, USA
7 Infectious Diseases Department, Caremeau University Hospital, 30029 Nîmes, France
* Correspondence: jean-pierre.moles@inserm.fr

Abstract: People who inject drugs (PWID) are a population exposed to many genotoxicants and with a high prevalence of HCV infection. Direct-acting antiviral (DAA) regimens are now widely used to treat chronic HCV infection. Although side effects to treatment are currently rare, the long-term effects such as suspicions of de novo hepatocellular carcinoma (HCC) occurrence or HCC recurrence and cardiac defects are still up for debate. Given the structure of DAAs, the molecules have a potential mitochondrial DNA (mtDNA) genotoxicity. We have previously reported acute mtDNA toxicity of three DAA regimens among PWID with a strong impact on the rate of mtDNA deletion, less on the quantity of mtDNA copy per cell at sustained viral response at 12 weeks (SVR12). Herein, we report the mtDNA parameters nine months after drug discontinuation. We observed that the percentage of the deleted mtDNA genome increased over time. No exposure to any other genotoxicants during this period was associated with a high deletion percentage, suggesting that the replicative advantage of the deleted molecules outweighed their elimination processes. Such observation calls for longer-term follow-up and may contribute to the molecular basis of subclinical side effects of DAA treatments.

Keywords: HCV; DAA; mitochondria; genotoxicity; side effect

Citation: Durand, M.; Nagot, N.; Nhu, Q.B.T.; Vizeneux, A.; Thuy, L.L.T.; Duong, H.T.; Thanh, B.N.; Rapoud, D.; Vallo, R.; Quillet, C.; et al. Long-Term Persistence of Mitochondrial DNA Instability among HCV-Cured People Who Inject Drugs. *Biomedicines* **2022**, *10*, 2541. https://doi.org/10.3390/biomedicines10102541

Academic Editor: Jinghua Wang

Received: 24 August 2022
Accepted: 7 October 2022
Published: 12 October 2022

1. Introduction

The availability of direct-acting antivirals (DAA) has revolutionized HCV therapy. Even though we lack sufficient hindsight on their long-term side effects, there are still controversial data on adverse cardiac side effects, higher extrahepatic and intrahepatic malignancies, accelerated hepatocellular carcinoma (HCC) recurrence and aggressiveness, as well as doubts of genotoxicity [1–3]. The molecular basis of these side effects has not been elucidated, however, DAAs that are nucleoside analogues could act as substrates for human polymerases, including mitochondrial RNA and DNA polymerases [4,5]. Unlike nuclear polymerases, mitochondrial DNA (mtDNA) polymerases are more sensitive to genotoxicants due to their lack of editing functions. Recent in vitro models showed that sofosbuvir (SOF) and daclatasvir (DCV) drugs impaired mitochondrial morphologies and lowered the mtDNA copy number in yeast [3]. Furthermore, the association of sofosbuvir and ribavirin (RBV) increased cytotoxicity in HepG2 cells [6]. We recently investigated mitochondrial genotoxicity among people who inject drugs (PWID) who were treated with a combination of SOF, DCV, and RBV drugs. This population is well known for its characteristically high prevalence of HCV infection and constitutes one of the key target populations to achieve HCV elimination, as stipulated by the World Health Assembly in the first Global Health Sector Strategy on Viral Hepatitis 2016–2021 [7]. Moreover, this population is continuously exposed to several other genotoxicants that might increase the risk of genetic instability [8]. Overall, we found that the variation in mtDNA copy per cell (MCN) did not differ significantly before and after treatment, while the proportion of detectable mtDNA deletions (MDD) increased after treatment. Combined exposition of DAA with other illicit drugs may explain some of these variations [8].

If mtDNA copy number can fluctuate with time, elimination of deleted DNA molecules or defective mitochondria is a complex process and could instead tend towards an accumulation over time, leading to bioenergetic defects, mito-ageing processes, and, possibly, to cell transformation [9]. Herein, we conducted an observational study by measuring the mitochondrial parameters nine months after the end of treatment among HCV-cured PWID. We then tested whether these parameters were similar to those of an HCV-seronegative PWID population.

2. Materials and Methods

2.1. Study Design and Study Population

The design of the study is a prospective cohort study. The study population was made up of HCV RNA-positive PWID who were successfully treated with combinations of sofosbuvir, daclatasvir, and/or ribavirin for 12 weeks (negative sustained viral response at 12 weeks, known as the SVR12 HCV viral load) from the DRIVE-C study (NCT03537196) [10]. An HCV-seronegative PWID control population was obtained from the initial HCV screening phase of the previously mentioned study. PWID were recruited during a respondent-driven sampling survey (RDSS) conducted by community workers in Hai Phong, Vietnam, in 2018. This RDSS enrolled a total of 1444 PWID [10].

2.2. MtDNA Genotoxicity Assays

A detailed description of the assays has previously been published [8]. Succinctly, blood samples were collected on dried blood spot cards (DBS, WhatmanTM 903, GE Healthcare Bio-Sciences Corp.) and DNA was extracted using QIAamp DNA Mini kit (Qiagen, Courtaboeuf, France). Mitochondrial copy number (MCN) was assessed by real-time quantitative PCR using QuickScanTM Mitox kit (Primagen©, Amsterdam, The Netherlands). The MCN is expressed as the number of mtDNA cp/cell. The percentage of MDD was obtained by relative quantification of two qPCRs ($2^{-\Delta\Delta Ct}$ method), one targeting the region which encompasses more than 85% of the known mtDNA deletions and one targeting a very constant region, using DNA extracted from plasma-rich platelets as a calibrator. The MDD rate is the ratio of mutated mtDNA to total mtDNA and is expressed as a percentage [8].

2.3. Statistical Analysis

Baseline characteristics are described as frequencies with percentages for categorical variables, or as means with their standard deviation for continuous variables. MtDNA parameters are expressed as raw values for MCN or as percentages of MDD, with their 95% confidence interval. Median MCN was calculated for each of the three time points and subsequently compared between time points, as well as median MCN of PWID with an initial HCV negative serology (n = 260). The threshold for statistical significance was set for a p value < 0.05.

For the risk factor analyses, variations in MCN and MDD for each PWID were calculated between the end of treatment and 36-weeks post treatment discontinuation. PWID were next stratified into two classes depending on their ΔMCN and their ΔMDD results, using a threshold set at the first tercile value of the pooled data, equivalent to $\leq -76.5\%$ for ΔMCN and to $\leq -32\%$ for ΔMDD. To construct multivariate models, we selected variables with a $p \leq 0.20$ in univariate analyses among demographic, drug consumption use, co-infections, and co-medication data. The final model was constructed in a stepwise manner and validated by considering the smallest AIC (Akaike information criteria). The threshold for statistical significance was set for a p value < 0.05. Statistical analyses were performed on SAS® studio (Copyright © 2012-2020, SAS Institute Inc., Cary, NC, USA).

2.4. Ethics Approvals

Participants signed an informed consent form at enrolment that included the use of their samples in ancillary studies related to HCV infection among PWID. The present study complies with the Declaration of Helsinki and Good Clinical Practice, was approved by the Scientific Advisory Board of DRIVE-C, and subsequently by the Institutional Review Board of the Haiphong University of Medicine and Pharmacy, Vietnam (#01/HPUMPRB).

3. Results

3.1. Study Population

Out of the 332 PWID with mitochondrial data at the end of treatment, 297 attended the 9-month follow-up visit and 295 had a full set of paired data (Supplementary Figure S1). Reasons for not attending the 9-month follow-up visit were primarily "being incarcerated". HCV-treated PWID included in these analyses (n = 295) differed from those not included (n = 37), with less frequent HIV-positive infection statuses and being less frequently engaged in a methadone program (data not shown). PWID were almost exclusively men (97.6%), with a mean age of 42.0 years, and were administered SOF400/DCV60 (n = 149), SOF400/DCV90 (n = 119), or SOF400/DCV/RBV (n = 27) (Table 1). At the end of the study, 121 (41.0%) PWID reported still injecting heroin, 243 (82.4%) being under methadone therapy, and 33 (11.2%) smoking methamphetamine. All HIV-infected PWID had received ARV treatment, and none had previously been treated for HCV infection. The HCV-seronegative PWID group was characterized by less HIV infection (2.3% vs. 46.4%), a more recent history of injection (injecting for less than 5 years: 22.3 % versus 4.4%), and a greater consumption of methamphetamine (72.7% vs. 64.6%) (Table 1).

Table 1. Baseline characteristics of PWID included in the analysis and compared to HCV- seronegative PWID.

	HCV-Cured PWID N= 295	HCV-Seronegative PWID N= 260	*p*-Values
DEMOGRAPHIC DATA			
Sex, Male or transgender, n (%)	288 (97.6)	246 (94.6)	0.06 *
Age, years, mean (SD)	42.0 (7.4)	41.7 (10.1)	0.74 #
VIRAL INFECTIONS, n (%)			
HIV coinfection	137 (46.4)	6 (2.3)	<0.001 *
HBV coinfection	18 (6.1)	N.A.	-
TREATMENTS DAA, n (%)			
SOF400/DCV60	149 (50.5)	N.A.	
SOF400/DCV90	119 (40.3)	N.A.	
SOF400/DCV/RBV	27 (9.1)	N.A.	-
ARV			
Receiving ARV treatment	137 (46.4)	3 (1.2)	< 0.001 *
SUBSTANCE USE—Heroin, n (%)			
Number of years of injection			
Less than 5 years	13 (4.4)	58 (22.3)	
5 to 10 years	57 (19.3)	80 (30.8)	
10 to 15 years	78 (26.4)	63 (24.2)	
Over 15 years	147 (49.8)	59 (22.7)	<0.001 *
Frequency of injection per month			
Less than once a day	88 (29.8)	90 (34.6)	
Daily	207 (70.2)	170 (65.4)	0.23 *

Table 1. *Cont.*

	HCV-Cured PWID N= 295	HCV-Seronegative PWID N= 260	p-Values
Methamphetamine			
Urinary test positive at baseline	79 (26.8)	93 (35.8)	0.02 *
Declaration of consumption	190 (64.4)	189 (72.7)	0.04 *
Frequency of consumption per month			
<4 times per month	142 (48.1)	121 (46.5)	
≥4 times per month	48 (16.3)	68 (26.1)	0.008 *
Tobacco smoking	286 (96.9)	N.A.	-
Hazardous drinking £	75 (25.4)	84 (32.3)	0.07 *

*: Chi-squared test; #: *t*-test; £: score above 4 for men or 3 for women on the AUDIT-C scale; N.A.: not available.

3.2. Long-Term Dynamics of the mtDNA Parameters

Nine months after the end of treatment, median MCN dropped from 568.7 copies/cell (95%CI: 494.5; 647.7) to 184.0 (95%CI: 168.6; 198.9), and median MDD increased from 0.35 (95%CI: 0.32; 0.39) to 0.49 (95%CI: 0.45; 0.52). These values were statistically different from both the baseline values of HCV-infected PWID and the baseline values of control HCV-seronegative PWID (Table 2).

Table 2. MtDNA parameters among HCV-treated PWID and control PWID.

Mitochondrial Outcomes	HCV-Treated PWID (n = 295)			Control PWID (n = 260)
	Baseline	End of Treatment	9-Month Follow-Up	
MCN (c/cell)	481.2 (448.6; 524.6)	568.7 (494.5; 647.7)	184.0 (168.6; 198.9)	439.1 (405.9; 466.8)
MDD	0.26 (0.23; 0.29)	0.35 (0.32; 0.39)	0.49 (0.45; 0.52)	0.31 (0.24; 0.34)

Values are medians with 95% confidence interval; MCN: mitochondrial DNA copy number; MDD: mitochondrial DNA deletion rate.

3.3. Determinants of Altered mtDNA Parameters

People who inject drugs were next stratified by those being in the highest tercile of MCN loss (with a threshold set at 76.5% loss or more) or those in the highest tercile of increase in MDD rate (with a threshold set a 32% loss or more) versus all those remaining. Multivariate analysis showed that none of the current exposure factors including medications, drug consumption, or viral co-infections are associated with an increased risk of being "PWID with high loss of MCN" or being "PWID with a high accumulation of MDD", in the 9-month period following the end of treatment. Furthermore, having been exposed to one DAA regimen compared to another was not associated with mitochondrial genomic instability (Supplementary Tables S1 and S2).

4. Discussion

A 9-month follow-up of DAA-treated PWID revealed that mitochondrial parameters are not yet stable; the percentage of mtDNA molecules with deletion increased, while the number of copies per cell dropped drastically. We recently reported an increased rate of MDD upon completion of DAA treatment, while remaining subclinical. The present data supported the long-term persistence of MDD, which even worsened, while once again remained below the clinical level. Even among infected PWID that were treated and cured from the HCV infection, nine months after DAA treatment discontinuation these parameters did not revert back to levels observed among uninfected individuals.

MtDNA mutations and deletions lead to mitochondrial dysfunctions. These processes participate in biological ageing and age-related diseases (such as neurodegenerative and cardiovascular pathologies and cancers [11,12]). They have already been well illustrated among people living with HIV (PLHIV) undergoing antiretroviral therapy. In fact, PLHIV have a shorter life expectancy than the general population and are more prone to age-related diseases [9]. Cellular processes exist to eliminate defective mitochondria [11,12].

Beyond a threshold which is not yet defined, and which may vary from one cell type to another, and most likely with age, the cells undergo cell death. The direct role of ARV in this toxicity has recently been demonstrated. Persons initiating post-exposure prophylaxis after a non-occupational sexual exposure to HIV showed mitochondrial toxicity, which was worsened for those having received one-month regimens containing zidovudine (AZT) molecules [13]. The clearance rate for these alterations has not yet been defined, but initial arguments suggest that it may be very slow. Exposure to ARV drugs during pregnancy was assessed in terms of mitochondrial toxicity in *Patas* monkey pups at specific time points from birth. Noticeably, mitochondrial toxicity was still detectable at three years of age, which corresponds to approximately 15 years of age in humans [14,15]. The same observation was conducted for the number of mtDNA copies in HIV-uninfected infants born to HIV-positive mothers undergoing ARV treatment. Aldrovrandi et al. showed that the mtDNA copy number was only able to return to baseline values at five years of age [16]. Given that DAAs are of the same class of polymerase inhibitors as ARVs, the mitochondrial genotoxicity reported herein could follow these same mechanisms.

It is noteworthy that slow cycling cells are known to accumulate more deleted mtDNA molecules than rapid cycling cells, such as blood cells, suggesting that the MDD rate in other cell types in DAA-treated patients may be even higher [11,17,18]. Given that we were not able to identify other exposures as risk factors for the observed mtDNA instability during the follow-up period, DAA treatments may have primed the acquisition of MDD, which then persists and continues to replicate.

MtDNA instability has been previously associated with HCC, but its role in the pathophysiology has not yet been established [19]. Reported side effects of DAA treatments are minimal so far, but HCC recurrence is currently under scrutiny. Further investigation is required regarding the level of MDD accumulation after DAA treatment compatible with HCC development.

This study has several limitations. First, it is a monocentric study. Secondly, the before–after study design allowed us to report observational data only. Analyses were conducted at the participant level, so that each participant was its own control. The risk factor analyses cannot be used to decipher the mechanism underlying the mitochondrial genotoxicity but rather addressed putative concomitant exposures. Thirdly, the PWID population analysed herein is almost exclusively men. Given the number of women, we were not able to conduct a stratified analysis to observe these effects specifically in women. In addition, our conclusions should only be applied to PWID. To increase the scope of our findings and be able to observe gender-specific effects, the present study deserves to be reproduced among non-drug users of both sexes. Fourthly, the integrity of the mtDNA molecules was only investigated through the search of their common deletion and not in terms of point mutation. Other regions of the mtDNA may also be targeted for deletions, given that the drug exposures were particular. The latter two aspects would require sequencing approaches.

Altogether, these findings strongly suggest the persistence of mitochondrial dysbiogenesis after HCV treatments among male PWID, which remained subclinical over the course of the 9-month follow-up. The presented data call for a longer follow-up of this mtDNA instability.

Supplementary Materials: The following supporting information can be downloaded at: https://www.mdpi.com/article/10.3390/biomedicines10102541/s1, Figure S1: Flowchart of the study population; Table S1: Baseline characteristics of PWID included in the analysis and compared to HCV-negative PWID; Table S2: Factors associated with high MCN loss; Table S3: Factors associated with high MDD accumulation.

Author Contributions: Conceptualization, N.N., P.V.P., D.L. and J.-P.M.; methodology, N.N. and K.P.M.; validation, M.D., Q.B.T.N., L.L.T.T., R.V. and J.-P.M.; investigation, H.T.D., A.V., B.N.T., D.R., C.Q., H.T.T. and T.N.T.T.; data curation, M.D. and J.-P.M.; writing—original draft preparation, M.D. and J.-P.M.; writing—review and editing, N.N., L.M., V.V.H., J.F., P.V.P., D.D.J. and D.R.; funding acquisition, H.T.D., O.K.T.H., D.D.J., N.N. and D.L. All authors have read and agreed to the published version of the manuscript.

Funding: This research was supported by the National Institute on Drug Abuse at the National Institutes of Health (Grant number R01DA041978) and France National Agency for Research on AIDS and hepatitis (Grant numbers ANRS 12353, ANRS 12380).

Institutional Review Board Statement: The present study complies with the Declaration of Helsinki and Good Clinical Practice, was approved by the Scientific Advisory Board of DRIVE-C, and subsequently by the Institutional Review Board of Haiphong University of Medicine and Pharmacy, Vietnam (#01/HPUMPRB).

Informed Consent Statement: All participants signed an informed consent form at enrolment that includes the use of their samples in ancillary studies related to HCV infection among PWID.

Data Availability Statement: The data presented in this study are available on request from the corresponding author.

Acknowledgments: We are grateful to all the participants and the peers of the DRIVE and DRIVE-C studies.

Conflicts of Interest: The authors declare no conflict of interest. The funders had no role in the design of the study; in the collection, analyses, or interpretation of data; in the writing of the manuscript, or in the decision to publish the results.

References

1. Kamal, A.; Elsheaita, A.; Abdelnabi, M. Association between Direct-Acting Antiviral Agents in Hepatitis C Virus Treatment and Hepatocellular Carcinoma Occurrence and Recurrence: The Endless Debate. *World J. Clin. Cases* **2022**, *10*, 1764–1774. [CrossRef] [PubMed]
2. Hayes, K.N.; Burkard, T.; Weiler, S.; Tadrous, M.; Burden, A.M. Global Adverse Events Reported for Direct-Acting Antiviral Therapies for the Treatment of Hepatitis C: An Analysis of the World Health Organization VigiBase. *Eur. J. Gastroenterol. Hepatol.* **2021**, *33*, e1017–e1021. [CrossRef] [PubMed]
3. Yahya, G.; Hashem Mohamed, N.; Pijuan, J.; Seleem, N.M.; Mosbah, R.; Hess, S.; Abdelmoaty, A.A.; Almeer, R.; Abdel-Daim, M.M.; Shulaywih Alshaman, H.; et al. Profiling the Physiological Pitfalls of Anti-Hepatitis C Direct-Acting Agents in Budding Yeast. *Microb. Biotechnol.* **2021**, *14*, 2199–2213. [CrossRef] [PubMed]
4. Ehteshami, M.; Zhou, L.; Amiralaei, S.; Shelton, J.R.; Cho, J.H.; Zhang, H.; Li, H.; Lu, X.; Ozturk, T.; Stanton, R.; et al. Nucleotide Substrate Specificity of Anti-Hepatitis C Virus Nucleoside Analogs for Human Mitochondrial RNA Polymerase. *Antimicrob. Agents Chemother.* **2017**, *61*, e00492-17. [CrossRef]
5. Jin, Z.; Kinkade, A.; Behera, I.; Chaudhuri, S.; Tucker, K.; Dyatkina, N.; Rajwanshi, V.K.; Wang, G.; Jekle, A.; Smith, D.B.; et al. Structure-Activity Relationship Analysis of Mitochondrial Toxicity Caused by Antiviral Ribonucleoside Analogs. *Antiviral. Res.* **2017**, *143*, 151–161. [CrossRef] [PubMed]
6. Librelotto, C.S.; DE SOUZA, A.P.; Álvares-Da-silva, M.R.; Simon, D.; Dihl, R.R. Evaluation of the Genetic Toxicity of Sofosbuvir and Simeprevir with and without Ribavirin in a Human-Derived Liver Cell Line. *An. Acad. Bras. Cienc.* **2021**, *93*. [CrossRef] [PubMed]
7. Pedrana, A.; Munari, S.; Stoové, M.; Doyle, J.; Hellard, M. The Phases of Hepatitis C Elimination: Achieving WHO Elimination Targets. *Lancet Gastroenterol. Hepatol.* **2021**, *6*, 6–8. [CrossRef]
8. Durand, M.; Nagot, N.; Nhu, Q.B.T.; Vallo, R.; Thuy, L.L.T.; Duong, H.T.; Thanh, B.N.; Rapoud, D.; Quillet, C.; Tran, H.T.; et al. Mitochondrial Genotoxicity of Hepatitis c Treatment among People Who Inject Drugs. *J. Clin. Med.* **2021**, *10*, 4824. [CrossRef] [PubMed]
9. Schank, M.; Zhao, J.; Moorman, J.P.; Yao, Z.Q. The Impact of HIV-and ART-Induced Mitochondrial Dysfunction in Cellular Senescence and Aging. *Cells* **2021**, *10*, 174. [CrossRef]
10. Rapoud, D.; Quillet, C.; Pham Minh, K.; Vu Hai, V.; Nguyen Thanh, B.; Nham Thi Tuyet, T.; Tran Thi, H.; Molès, J.P.; Vallo, R.; Michel, L.; et al. Towards HCV Elimination among People Who Inject Drugs in Hai Phong, Vietnam: Study Protocol for an Effectiveness-Implementation Trial Evaluating an Integrated Model of HCV Care (DRIVE-C: DRug Use & Infections in ViEtnam-Hepatitis C). *BMJ Open* **2020**, *10*, e039234. [CrossRef]
11. Jang, J.Y.; Blum, A.; Liu, J.; Finkel, T. The Role of Mitochondria in Aging. *J. Clin. Invest.* **2018**, *128*, 3662–3670. [CrossRef] [PubMed]
12. Fontana, G.A.; Gahlon, H.L. Mechanisms of Replication and Repair in Mitochondrial DNA Deletion Formation. *Nucleic Acids Res.* **2020**, *48*, 11244–11258. [CrossRef] [PubMed]
13. Bañó, M.; Morén, C.; Barroso, S.; Juárez, D.L.; Guitart-Mampel, M.; González-Casacuberta, I.; Canto-Santos, J.; Lozano, E.; León, A.; Pedrol, E.; et al. Mitochondrial Toxicogenomics for Antiretroviral Management: HIV Post-Exposure Prophylaxis in Uninfected Patients. *Front. Genet* **2020**, *11*, 497. [CrossRef]

14. Divi, R.L.; Einem, T.L.; Fletcher, S.L.L.; Shockley, M.E.; Kuo, M.M.; St Claire, M.C.; Cook, A.; Nagashima, K.; Harbaugh, S.W.; Harbaugh, J.W.; et al. Progressive Mitochondrial Compromise in Brains and Livers of Primates Exposed in Utero to Nucleoside Reverse Transcriptase Inhibitors (NRTIs). *Toxicol. Sci.* **2010**, *118*, 191–201. [CrossRef] [PubMed]
15. Liu, Y.; Shim Park, E.; Gibbons, A.T.; Shide, E.D.; Divi, R.L.; Woodward, R.A.; Poirier, M.C. Mitochondrial Compromise in 3-Year Old Patas Monkeys Exposed in Utero to Human-Equivalent Antiretroviral Therapies. *Environ. Mol. Mutagen* **2016**, *57*, 526–534. [CrossRef] [PubMed]
16. Aldrovandi, G.M.; Chu, C.; Shearer, W.T.; Li, D.; Walter, J.; Thompson, B.; McIntosh, K.; Foca, M.; Meyer, W.A.; Ha, B.F.; et al. Antiretroviral Exposure and Lymphocyte MtDNA Content Among Uninfected Infants of HIV-1-Infected Women. *Pediatrics* **2009**, *124*, e1189–e1197. [CrossRef]
17. Picard, M.; Vincent, A.E.; Turnbull, D.M. Expanding Our Understanding of MtDNA Deletions. *Cell Metab.* **2016**, *24*, 3–4. [CrossRef]
18. Lawless, C.; Greaves, L.; Reeve, A.K.; Turnbull, D.M.; Vincent, A.E. The Rise and Rise of Mitochondrial DNA Mutations. *Open Biol.* **2020**, *10*, 200061. [CrossRef]
19. Zekri, A.R.N.; Salama, H.; Medhat, E.; Hamdy, S.; Hassan, Z.K.; Bakr, Y.M.; Youssef, A.S.E.-D.; Saleh, D.; Saeed, R.; Omran, D. Potential Diagnostic and Prognostic Value of Lymphocytic Mitochondrial DNA Deletion in Relation to Folic Acid Status in HCV-Related Hepatocellular Carcinoma. *Asian Pac. J. Cancer Prev.* **2017**, *18*, 2451–2457. [CrossRef]

biomedicines

MDPI

Article

Comparable Outcomes in Early Hepatocellular Carcinomas Treated with Trans-Arterial Chemoembolization and Radiofrequency Ablation

Benjamin Wei Rong Tay [1,†], Daniel Q. Huang [1,2,†], Muthiah Mark [1], Neo Wee Thong [3], Lee Guan Huei [1,2], Lim Seng Gee [1,2], Low How Cheng [1], Lee Yin Mei [1], Prem Thurairajah [1], Lim Jia Chen [1], Cheng Han Ng [2], Wen Hui Lim [2], Darren Jun Hao Tan [2], Da Costa Maureen [4], Kow Wei Chieh Alfred [4], Iyer Shridar Ganpathi [4], Tan Poh Seng [1] and Dan Yock Young [1,2,*]

1 Division of Gastroenterology and Hepatology, National University Health System, Singapore 119228, Singapore
2 Department of Medicine, Yong Loo Yin School of Medicine, National University of Singapore, Singapore 119077, Singapore
3 Department of Diagnostic Imaging, National University Health System, Singapore 119228, Singapore
4 Division of Hepatobiliary Surgery, National University Health System, Singapore 119228, Singapore
* Correspondence: mdcdyy@nus.edu.sg
† These authors contributed equally to the work.

Citation: Tay, B.W.R.; Huang, D.Q.; Mark, M.; Thong, N.W.; Guan Huei, L.; Gee, L.S.; Cheng, L.H.; Mei, L.Y.; Thurairajah, P.; Chen, L.J.; et al. Comparable Outcomes in Early Hepatocellular Carcinomas Treated with Trans-Arterial Chemoembolization and Radiofrequency Ablation. *Biomedicines* **2022**, *10*, 2361. https://doi.org/10.3390/biomedicines10102361

Academic Editor: Jinghua Wang

Received: 1 August 2022
Accepted: 18 September 2022
Published: 22 September 2022

Publisher's Note: MDPI stays neutral with regard to jurisdictional claims in published maps and institutional affiliations.

Abstract: The guidelines recommend radiofrequency ablation (RFA) for early hepatocellular carcinomas that are less than 3 cm and trans-arterial chemoembolization (TACE) for intermediate-stage tumors. Real-world patient and tumor factors commonly limit strict adherence to the guidelines. We aimed to compare the clinical outcomes for TACE and RFA in early HCC. All consecutive patients from 2010 to 2014 that were treated with locoregional therapy at our institution were enrolled. The decision for TACE or RFA was based on tumor location, stage and technical accessibility for ablation. A subgroup analysis was performed for patients with tumors less than 3 cm. A total of 168 patients underwent TACE while 56 patients underwent RFA. Patients treated with TACE and RFA had 1- and 5-year survival rates of 84.7% and 39.8% versus 91.5% and 51.5%, respectively ($p = 0.28$). In tumors less than 3 cm, there was no significant difference in overall survival ($p = 0.69$), time to progression ($p = 0.55$), or number of treatment sessions required ($p = 0.12$). Radiofrequency ablation had a significantly higher chance of a complete response ($p = 0.004$). In conclusion, TACE may be selectively considered for early-stage hepatocellular carcinoma in patients unsuitable for other modalities.

Keywords: transarterial chemoembolization; radiofrequency ablation; hepatocellular carcinoma

1. Introduction

Hepatocellular carcinoma (HCC) is the third leading cause of cancer-related death worldwide [1,2]. The optimal treatment for HCC is oncologic resection or liver transplant [3–6]. Unfortunately, this is often limited by poor liver function precluding a safe resection and a shortage of donor livers. In situations when a resection or transplant is not possible and the disease is confined to the liver, locoregional therapies for HCC are recommended, including radiofrequency ablation (RFA) and transarterial chemoembolization (TACE) [7,8].

RFA delivers a high-frequency alternating current via a catheter tip, producing thermal-energy-induced area necrosis to tissue within a 1.5 cm radius. RFA is best used in tumors with a diameter of less than 3 cm and can provide sustained recurrence-free survival in these patients. In major society guidelines, RFA is recommended for small HCCs less than 3 cm in size, especially if resection is not feasible [7–9]. RFA is generally avoided in tumors that are near the dome of the diaphragm or next to bowel lumen, for fear of diaphragmatic injury or bowel perforation [10,11].

TACE delivers chemotherapy-infused particles via the hepatic artery, inducing ischemia in the tumor and delivering the local chemotherapeutic agent. Previously, a Taiwanese study showed that TACE and RFA resulted in similar overall survival for HCC patients within the Milan criteria, although RFA still showed significantly better survival in small tumors with a total tumor volume < 11 cm^3 [12]. However, Kim et al. compared TACE and RFA for small tumors less than 2 cm and showed a similar overall survival in both groups, and another study comparing single small tumors less than 3 cm showed a similar tumor response and recurrence [13,14]. The current practice guidelines recommend ablation in HCCs less than 3 cm. Considering the conflicting literature with regards to the use of TACE in small tumors, and the current clinical practice guidelines recommending ablation in HCCs less than 3 cm, we aimed to compare the outcomes of TACE and RFA in patients with HCCs less than 3 cm.

2. Materials and Methods

2.1. Patients

This was a single-center retrospective cohort study. We enrolled all consecutive patients between 1 January 2010 to 31 December 2014 treated with either TACE or RFA as the first line monotherapy for Barcelona Clinic Liver Cancer (BCLC) stage 0, A or B HCC. Patients with evidence of vascular invasion or metastatic disease were excluded. This study was approved by the Investigation and Ethics Committee of the National University Hospital (Singapore), according to the standards of the Declaration of Helsinki. Written informed consent was obtained from each patient before treatment.

2.2. Selection of Primary Treatment Modality

The diagnosis of HCC was in accordance with major society guidelines [7,8,15]. The selection of the locoregional modality was made by a multidisciplinary hepatobiliary tumor board consisting of hepatobiliary surgeons, hepatologists, interventional radiologists, medical/radiation oncologists and pathologists. Locoregional therapy was offered to patients who were not surgical candidates due to a combination of poor liver function, poor functional status and/or multiple comorbidities. The decision between RFA and TACE depended on factors such as tumor location, size, number of nodules and technical feasibility.

2.3. Trans-Arterial Chemoembolization

Dynamic multiphasic cross-sectional imaging of the liver via magnetic resonance imaging (MRI) or computed tomography (CT) was performed prior to the procedure to guide the approach to the tumor. Catheterization of the hepatic artery and identification of the tumor feeding vessel was performed, followed by administration of Cisplatin, Doxorubicin or Adriamycin.

2.4. Radiofrequency Ablation

A triphasic CT scan was performed prior to the procedure to guide the approach to the tumor. An ultrasound-guided percutaneous approach was used for the placement of a 14-gauge needle electrode into the target area. Radiofrequency current was then emitted for 12 to 15 min by a 200 W generator.

2.5. Patient Follow-Up

A CT or MRI scan was obtained from all patients one month following the procedure to document treatment response. Treatment response was assessed using the modified RECIST criteria [16]. Clinical evaluation, surveillance liver scans, and laboratory investigations were subsequently performed every 3–6 months to monitor for progressive disease or recurrence. Repeat treatment was performed for patients with an inadequate response to the initial therapy and for those with recurrence or a progressive disease.

2.6. Evaluation of Data

The primary outcome evaluated was overall survival, which was defined as the time between HCC diagnosis and death. Secondary endpoints included treatment response in accordance with the modified RECIST criteria, recurrence, and time to progression (TTP). Recurrence was defined as any new onset lesion or progression of lesions originally considered suspicious or metastasis in patients who had demonstrated a complete response at any time during the follow-up. TTP was defined as the time between primary treatment and the first evidence of radiological progression as defined by the modified RECIST criteria. Outcome measures were evaluated for the whole study population followed by subgroup analysis on tumors less than 3 cm. Adverse effects of treatment were monitored throughout the period of admission and recorded.

2.7. Statistical Analysis

All statistical analysis was performed using the Statistical Packages for Social Sciences version 25.0 (SPSS Inc., Chicago, IL, USA). A two-sided p-value of <0.05 was considered to be statistically significant. The chi-squared test was used for categorical data comparison and the Mann–Whitney test was used for continuous data. The Kaplan–Meier method with log-rank testing was used for the analysis of survival and time to progression.

3. Results

3.1. Baseline Charateristics

Between March 1989 and September 2013, 224 patients met the inclusion criteria and were entered in the study. TACE was performed for 168 patients while RFA was performed for 56 patients. Patients were predominantly male and Chinese, with a median age of 65 years at the point of diagnosis. About 86% of patients were cirrhotic with the majority being Child-Pugh A. The main etiology of the underlying liver disease was hepatitis B for both groups. Multiple etiologies of chronic liver disease were noted in 11 patients. No significant differences were noted in the background hepatic function or alpha-fetoprotein levels between both cohorts.

The size of tumor was significantly larger ($p < 0.001$) in the cases treated with TACE compared to RFA. The median size of the primary tumor nodule in the cases treated with TACE was 3.8 cm (interquartile range (IQR) 2.2–6.2 cm) while the median size of the primary nodule in cases treated with RFA was 2.1 cm (IQR 1.5–2.7 cm). The baseline characteristics of all the patients treated with TACE and RFA are shown in Table 1.

There were significant differences between the TACE and RFA subpopulations with regard to ethnicity ("Chinese" and "Others") and primary diagnosis ("Non-Alcoholic Fatty Liver Disease (NAFLD)"). All differences in sociodemographics and baseline hepatic and clinical factors were resolved by the stratification to a tumor size less than 3 cm, as shown in Table 2.

Table 1. Baseline characteristics of all 224 study subjects.

	TACE		RFA		p Value
Number of patients	168		56		
Age, median (IQR)	68	(57–75)	65	(59–70)	0.173
		Gender (%)			
Male	123	(73.2%)	43	(76.8%)	0.597
Female	45	(26.8%)	13	(23.2%)	
		Ethnicity (%)			
Chinese	95	(56.5%)	45	(80.4%)	
Malay	9	(5.4%)	2	(3.5%)	0.012
Indian	6	(3.6%)	0	-	
Others	58	(34.5%)	9	(16.1%)	

Table 1. *Cont.*

	TACE		RFA		*p* Value
Cirrhosis (%)					
Yes	167	(86.8%)	47	(83.9%)	0.564
No	22	(13.1%)	8	(14.3%)	
Unknown	1	(0.6%)	1	(1.8%)	
Etiology of underlying liver disease (% of total etiologies) 213 cases have a single etiology while 11 cases have multiple etiologies.					
Hepatitis B	78		23		0.002
Hepatitis C	34		13		
Alcoholic Cirrhosis	11		12		
NAFLD	12		8		
Autoimmune Hepatitis	1		1		
Wilson's disease	2		0		
Primary Biliary Cirrhosis	0		2		
Etiology not known	35		4		
Biochemistry					
Alpha-fetoprotein (ng/mL)	18.0	(5.0–122.0)	12.5	(7.0–58.0)	0.460
Prothrombin Time (s)	14.0	(13.0–16.0)	15.0	(14.0–16.0)	0.193
Platelet $\times 10^9$/L	128.0	(91.0–211.0)	132.5	(82.5–171.3)	0.339
Total Bilirubin (umol/L)	16.0	(10.0–26.25)	17.0	(11.0–33.75)	0.283
Albumin (g/L)	36.0	(31.0–40.0)	36.0	(31.0–40.0)	0.870
Child-Pugh Score (%)					
A	124	(73.8%)	41	(73.2%)	0.930
B	44	(26.2%)	15	(26.8%)	
Tumor Nodularity					
Uninodular	95	(56.5%)	34	(60.7%)	0.748
Multinodular	71	(43.5%)	22	(39.3%)	
Diffuse	2	(1.2%)	0	-	
Primary nodule characteristics					
Median Size (cm)	3.8	(2.2–6.2)	2.10	(1.5–2.7)	<0.001

Continuous variables are presented as median (IQR) and categorical variables as n (%).

Table 2. Baseline characteristics of patients with primary HCC tumor <3 cm.

	TACE		RFA		*p* Value
Number of patients	62		45		0.100
Age	64	(57–72)	65	(59–70)	0.880
Gender (%)					
Male	40	(64.5%)	34	(75.6%)	0.222
Female	22	(35.5%)	11	(24.4%)	
Ethnicity (%)					
Chinese	34	(54.8%)	37	(82.2%)	0.018
Malay	3	(4.8%)	2	(4.4%)	
Indian	3	(4.8%)	0	-	
Others	22	(35.5%)	6	(13.3%)	
Etiology of underlying liver disease (% of total etiologies) 101 cases had single etiology while 6 cases had multiple etiologies					
Hepatitis B	24		19		0.2184
Hepatitis C	18		10		
Alcoholic Cirrhosis	7		10		
NAFLD	6		6		
Autoimmune Hepatitis	0		1		
Wilson's disease	1		0		
Primary Biliary Cirrhosis	0		2		
Etiology not known	6		1		
Biochemistry					
Alpha-fetoprotein (ng/mL)	16.5	(5.8–99.0)	12.0	(7.0–46.0)	0.781
Prothrombin Time (s)	14.0	(13.0–15.0)	15.0	(14.0–15.0)	0.229
Platelet $\times 10^9$/L	108.0	(73.5–160.5)	137.0	(91.0–169.5)	0.100
Total Bilirubin (umol/L)	15.0	(11.75–27.0)	15.0	(10.0–27.0)	0.865
Albumin (g/L)	37.0	(31.5–40.5)	36.4	(32.5–40.0)	0.597
Tumor Nodularity					
Uninodular	34	(54.8%)	26	(57.8%)	0.762
Multinodular	28	(45.2%)	19	(42.2%)	

Continuous variables are presented as median (IQR) and categorical variables as n (% of total population).

3.2. Survival

Overall survival rates at 1, 3 and 5 years in the RFA and TACE groups were 91.5%, 72.8%, 51.5% and 84.7%, 57.6%, 39.8%, respectively. There was no statistical significance between the two groups (Figure 1, $p = 0.28$). When overall survival was stratified by a size of the HCC of less than 3 cm, the median survival for TACE and RFA groups was 48.0 (IQR 21.0–75.0) and 54.0 (IQR 42.0–67.0) months, respectively, with no significant difference between the groups (Figure 2, $p = 0.69$). The main cause of death was due to hepatic failure from the progression of hepatocellular carcinoma.

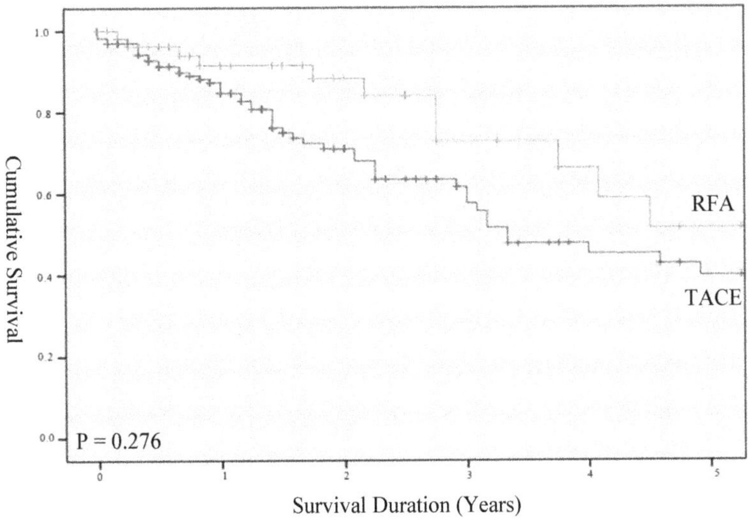

Figure 1. Overall survival in unstratified cohort.

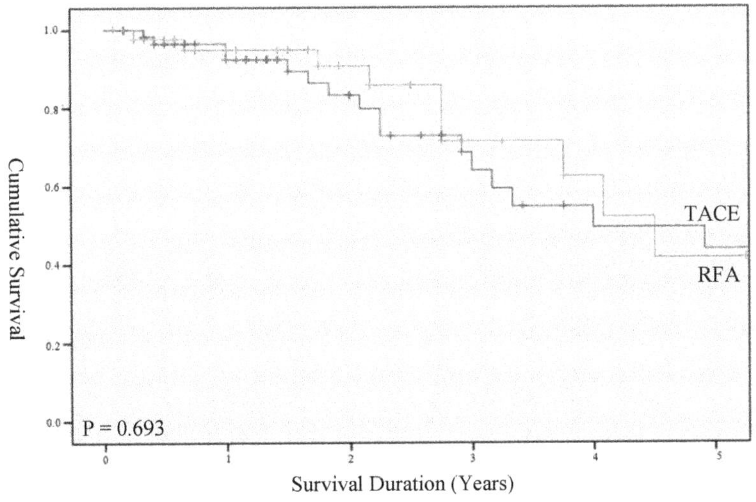

Figure 2. Survival duration stratified for HCC < 3 cm.

3.3. Time to Progression

Patients treated with RFA had a significantly longer TTP than those treated with TACE, with a median TTP of 9.0 months (IQR 4.0–19.0) and 13.0 months (IQR 8.0–29.0) ($p = 0.02$), respectively (Figure 3). However, in a subgroup of patients with HCCs less than 3 cm, there was no significant difference in TTP between the TACE (median TTP 13.0 months; IQR 4.0–28.0 months) and RFA groups (median TTP 13.0 months; IQR 9.0–22.0 months) (p = 0.55, Figure 4).

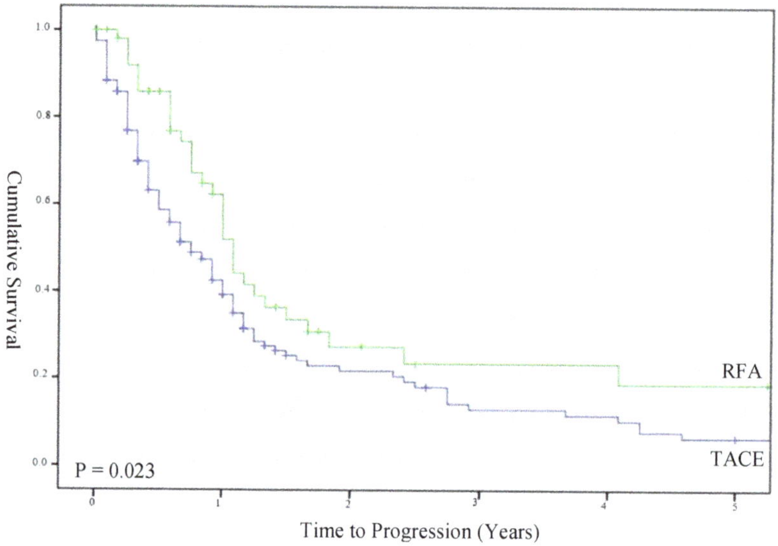

Figure 3. Time to progression in unstratified cohort.

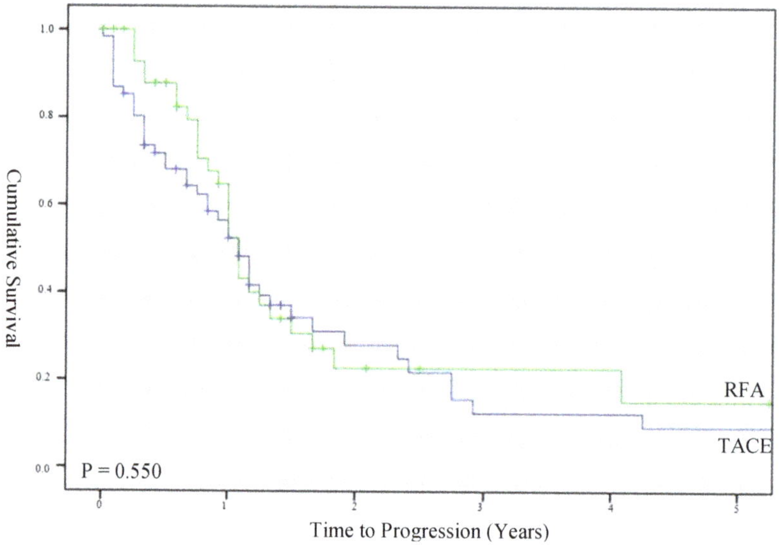

Figure 4. Time to progression stratified for HCC < 3 cm.

3.4. Chance of Complete Response

HCC treated with RFA was associated with a significantly higher chance of complete response (CR) compared to TACE (83.9% vs. 32.7%, $p < 0.001$). When stratified by size, RFA-treated HCCs again had a significantly higher CR rate for lesions less than 3 cm compared to TACE (82.2% vs. 55.7%, $p = 0.004$).

3.5. Recurrence

Recurrence rates were similar between the TACE- and RFA-treated cases in the overall cohort including both large and small hepatomas (40.3% vs. 58.2%, $p = 0.21$). When stratified to HCCs less than 3 cm, there was a significantly lower recurrence rate in patients that were treated by TACE compared to RFA (39.7% vs. 61.3%, $p = 0.03$).

3.6. Number of Treatments

The total number of treatment sessions did not differ significantly ($p = 0.22$) between TACE (median = 2.0, IQR 1.0–3.0) and RFA (median = 2.0, IQR 1.0–3.0). Among hepatomas less than 3 cm, the total number of treatment sessions likewise did not differ significantly ($p = 0.12$), with a median of 2 sessions for TACE (IQR 1.0–2.0) and RFA (IQR 1.0–2.0).

3.7. Adverse Events

TACE resulted in an adverse event rate of 37% with 7.4% of TACE patients having a greater number of multiple complications. RFA resulted in single adverse events in 16.1% of patients. Of these, the majority were minor adverse events such as pyrexia, nausea, vomiting, abdominal discomfort and elevated transaminases. For tumors <3 cm, adverse events occurred in 17.7% of TACE patients while RFA patients had adverse events 13.3% of the time. Three episodes of major adverse events were associated with TACE of tumors >3 cm, namely one case of hepatorenal syndrome and two cases tumor rupture. RFA resulted in one major adverse event of pneumothorax in a patient with an HCC <3 cm. Three patients died soon after receiving TACE (1.6%), while no patients died after receiving RFA.

4. Discussion

A substantial proportion of HCC patients presenting to tertiary hospitals require loco-regional therapy. Our study shows that treatment with either TACE or RFA for tumors less than 3 cm did not result in a significant difference in overall survival. This is despite a significantly favorable chance of a complete response following RFA therapy.

In accordance with guidelines, patients in our center with larger tumors and a more advanced BCLC stage tend to be treated with chemoembolization while the smaller tumors are primarily managed with RFA. Even so, there exist factors limiting the use of RFA in these patients: central tumors close to the hepatic hilum are at an increased risk of damage to major biliary structures while those peripherally situated adjacent to extrahepatic organs are liable to heat injuries, such as pleural effusion and intestinal perforation [17]. Incomplete ablation may occur in tumors contiguous to large vessels due to tissue cooling caused by increased circulation [18]. Needle-track seeding is a further consideration that has yet to be addressed convincingly [19]. In these cases, patients were treated with TACE. This trend is especially relevant in Asia where TACE has traditionally been favored as the primary anticancer therapy, and hence is even utilized in treating lesions outside the current guidelines [19].

The outcomes at our center were comparable to published studies [20,21]. Our 3-year overall survival rate of 72.8% for RFA and 57.6% for TACE is in line with the pooled 3-year survival rate of 50.8% described in a systematic review by Singal et al. [20]. TACE was used for patients with a larger tumor load, which could explain the difference in overall survival between TACE and RFA. After stratification for smaller tumors less than 3 cm there was resolution of the survival disparity, with no significant difference seen in median survival between patients treated with TACE and RFA.

The examination of secondary clinical outcomes in the subgroup analysis of hepatomas less than 3 cm provides a possible explanation for the comparable survival between RFA and TACE in small tumors. RFA in small tumors has a higher chance of a complete response compared to TACE, though patients who respond to TACE benefit from a lower recurrence. RFA offers a high chance of a complete response in small tumors due to the ability to completely ablate liver tissue and all tumoral residues in the area of the burn. There are, however, risks of tumor seeding, which may increase recurrence [19]. In contrast, the efficacy of TACE depends on arterial supply, and incomplete response may occur if there is more than a single supply and incomplete embolization. This effect is higher in larger and multinodular tumors. There have been concerns that the hypoxia induced by TACE induces vascular endothelial growth factor (VEGF) expression, promoting neovascularization and tumor recurrence in patients incompletely treated by TACE [22]. However, in patients who do respond to TACE, the lower recurrence rates in patients could be due to several reasons: (1) Early recurrence would primarily come from microsatellite and microvascular invasion before treatment [23,24]. Many of these are too small to be identified even with high-resolution imaging and may extend past the safety margin of ablation [25,26]. In such a setting, TACE is able to control these micro-metastases missed by radiofrequency ablation; (2) De novo tumors do arise in cirrhotic livers and may occur in the vicinity of previously treated areas, reflecting a milieu that is favorable for carcinogenesis [24,27–29]. The inadvertent spill-over treatment of these high-risk regions with a field change effect downstream of the intended TACE-targeted area may decrease the chance of de novo tumorigenesis and thus explain the longer TTP.

In the era of individualized HCC therapy, there are implications for our results on the treatment of early-stage HCC. The current guidelines advocate for RFA over TACE for the management of HCCs smaller than 3 cm [7,8]. Our study showed that for HCCs less than 3 cm, TACE could lead to a comparable overall survival and TTP compared to RFA. There have been three other retrospective comparative studies of RFA and TACE in small tumors <3 cm or within the Milan criteria, which showed similar overall survival in both groups [12–14]. However, the study by Hsu et al. reported a poorer long-term survival in the subgroup undergoing TACE with a total tumor volume <11 cm^3 [12]. In this study, the patients who underwent TACE had a very high mean AFP of 3175 (ng/mL) compared to 320 in the RFA group. Therefore, the TACE group in the study by Hu et al. may have included tumors with a more aggressive biology.

We acknowledge that limitations exist in this study. All the patients in our study had low AFP, which may suggest favorable biology and impact tumor response. This could also explain the differing findings from Hsu et al. and our results have to be cautiously applied to patients with significantly elevated AFP [12]. Due to its retrospective nature and lack of randomization, our study is unable to provide as strong a conclusion as a randomized controlled trial. Our study is also limited by the small numbers in the subgroup analysis. Even so, a direct comparison between TACE and RFA through a randomized trial has been difficult due to the ethical implications imposed by the present treatment guidelines. We hence hope that our study adds to the body of literature supporting the feasibility of TACE in small HCCs less than 3 cm, especially when other options are unfeasible.

5. Conclusions

In summary, we found that in patients with early-stage HCC, both TACE and RFA led to similar overall survival and recurrence rates. This suggests that TACE may be considered as an alternative treatment option in patients unsuitable for surgery and/or RFA.

Author Contributions: Conceptualization, B.W.R.T., D.Q.H., L.J.C. and D.Y.Y.; methodology, B.W.R.T., D.Q.H., L.J.C. and D.Y.Y.; software, B.W.R.T., D.Q.H., L.J.C. and D.Y.Y.; validation, K.W.C.A., I.S.G., T.P.S., D.Y.Y., L.G.H., N.W.T., L.H.C. and M.M.; formal analysis, B.W.R.T., D.Q.H., L.J.C. and D.Y.Y.; investigation, K.W.C.A., I.S.G., T.P.S., D.Y.Y., L.G.H., L.Y.M., P.T., L.S.G., D.C.M., N.W.T., L.H.C. and M.M.; resources, K.W.C.A., I.S.G., T.P.S., D.Y.Y., L.G.H., M.M., L.H.C., L.Y.M., P.T., L.S.G., D.C.M., N.W.T. and M.M.; data curation, B.W.R.T. and L.J.C.; writing—original draft preparation, B.W.R.T., D.Q.H. and L.J.C.; writing—review and editing, B.W.R.T., D.Q.H., L.J.C., P.T., W.H.L., C.H.N., D.J.H.T. and D.Y.Y.; visualization, B.W.R.T. and D.Q.H.; supervision, D.Y.Y.; project administration, D.C.M. and B.W.R.T. All authors have read and agreed to the published version of the manuscript.

Funding: This research received no external funding.

Institutional Review Board Statement: This study was approved by the Investigation and Ethics Committee of the National University Hospital (Singapore), according to the standards of the Declaration of Helsinki. 2016/00086-AMD0001.

Informed Consent Statement: Informed consent was obtained from all subjects involved in the study.

Data Availability Statement: Kindly contact corresponding author for information requests.

Conflicts of Interest: The authors declare no conflict of interest.

References

1. Cancer. Available online: https://www.who.int/news-room/fact-sheets/detail/cancer (accessed on 14 September 2022).
2. Global Cancer Observatory. Available online: https://gco.iarc.fr/ (accessed on 14 September 2022).
3. Reveron-Thornton, R.F.; Teng, M.L.P.; Lee, E.Y.; Tran, A.; Vajanaphanich, S.; Tan, E.X.; Nerurkar, S.N.; Ng, R.X.; Teh, R.; Tripathy, D.P.; et al. Global and regional long-term survival following resection for HCC in the recent decade: A meta-analysis of 110 studies. *Hepatol. Commun.* **2022**. [CrossRef] [PubMed]
4. Koh, J.H.; Tan, D.J.H.; Ong, Y.; Lim, W.H.; Ng, C.H.; Tay, P.W.L.; Yong, J.N.; Muthiah, M.D.; Tan, E.X.; Pang, N.Q.; et al. Liver resection versus liver transplantation for hepatocellular carcinoma within Milan criteria: A meta-analysis of 18,421 patients. *Hepatobiliary Surg. Nutr.* **2022**, *11*, 78–93. [CrossRef] [PubMed]
5. Tan, D.J.H.; Lim, W.; Yong, J.N.; Ng, C.H.; Muthiah, M.D.; Tan, E.X.; Xiao, J.; Lim, S.Y.; Tang, A.S.P.; Pan, X.H.; et al. UNOS Down-Staging Criteria for Liver Transplantation of Hepatocellular Carcinoma: Systematic Review and Meta-Analysis of 25 Studies. *Clin. Gastroenterol. Hepatol.* **2022**. [CrossRef]
6. Huang, D.Q.; Muthiah, M.D.; Zhou, L.; Jumat, H.; Tan, W.X.; Lee, G.H.; Lim, S.G.; Kow, A.; Bonney, G.; Shridhar, I.; et al. Predicting HCC Response to Multikinase Inhibitors With In Vivo Cirrhotic Mouse Model for Personalized Therapy. *Cell. Mol. Gastroenterol. Hepatol.* **2020**, *11*, 1313–1325. [CrossRef] [PubMed]
7. Heimbach, J.K.; Kulik, L.M.; Finn, R.S.; Sirlin, C.B.; Abecassis, M.M.; Roberts, L.R.; Zhu, A.X.; Murad, M.H.; Marrero, J.A. AASLD Guidelines for the Treatment of Hepatocellular Carcinoma. *Hepatology* **2018**, *67*, 358–380. [CrossRef]
8. European Association for the Study of the Liver. Electronic address: Easloffice@easloffice.eu; European Association for the Study of the Liver EASL Clinical Practice Guidelines: Management of Hepatocellular Carcinoma. *J. Hepatol.* **2018**, *69*, 182–236. [CrossRef] [PubMed]
9. Feng, Y.; Wu, H.; Huang, D.Q.; Xu, C.; Zheng, H.; Maeda, M.; Zhao, X.; Wang, L.; Xiao, F.; Lv, H.; et al. Radiofrequency ablation versus repeat resection for recurrent hepatocellular carcinoma ($\leq$ 5 cm) after initial curative resection. *Eur. Radiol.* **2020**, *30*, 6357–6368. [CrossRef]
10. Teratani, T.; Yoshida, H.; Shiina, S.; Obi, S.; Sato, S.; Tateishi, R.; Mine, N.; Kondo, Y.; Kawabe, T.; Omata, M. Radiofrequency Ablation for Hepatocellular Carcinoma in So-Called High-Risk Locations. *Hepatology* **2006**, *43*, 1101–1108. [CrossRef] [PubMed]
11. Komorizono, Y.; Oketani, M.; Sako, K.; Yamasaki, N.; Shibatou, T.; Maeda, M.; Kohara, K.; Shigenobu, S.; Ishibashi, K.; Arima, T. Risk Factors for Local Recurrence of Small Hepatocellular Carcinoma Tumors after a Single Session, Single Application of Percutaneous Radiofrequency Ablation. *Cancer* **2003**, *97*, 1253–1262. [CrossRef]
12. Hsu, C.-Y.; Huang, Y.-H.; Chiou, Y.-Y.; Su, C.-W.; Lin, H.-C.; Lee, R.-C.; Chiang, J.-H.; Huo, T.-I.; Lee, F.-Y.; Lee, S.-D. Comparison of Radiofrequency Ablation and Transarterial Chemoembolization for Hepatocellular Carcinoma within the Milan Criteria: A Propensity Score Analysis. *Liver Transpl.* **2011**, *17*, 556–566. [CrossRef]
13. Kim, J.W.; Kim, J.H.; Sung, K.-B.; Ko, H.-K.; Shin, J.H.; Kim, P.N.; Choi, H.-K.; Ko, G.-Y.; Yoon, H.-K.; Chun, S.-Y.; et al. Transarterial Chemoembolization vs. Radiofrequency Ablation for the Treatment of Single Hepatocellular Carcinoma 2 Cm or Smaller. *Am. J. Gastroenterol.* **2014**, *109*, 1234–1240. [CrossRef] [PubMed]
14. Kim, T.H.; Kim, N.H.; Kim, J.D.; Kim, Y.N.; Kim, Y.J.; Kim, E.J.; Yoo, K.D.; Ryu, C.H.; Song, H.H.; Kim, H. Transarterial Chemoembolization Using Drug-Eluting Bead Compared with Radiofrequency Ablation for Treatment of Single Small Hepatocellular Carcinoma: A Pilot Non-Randomized Trial. *J. Liver Cancer* **2021**, *21*, 146–154. [CrossRef]
15. Attwa, M.H.; El-Etreby, S.A. Guide for Diagnosis and Treatment of Hepatocellular Carcinoma. *World J. Hepatol.* **2015**, *7*, 1632–1651. [CrossRef] [PubMed]
16. Eisenhauer, E.A.; Therasse, P.; Bogaerts, J.; Schwartz, L.H.; Sargent, D.; Ford, R.; Dancey, J.; Arbuck, S.; Gwyther, S.; Mooney, M.; et al. New Response Evaluation Criteria in Solid Tumours: Revised RECIST Guideline (Version 1.1). *Eur. J. Cancer* **2009**, *45*, 228–247. [CrossRef] [PubMed]
17. Curley, S.A.; Marra, P.; Beaty, K.; Ellis, L.M.; Vauthey, J.N.; Abdalla, E.K.; Scaife, C.; Raut, C.; Wolff, R.; Choi, H.; et al. Early and Late Complications After Radiofrequency Ablation of Malignant Liver Tumors in 608 Patients. *Ann. Surg.* **2004**, *239*, 450–458. [CrossRef]
18. Huang, H.-W. Influence of Blood Vessel on the Thermal Lesion Formation during Radiofrequency Ablation for Liver Tumors. *Med. Phys.* **2013**, *40*, 073303. [CrossRef]
19. Llovet, J.M.; Vilana, R.; Brú, C.; Bianchi, L.; Salmeron, J.M.; Boix, L.; Ganau, S.; Sala, M.; Pagès, M.; Ayuso, C.; et al. Increased Risk of Tumor Seeding after Percutaneous Radiofrequency Ablation for Single Hepatocellular Carcinoma. *Hepatology* **2001**, *33*, 1124–1129. [CrossRef]

20. Singal, A.G.; Pillai, A.; Tiro, J. Early Detection, Curative Treatment, and Survival Rates for Hepatocellular Carcinoma Surveillance in Patients with Cirrhosis: A Meta-Analysis. *PLoS Med.* **2014**, *11*, e1001624. [CrossRef]
21. Park, J.-W.; Chen, M.; Colombo, M.; Roberts, L.R.; Schwartz, M.; Chen, P.-J.; Kudo, M.; Johnson, P.; Wagner, S.; Orsini, L.S.; et al. Global Patterns of Hepatocellular Carcinoma Management from Diagnosis to Death: The BRIDGE Study. *Liver Int.* **2015**, *35*, 2155–2166. [CrossRef]
22. Liu, K.; Min, X.-L.; Peng, J.; Yang, K.; Yang, L.; Zhang, X.-M. The Changes of HIF-1α and VEGF Expression After TACE in Patients With Hepatocellular Carcinoma. *J. Clin. Med. Res.* **2016**, *8*, 297–302. [CrossRef]
23. Sumie, S.; Kuromatsu, R.; Okuda, K.; Ando, E.; Takata, A.; Fukushima, N.; Watanabe, Y.; Kojiro, M.; Sata, M. Microvascular Invasion in Patients with Hepatocellular Carcinoma and Its Predictable Clinicopathological Factors. *Ann. Surg. Oncol.* **2008**, *15*, 1375–1382. [CrossRef] [PubMed]
24. Shah, S.A.; Greig, P.D.; Gallinger, S.; Cattral, M.S.; Dixon, E.; Kim, R.D.; Taylor, B.R.; Grant, D.R.; Vollmer, C.M. Factors Associated with Early Recurrence after Resection for Hepatocellular Carcinoma and Outcomes. *J. Am. Coll Surg.* **2006**, *202*, 275–283. [CrossRef]
25. Shi, M.; Zhang, C.; Feng, K.; Zhang, Y.; Chen, M.; Guo, R.; Lin, X.; Li, J. Micrometastasis distribution in liver tissue surrounding hepatocellular carcinoma. *Zhonghua Zhong Liu Za Zhi* **2002**, *24*, 257–260. [PubMed]
26. Chen, M.-S.; Li, J.-Q.; Zheng, Y.; Guo, R.-P.; Liang, H.-H.; Zhang, Y.-Q.; Lin, X.-J.; Lau, W.Y. A Prospective Randomized Trial Comparing Percutaneous Local Ablative Therapy and Partial Hepatectomy for Small Hepatocellular Carcinoma. *Ann. Surg.* **2006**, *243*, 321–328. [CrossRef]
27. Dehn, T. Optimal Treatment for Hepatocellular Carcinoma in the Cirrhotic Liver. *Ann. R Coll Surg. Engl.* **2009**, *91*, 545–550. [CrossRef] [PubMed]
28. Imamura, H.; Matsuyama, Y.; Tanaka, E.; Ohkubo, T.; Hasegawa, K.; Miyagawa, S.; Sugawara, Y.; Minagawa, M.; Takayama, T.; Kawasaki, S.; et al. Risk Factors Contributing to Early and Late Phase Intrahepatic Recurrence of Hepatocellular Carcinoma after Hepatectomy. *J. Hepatol.* **2003**, *38*, 200–207. [CrossRef]
29. Hernandez-Gea, V.; Turon, F.; Berzigotti, A.; Villanueva, A. Management of Small Hepatocellular Carcinoma in Cirrhosis: Focus on Portal Hypertension. *World J. Gastroenterol.* **2013**, *19*, 1193–1199. [CrossRef]

MDPI
St. Alban-Anlage 66
4052 Basel
Switzerland
Tel. +41 61 683 77 34
Fax +41 61 302 89 18
www.mdpi.com

Biomedicines Editorial Office
E-mail: biomedicines@mdpi.com
www.mdpi.com/journal/biomedicines

www.ingramcontent.com/pod-product-compliance
Lightning Source LLC
LaVergne TN
LVHW070706100526
838202LV00013B/1039